NANDA Approved Diagnosis Labels (1999–2000)
Grouped by Gordon's Functional Health Patterns

HEALTH PERCEPTION-HEALTH MANAGEMENT

Health maintenance, altered
Health seeking behaviors (specify)
Infection, risk for
Injury, risk for
Latex allergy response
Latex allergy response, risk for
Management of therapeutic regimen: community, ineffective
Management of therapeutic regimen: families, ineffective
Management of therapeutic regimen: individual, effective
Management of therapeutic regimen: individual, ineffective
Noncompliance (specify)
Trauma, risk for
Poisoning, risk for
Protection, altered
Suffocation, risk for

NUTRITIONAL-METABOLIC

Adaptive capacity: intracranial, decreased
Aspiration, risk for
Body temperature, risk for altered
Breastfeeding, effective
Breastfeeding, ineffective
Breastfeeding, interrupted
Dentition, altered
Failure to thrive, adult
Fluid volume deficit
Fluid volume deficit, risk for
Fluid volume excess
Fluid volume imbalance, risk for
Hyperthermia
Hypothermia
Infant feeding pattern, ineffective
Nutrition: less than body requirements, altered
Nutrition: more than body requirements, altered
Nutrition: risk for more than body requirements, altered
Oral mucous membrane, altered
Skin integrity, impaired
Skin integrity, risk for impaired
Surgical recovery, delayed
Swallowing, impaired
Thermoregulation, ineffective
Tissue integrity, impaired

ELIMINATION

Constipation
Constipation, perceived
Constipation, risk of
Diarrhea
Incontinence, bowel
Incontinence, urinary, functional
Incontinence, urinary, reflex
Incontinence, urinary, stress
Incontinence, urinary, total
Incontinence, urinary, urge
Incontinence, urinary, urge, risk for
Urinary elimination, altered
Urinary retention

ACTIVITY-EXERCISE PATTERN

Activity intolerance
Activity intolerance, risk for
Airway clearance, ineffective
Breathing pattern, ineffective
Cardiac output, decreased
Development, risk for altered
Disuse syndrome, risk for
Diversional activity deficit
Dysreflexia
Dysreflexia, risk for autonomic
Fatigue
Gas exchange, impaired
Growth, risk for altered
Growth and development, altered
Home maintenance management, impaired
Mobility: bed, impaired
Mobility: physical, impaired
Mobility: wheelchair, impaired
Perioperative positioning injury, risk for
Peripheral neurovascular dysfunction, risk for
Self care deficit: bathing/hygiene
Self care deficit: dressing/grooming
Self care deficit: feeding
Self care deficit: toileting
Spontaneous ventilation, inability to sustain
Tissue perfusion, altered (specify: cardiopulmonary, cerebral, gastrointestinal, renal)
Tissue perfusion, altered (peripheral)
Ventilatory weaning response, dysfunctional
Walking, impaired

SLEEP-REST

Sleep deprivation
Sleep pattern disturbance

COGNITIVE-PERCEPTUAL

Confusion, acute
Confusion, chronic
Decisional conflict (specify)
Environmental interpretation syndrome, impaired
Infant behavior: disorganized
Infant behavior: disorganized, risk for
Infant behavior: organized, potential for enhanced
Knowledge deficit (specify)
Memory, impaired
Nausea
Pain
Pain, chronic
Sensory/perceptual alterations (specify: auditory, gustatory, kinesthetic, olfactory, tactile, visual)
Thought processes, altered
Unilateral neglect

SELF-PERCEPTION/SELF-CONCEPT

Anxiety
Anxiety, death
Body image disturbance
Energy field disturbance
Fear
Hopelessness
Personal identity disturbance
Powerlessness
Self esteem, chronic low
Self esteem disturbance
Self esteem, situational low
Self-mutilation, risk for
Violence: self-directed, risk for

ROLE-RELATIONSHIP

Caregiver role strain
Caregiver role strain, risk for
Communication, impaired verbal
Family processes: alcoholism, altered
Family processes, altered
Grieving, anticipatory
Grieving, dysfunctional
Loneliness, risk for
Parent/infant/child attachment, risk for altered
Parental role conflict
Parenting, altered
Parenting, risk for altered
Relocation stress syndrome
Role performance, altered
Social interaction, impaired
Social isolation
Sorrow, chronic
Violence: directed at others, risk for

SEXUALITY-REPRODUCTIVE

Rape-trauma syndrome
Rape-trauma syndrome: compound reaction
Rape-trauma syndrome: silent reaction
Sexual dysfunction
Sexuality patterns, altered

COPING/STRESS-TOLERANCE

Adjustment, impaired
Coping: community, ineffective
Coping: community, potential for enhanced
Coping, defensive
Coping: family, ineffective, compromised
Coping: family, ineffective, disabling
Coping: family, potential for growth
Coping: individual, ineffective
Denial, ineffective
Post-trauma syndrome
Post-trauma syndrome, risk for

VALUE-BELIEF

Spiritual distress
Spiritual distress, risk for
Spiritual well-being, potential for enhanced

Nursing Process and Critical Thinking

THIRD EDITION

Judith M. Wilkinson, PhD, ARNP, RNC

Prentice Hall, Upper Saddle River, New Jersey   07458

Library of Congress Cataloging-in-Publication Data

Wilkinson, Judith M., 1946–
    Nursing process and critical thinking / Judith M. Wilkinson.—3rd ed.
        p. cm.
    Includes bibliographical references and index.
    ISBN 0-8053-9176-2
    1. Nursing.   2. Critical thinking.   I. Title.
RT41.W57 2001
610.73—dc21
                                                    00-058041
                                                        CIP

Publisher: Julie Alexander
Executive Editor: Maura Connor
Acquisitions Editor: Nancy Anselment
Production Editor: Clarinda Publication Services
Director of Manufacturing
    and Production: Bruce Johnson
Managing Editor: Patrick Walsh
Production Liaison: Janet Bolton
Manufacturing Buyer: Ilene Sanford
Art Director: Marianno Frasco
Marketing Manager: Kristin Walton
Editorial Assistant: Beth Ann Romph
Cover Design: Rhonda N. Merider
Interior Design: John Edeen
Compositor: Rainbow Graphics
Printing and Binding: R.R. Donnelley, Harrisonburg
Prentice-Hall International (UK) Limited, *London*
Prentice-Hall of Australia Pty. Limited, *Sydney*
Prentice-Hall Canada, Inc., *Toronto*
Prentice-Hall Hispanoamericana, S.A., *Mexico*
Prentice-Hall of India Private Limited, *New Delhi*
Prentice-Hall of Japan, Inc., *Tokyo*
Prentice-Hall Singapore Pte. Ltd.
Editora Prentice-Hall do Brasil Ltda., *Rio de Janeiro*

Care has been taken to confirm the accuracy of information presented in this book. The author, editors, and the publisher, however, cannot accept any responsibility for errors or omissions or for the consequences from application of the information in this book and make no warranty, express or implied, with respect to its contents.

The author and publisher have exerted every effort to ensure that drug selections and dosages set forth in this text are in accord with current recommendation and practice at time of publication. However, in view of ongoing research, changes in government regulations, and the constant flow of information relating to drug therapy and drug reactions, the reader is urged to check the package inserts of all drugs for any change in indications of dosage and for added warnings and precautions. This is particularly important when the recommended agent is a new and/or infrequently employed drug.

10 9 8
ISBN 0-8053-9176-2

Contents

1

Overview of Nursing Process   1

2
Critical Thinking 33

3

Assessment 75

4

Diagnostic Reasoning 143

5

Diagnostic Language   197

6

Planning: Overview and Outcomes

7

Planning: Interventions   303

8
Implementation   341

Preface

Students find this text easy, even enjoyable to use. Nevertheless, it is a serious text, with in-depth treatment of concepts. Because nurses need conceptual understanding of nursing process as well as the practical ability to plan and implement nursing care, this text balances conceptual and practical aspects. For example, Chapter 4 describes a diagnostic process, and Chapter 5 explains how to write diagnostic statements; Chapters 6 and 10 contain detailed explanations of how to create working care plans for real patients, while Chapters 6 and 7 discuss concepts related to choosing outcomes and interventions.

■ CONTENT

The nursing process provides a basic framework within which nurses apply the unique combination of knowledge, skills, and caring that constitute the art and science of nursing. The purpose of this book is to promote professional practice through effective use of the nursing process. To that end, the text integrates the following topics into the discussion of each nursing process step:

- **Collaborative Practice and Delegation**. The text acknowledges the changing face of nursing and healthcare by emphasizing collaborative practice and expanding discussion of work delegation by nurses. Case management and critical pathways are treated extensively, as well.
- **Critical Thinking**. Critical thinking is important for nurses—perhaps in different degrees and for different uses, but at all levels of practice. The nursing process provides an excellent vehicle for encouraging critical thinking. Chapter 2 presents concepts of critical thinking as it relates to nursing, and subsequent chapters integrate critical thinking into assessment, diagnosis, planning, implementation, and evaluation. In addition, the "Nursing Process Practice" exercises are designed to foster critical thinking while learning nursing process. Each chapter includes special "Critical Thinking Practice" exercise, designed to teach a specific critical thinking skill. These are excellent for class discussion or small-group projects. The "Case Studies" at the end of each chapter provide opportunity

for students to use *both* critical thinking and the nursing process to practice clinical decision-making safely in simulated situations.

- **Standardized Nursing Language**. Standardized language for problems, outcomes, and interventions is introduced and integrated throughout each chapter in order to help students prepare to use computerized information systems. The text includes discussions and illustrations of NANDA, NIC, NOC, the Omaha System, and the Home Health Care Classification.
- **Culture and Spirituality**. In order to reflect our multicultural society and promote holistic care, cultural and spiritual dimensions of each step of the nursing process are explored. For example, the Assessment chapter includes tools for both cultural and spiritual assessment.
- **Ethical and Legal Issues**. In order to increase awareness of ethical issues embedded in the practice of nursing, each chapter includes ethical and legal principles and considerations pertinent to that particular nursing process phase (eg, maintaining confidentiality of client data in the assessment phase).
- **Home, Family, and Community Care**. Examples and discussions are greatly expanded in this edition, reflecting the expanding role of nursing in homes and other community settings.
- **Nursing Frameworks/Theories**. Nursing models are integrated into the explanation of each nursing process phase in order to encourage theory-based practice. For example, assessment tools and nursing diagnoses are categorized according to different frameworks. In order to maintain flexibility, a single model was not chosen. Instead, several nursing frameworks are summarized and used. For some courses, teachers may choose to not use the nursing theories; for others, a particular framework could be chosen and emphasized.
- **Professional Standards of Care**. Nurses are more than just the means to organizational ends. Even in a bottom-line, outcomes-driven environment, nurses are accountable for the quality of the care they give: for what they know and what they do. To this end, the American Nurses Association (ANA) Standards of Clinical Nursing Practice are linked to each phase of the nursing process. These standards enable nurses to evaluate their own behaviors—not merely the patient outcomes they help produce.
- **Wellness Concepts**. Wellness language and examples are used throughout the text in order to promote awareness of health promotion as a vital part of nursing practice. Most chapters include a section in which wellness concepts are related to the chapter material; the end-of-chapter exercises also include wellness examples.

■ TEACHING/LEARNING FEATURES

I have used these chapters as learning units to teach nursing process to students of various levels, as well as in continuing education for practicing nurses. Student response has been overwhelmingly positive.

- **Interactive Format**. Neither nursing process nor critical thinking can be mastered by memorizing facts and principles. Students need to practice applying the concepts; they need to "work problems," just as they do in a math class. This text provides many practice problems. The exercises are not just "recall and fill in the blanks." They are application exercises, designed to promote high-level thinking skills. In addition to end-of-chapter exercises, "Thinking Points" are integrated within the chapters to help students reflect on their reading.

- **Learning Aids**. Each chapter begins with Learning Outcomes and a figure that serves as a visual guide to chapter content. "Key Point" boxes summarize selected content in easily remembered lists. Each chapter ends with a Summary of chapter content.

- **Case Studies**. In addition to the "Nursing Process Practice" and "Critical Thinking Practice" features, each chapter also contains a case study ("Applying Nursing Process and Critical Thinking") to allow students to use critical thinking within the framework of the nursing process. These cases focus on critical thinking and nursing process. They are *not* intended to teach in-depth content about medical conditions and pathophysiology. Even beginning students can use the case studies.

- **Detailed Answer Keys**. For the "Nursing Process Practices," the answer keys give the rationale for both correct and incorrect answers and frequently demonstrate the thinking process used to arrive at the answers. This detailed feedback provides for truly interactive learning, as well as the kind of student–instructor dialogue that is so important for learning nursing process. Students are easily frustrated by the many ambiguities and seeming contradictions that arise when applying abstract nursing process concepts to concrete/specific situations. The answer key discussions are vital for easing this frustration and modeling the thinking inherent in the process. Because answers can vary widely, the answer keys for "Critical Thinking Practices" and the "Case Studies" provide suggested, not comprehensive, answers.

- **Versatility**. This text is suitable for nursing students as an introduction to nursing process or for use in the continuing education of professionals who may need refresher information and practice. It is effective for students who have had nursing process early in the curriculum and who later have difficulty applying it in a clinical course—simply assign a chapter and exercises to remediate the difficulty. The text is organized to accommodate the instructor's professional judgment—that is, it can be used in whole or in part, and for students of different levels, depending on what the instructor chooses to assign or emphasize. For example, for instructors who believe the concept of "possible problems" is too difficult for beginning students, that portion of Chapter 4 could be omitted without damaging the continuity of the material. Some teachers may choose to present Chapter 5 before Chapter 4. Some use Chapter 10 as a sort of "road map," presenting it after Chapter 2; others prefer to use it at the end of the course, after all the phases of the nursing process have been taught. All approaches are workable.

- **Independent Study**. This text can be used for independent study and for distance learning, but it is in no way limited to that approach. It can be used as a text to supplement lectures, either in a separate course or when the nursing process is integrated in the curriculum.
- **Care Plans—or not**. This text makes clear that nursing process and a written care plan are *not* one and the same. For teachers who question the exclusive use of written care plans as a teaching strategy, this text will be helpful. I have found that the time I previously allotted to lecture can be used to discuss student questions about nursing process and patient care. Even more exciting, I assign fewer traditional care plans, and I need to make fewer comments on the plans they do write. I also spend less time in remedial conferences helping students with nursing process.
- **Terminology**. I use both *client* and *patient* in this book. Either can be appropriate, depending on the context. *Client* implies that nurses have independent functions, are increasingly accountable to individuals rather than institutions, and are not setting-bound; it also stresses that people are increasingly active in managing their own healthcare. On the other hand, most nursing still does occur in hospitals, and with ill people who are in a dependent state. Furthermore, most nurses are paid by an employing health agency, rather than directly by a client. In these situations, the term *patient* seems more accurate.

- I use a similar approach for denoting gender. I acknowledge and welcome the presence of men in nursing and, further, realize that patients are both men and women. However, terms like *s/he* and *she/he* are artificial and awkward to read, so I do not use them. Both nurses and patients are arbitrarily assigned gender and referred to either as *he* or *she*.

- In this text I often speak to the reader as "you" instead of "the nurse" or "the student." For one thing, this suits my informal nature. But more importantly, I hope this will empower and engage the reader personally, promoting active involvement with the text.

I welcome your comments.

Judith Wilkinson
11959 West 66th Street
Shawnee, KS 66216
(913) 631-1089
judithwilkins@att.net
http://judithwilkinson.com

Reviewers

I am grateful to the following for their comments and suggestions provided in their review of the manuscript:

Indeborg DiGiacomo, EdD, MA, BS
Department of Nursing & Allied Health
County College of Morris
Randolph, NJ

Carolyn J. Green-Nigro, PhD, RN
Department of Nursing
Johnson County Community College
Overland Park, KS

Judith Harmer
Health Professions Division
Golden West College
Huntington Beach, CA

Allen Hamilton
Department of Nursing
McLennan Community College
Waco, TX

Janene Jeffery, RN, MSN, PDE
Department of Nursing
Austin Community College
Austin, TX

Mary Moser-Gautreaux
Department of Nursing
Albuquerque Technical Vocational Institute
Albuquerque, NM

Janet A. Sipple, RN, EdD
St. Luke's Hospital
School of Nursing
Bethlehem, PA

STUDENTS: Getting the Most from Your Reading

The following suggestions should help you make best use of this text. Because people learn in different ways, you should adapt them to fit your particular learning style.

1. **Read the chapter learning outcomes first**. These give you a blueprint of the chapter and direct your reading.
2. **Key terms** are in bold print in the chapter text. Be sure you can recognize and define these terms.
3. **Read the chapter content**.
    A. Pay attention to headings and subheadings. Because they give you a concept label for the paragraphs that follow them, they can focus your thinking and help you to remember what you have read.
    B. Make notes in the margins. Writing reinforces your learning.
4. **Work the exercises in "Nursing Process Practice" at the end of each chapter**. In order to learn the nursing process, you must apply it, not simply memorize what you read about it. As a nurse, you will be applying the nursing process, not simply recalling facts about it, so begin learning to do that now.
    A. Write the answers in the text to reinforce your learning.
    B. Work the exercises before you look at the answer keys. Be sure you understand the rationale provided in the answer keys, and refer back to the chapter text as you need to.
5. **Do the Critical Thinking Practice at the end of the chapter.** Write your answers, make notes, and discuss these with your instructor or your classmates to be sure you are on the right track. Discuss your thinking processes—*how* you arrived at your answers. Answer keys for the critical thinking exercises provide a few suggestions, but they focus on correct use of the *thinking skill*, not on the *correct answer*. Critical thinking skills are best acquired through discussion with others, either individually or in class.
6. **Work the case study at the end of each chapter**. The case studies provide practice in applying critical thinking and nursing process together. They are a safe way for you to practice making clinical judgments before you actually need to do so in a clinical setting.

If you have difficulty with any of the exercises, reread the chapter and try again. If you are still having trouble, ask your instructor to suggest additional exercises, audiovisual materials, or further readings.

1
Overview of Nursing Process

Learning Outcomes

After completing this chapter, you should be able to do the following:

- Define *human responses* in the context of nursing.
- Compare and contrast the concerns of nursing and medicine.
- Define *nursing process* in terms of purpose, characteristics, and organization.
- Name and describe the six phases of the nursing process.
- Describe qualities a nurse needs in order to use the nursing process successfully.
- Explain the importance of the nursing process to patients and nurses.
- Discuss the use of the nursing process in wellness/health promotion.

■ INTRODUCTION

Because nursing process texts (and teachers) talk about *concepts, ideas,* and *processes,* students sometimes wonder what all this has to do with taking care of patients—with the "real world," as you may hear nurses refer to it. In this book you will learn that the **nursing process** is a special way of thinking that nurses use. It is also what nurses *do* when giving patient care. In other words, the nursing process is a thinking/doing *approach* that nurses use in their work. Keeping this general idea in mind will help you as you work through the more detailed explanation developed in this chapter. The six phases (processes) of the nursing process are shown in Figure 1–1.

■ WHAT IS NURSING?

A good understanding of nursing will help you to understand the nursing process and place it in proper perspective. **Nursing** is a unique blend of art and science applied within the context of interpersonal relationships for the purpose of promoting wellness, preventing illness, and restoring health

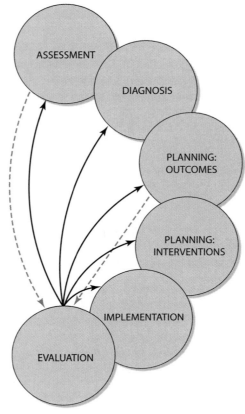

Figure 1–1
The basic phases of the nursing process

in individuals, families, and communities. According to Johnson (1994), **art** in nursing means the ability to:

1. develop meaningful connections with clients
2. grasp the meaning in client encounters
3. perform nursing activities skillfully
4. use rational thinking to choose appropriate courses of action
5. conduct one's nursing practice ethically.

Many professional organizations and leaders have defined nursing. Florence Nightingale (1969, p. 133), the first nurse theorist, said that what nurses do "is to put the patient in the best condition for nature to act upon him." This fits with the idea that people have innate abilities for growth and self-healing, and that the nurse's role is to nurture and support these abilities (Bryant 1998). In 1980, the American Nurses Association, the professional organization for all United States nurses, said that nursing is "the diagnosis and treatment of human responses to actual or potential health problems" (ANA p. 9). More recently, they have said that four essential features of contemporary nursing practice are as follows (ANA 1995, p. 6). Nursing:

1. is not restricted to a focus on problems—it includes health promotion.
2. integrates patients' subjective experience with objective data.
3. applies scientific knowledge to diagnosis and treatment processes.
4. provides a caring relationship that facilitates health and healing.

Nursing Theory

A **theory** offers a way of looking at a discipline in clear, explicit terms that can be communicated to others. Nursing theories help to explain the unique place of nursing in the multidisciplinary team. Theories are based on the theorist's values and assumptions about health, patients, nursing, and the environment. Each theory describes those concepts and explains how they are related. Think of a theory as a lens through which to view nursing and patients: the color and shape of the lens affect what you see. That is why there are so many definitions of nursing (see Table 1–1 on page 4), and that is how a nurse's theory affects his or her use of the nursing process.

Although definitions and theories vary, there is general agreement that even though nurses care for patients with health problems, nursing is not limited to disease processes, and that nursing phenomena of concern are different from those of medicine. Overall, nursing models (theories) describe nursing as:

- an art and a science with its own evolving, scientific body of knowledge,
- holistic, or concerned with the client's physical, psychosocial, cultural, and spiritual needs,
- involving caring,
- occurring in a variety of settings, and
- concerned with health promotion, disease prevention, and care during illness.

The act of nursing is special and unique because it blends art (caring) and science (knowledge and problem-solving processes) within person-to-person relationships.

Human Responses

According to the ANA, nurses, viewing the patient holistically, are concerned with **human responses**—the biological, psychological, social, and spiritual reactions to an event or a stressor such as disease or injury. Nurses diagnose, treat, and prevent the patient's *responses* to diseases, such as diabetes (eg, lack of knowledge about diet, loss of self-esteem), rather than the disease itself (eg, prescribing insulin).

KEY POINT
Nursing is a unique blend of art and science applied within the context of interpersonal relationships for the purpose of promoting wellness, preventing illness, and restoring health in individuals, families, and communities.

Table 1–1   Definitions of Nursing by Nurse Theorists

Theorist	Definition of Nursing
Hildegarde Peplau Interpersonal model (1952)	"A significant therapeutic interpersonal process which functions cooperatively with other human processes that make health possible for individuals" (p. 16). "A maturing force and educative instrument" (p. 8). A practice discipline.
Martha Rogers Unitary Man model (1970, 1980)	Nursing is both art and science; a learned profession. It promotes achievement of maximum health potential by promoting "symphonic interaction between man and environment, to strengthen the coherence and integrity of the human field" (1970, p. 122). Nurses promote health, prevent illness, and care for and rehabilitate the sick and disabled (1970, p. vii).
Sister Callista Roy Adaptation model (1970, 1976, 1980)	Nursing is "a theoretical system of knowledge which prescribes a process of analysis and action related to care of the ill or potentially ill person" (1976, p. 31). Nurses promote adaptation of the client in the physiologic, self-concept, role-function, and interdependence modes by manipulating stimuli (or stressors).
Dorothea Orem Self-Care model (1971)	Nursing is a human service concerned with the need for continuous self-care action in order to sustain life and health or to recover from disease or injury. Nursing has both health and illness dimensions. Nurses help clients (mainly individuals) to achieve self-care agency and maintain an optimal state of health.
Betty Neuman Health-Care Systems model (1972, 1980)	The nurse helps the client to attain and maintain system equilibrium. Nursing is concerned with all variables that affect a person's response to stressors. The nurse attempts to help the client avoid or defend against stressors. Both client and nurse are active, but the nurse is more so.
Rosemarie Parse Human-Living-Health model (1974, 1981, 1987)	"Nursing is a human science profession concerned with the care of unitary man as he evolves from conception to death" (1974, p. 7). Nursing is a science and an art concerned with exploring personal meanings of lived experiences. The nurse guides clients in assuming responsibility for their health.

EXAMPLE: Consider the following possible patient responses to a heart attack:

Physical response	Pain
Psychological response	Fear
Sociological response	Returning to work before she is well
Spiritual response	Praying

An infinite variety of possible human responses occurs at all levels: cells, organs, systems, interpersonal, cultural, and so on. Note, too, that the stressors that cause health problems are not always diseases or microorganisms. They can be environmental (eg, too much exposure to the sun produces a sunburn), interpersonal (eg, the stress of adapting to parenthood when a new baby is born), or spiritual (eg, guilt from falling away from one's religion may lead to depression).

Nursing, Medicine, and Multidisciplinary Practice

Increasingly, multidisciplinary teams are delivering healthcare. This is also referred to as *collaborative practice* and *interdisciplinary practice*. This means that nurses, physicians, and other professionals work together to plan and provide patient care (see Box 1–1). This does not mean that nurses must become invisible; each discipline retains its identity, even as they collaborate (Maas 1998).

Although some functions may be shared, nursing is different from medicine. Physicians focus on diagnosis and treatment of disease; nurses focus on giving care during the cure. This is sometimes referred to as "curing versus caring." Caring in this sense refers to the activities that nurses perform in *taking care of* patients, not the subjective feeling of *caring about* patients. That feeling may, of course, be involved, but it does not necessarily differentiate nursing from medicine. Table 1–2, on page 6, summarizes the differences between nursing and medicine. In reality, all health team members contribute to implement a plan of care. Box 1–2, on page 6, describes strategies for improving relationships among health professionals.

Nursing in Wellness and Illness

Nursing is concerned with the whole person, ill or well. Nurses support ill people and help them to solve or reduce their health problems; they help patients to adapt to and accept problems that cannot be treated; and they help

---

BOX 1–1

Collaborative (Multidisciplinary) Practice

Collaboration means a collegial working relationship with another health care provider in the provision of (to supply) patient care. Collaborative practice requires (may include) the discussion of patient diagnosis and cooperation in the management and delivery of care. (American Nurses Association 1992)

. . . members of various professions cooperate by exchanging knowledge and ideas about how to deliver high quality health care. Collaboration among health care professions involves recognition of the expertise of others within and outside one's profession and referral to those providers when appropriate. Collaboration also involves some shared functions and a common focus on the same overall mission. (American Nurses Association 1995)

Table 1–2   Comparison of Nursing and Medicine

Medical Focus	Nursing Focus
1. Diagnose and treat disease 2. Cure disease 3. Pathophysiology, biological, physical effects 4. Teach patients about the treatments for their disease or injury	1. Diagnose, treat, and prevent human responses 2. Care for the patient 3. Holistic—effects on whole person (biological, psychosocial, cultural, spiritual) 4. Teach clients self-care strategies to increase independence in daily activities 5. Promote wellness activities

BOX 1–2

Strategies for Collaboration

1. Address difficult situations immediately. Don't remain silent to avoid conflict; this only prolongs the inevitable friction.
2. Avoid angry or sarcastic remarks.
3. Be assertive, but not aggressive or hostile.
4. Use an empathetic, non-defensive, but persistent approach.
5. Realize that individuals have the right to feel however they choose. Acknowledge feelings, then focus your interactions on the matter at hand.
6. Find a mentor—an experienced nurse who collaborates successfully with physicians.
7. Strive to reach an agreeable solution using input from everyone involved.
8. Cultivate and demonstrate mutual respect. Recognize, compliment, and praise positive attributes and actions.
9. Seek a free exchange of patient care information between disciplines.
10. Be holistically patient oriented, not task oriented.
11. Strive for professional excellence in organizational and prioritizing skills, knowledge, and clinical performance.
12. Think ahead and anticipate needs, particularly in emergency situations.
13. Recognize that nursing has power to impact healthcare. Become involved with policy making and decision making; become politically active in and for the nursing profession.

Source: Adapted from S. Pavlovich-Danis, H. Forman, and P. O. Simek (1998). The nurse-physician relationship. Can it be saved? *Journal of Nursing Administration* 28(7–8):17–20.

those who are terminally ill to achieve a peaceful death. For well people, nurses aim to prevent illness and promote wellness. This may involve a variety of activities, such as role modeling a healthy lifestyle, being an advocate for community environmental changes, or teaching self-care strategies, decision making, and problem solving.

EXAMPLE: Cara Wolinski is a nurse in a factory. She promotes health by organizing and supervising a daily exercise class for employees. Cara also provides nutrition counseling for those who request it.

> Why did you decide to become a nurse instead of a physician? Or a respiratory therapist? Or any other healthcare worker? Who influenced you in this decision? Do you think you made a good decision?

???
THINKING POINT

■ WHY IS THE NURSING PROCESS IMPORTANT?

There are many reasons for learning and using the nursing process. Because the client is the focus of nursing, the most important reasons are the ways in which it benefits clients. However, the nursing process is good for nurses and the nursing profession as well. The nursing process:

- **Promotes collaboration**. When all team members value a systematic, organized approach, communication improves. Each feels satisfaction from delivering effective, individualized care, and the work atmosphere becomes more positive.
- **Is cost-efficient**. By improving communication, the nursing process prevents errors and expedites diagnosis, treatment, and prevention of patient problems. This means shorter hospital stays and lower costs for healthcare agencies.
- **Helps people understand what nurses do**. Because nursing is complex, it is sometimes difficult for nurses to define their role to others. In order to be valued by employers and patients, nurses must show that they contribute to better outcomes and decreased costs. A record of nursing assessments and interventions can be used to show how nurses prevent complications and hasten recovery.
- **Is required by professional standards of practice**. Successful use of the nursing process will help you to meet the professional standards of practice, to which nurses are held accountable (eg, see Box 1–3 on page 8).
- **Increases client participation in care and promotes client autonomy**. Self-care is very important in our cost-driven healthcare environment. Clients are often discharged from the hospital while still in need of care and treatment. Involving clients at each step of the nursing

---

BOX 1–3

ANA Standards of Care

I. Assessment	The nurse collects patient health data.
II. Diagnosis	The nurse identifies nursing diagnoses individualized to the client.
III. Outcome Identification	The nurse identifies expected outcomes individualized to the client.
IV. Planning	The nurse develops a plan of care that prescribes interventions to attain expected outcomes.
V. Implementation	The nurse implements the interventions identified in the plan of care.
VI. Evaluation	The nurse evaluates the client's progress toward attainment of outcomes.

Source: Reprinted with permission from American Nurses Association, *Standards of Clinical Nursing Practice*. 2nd ed. © 1998. American Nurses Publishing, American Nurses Foundation/American Nurses Association, 600 Maryland Ave. SW, Suite 100W, Washington, DC.

---

process helps them to realize the importance of their contributions, learn more about their bodies, improve their health decisions, and regain independence more quickly.

- **Promotes individualized care**. Human responses (eg, to a disease) are infinitely variable. With a care plan to point out specific, unique needs, nurses can avoid the tendency to categorize and give standardized care based solely on a patient's medical diagnosis.

EXAMPLE: The standardized care plan for a patient with a hysterectomy includes monitoring for complications and teaching for self-care. Because Carol Wu's care plan also stated that she has a hearing problem, the nurses were careful to position themselves so that Ms. Wu could read their lips and understand the discharge teaching.

Notice that the interventions for Ms. Wu's hearing deficit were not related to her surgical diagnosis (hysterectomy). Because nurses focused on the person instead of her surgical diagnosis, Ms. Wu's needs were successfully met.

- **Promotes efficiency**. Duplication wastes time and can be tiring and irritating for patients. A systematic approach prevents omissions and duplications.

EXAMPLE: Melissa Carpenter has just had a baby and is on a unit that uses care plans with a checklist for teaching needs. When the evening nurse arrives, she sees that the day nurse has checked off "episiotomy care," so she does not reteach that information. Instead, she spends her time helping Ms. Carpenter learn to bathe her baby.

- **Promotes continuity and coordination of care**. A written care plan ensures that all caregivers are informed of patient needs. Hospitals are staffed 24 hours a day, so a patient usually receives care from two or three registered nurses each day. Each nurse may be competent, but if they do not function in a coordinated manner, patients may doubt their competence and lose confidence that their needs will be met.

  EXAMPLE: A new mother is having difficulty breastfeeding her baby. The day nurse has told her she should wake the baby and try to feed him every two hours. The evening nurse tells her to feed the baby on demand because he will wake up when he is hungry. The mother is becoming confused and discouraged. She says to her partner, "Maybe we should bottle feed the baby; this is really too hard to do."

- **Increases your job satisfaction**. Many of the rewards in nursing come from realizing that you have helped someone. As you begin to see how the nursing process increases your ability to help, you will take satisfaction in a job well done. Good care plans also save you time, energy, and frustration, thereby increasing your ability to find creative solutions to client problems. Creativity helps prevent the burnout that can result from a repetitive, "cookbook" approach to your daily work.

■ WHAT IS NURSING PROCESS?

Nursing process is a special way of thinking and acting. It is a systematic, creative approach used to identify, prevent, and treat actual or potential health problems; to identify patient strengths; and to promote wellness. It provides the framework in which nurses use their knowledge and skills to express human caring. The nursing process can be more completely explained by describing its relationship to nursing and caring, as well as its background, purpose, characteristics, and six-step organization.

Relationship to Nursing and Caring

You may have noticed that the definitions of nursing and nursing process are similar. They are certainly interrelated, but nursing is more than just nursing process. A nurse may have an organized, systematic, deliberate approach that is, nevertheless, mechanical and lacking in warmth and caring. On the other hand, a nurse can feel deeply for a patient, want to help, and yet not have the necessary problem-solving skills to do so. Although the nursing process is systematic and logical, its use does not negate the caring aspect of nursing. As you master the nursing process, it will become second nature to you and actually facilitate your caring.

KEY POINT
Nursing process
1. involves creativity and intuition.
2. is a special way of thinking and acting.
3. is a systematic problem-solving approach.
4. is used to identify, prevent, and treat health problems.
5. is used to promote wellness.
6. provides a framework in which nurses use their knowledge and skills to express human caring.

Nurses view caring in various ways; for example, as comforting, involvement, kindness, nurturing, tenderness, and concern. Leininger (1978) states that care is the essence of nursing and that there can be no cure without caring. Watson's (1988, p. 75) nursing theory describes nursing interventions that are related to human care (see Box 1–4 below). Caring "sets up the conditions of trust that enable the [patient] to accept the help offered and to *feel cared for*" (Benner and Wrubel 1989, p. 1–4).

Background

Hall (1955) first described nursing as a *process*. Among those who first used the term *nursing process* were Johnson (1959), Orlando (1961), and Wiedenbach

---

BOX 1–4

Watson's Carative Factors: Interventions Related to Human Care

1. *Forming a humanistic-altruistic system of values.* Obtaining satisfaction through giving and extending the sense of self.
2. *Instilling faith and hope* through development of an effective nurse-client relationship.
3. *Cultivating sensitivity to one's self and others.* This includes the ability to recognize and express your own feelings.
4. *Developing a helping-trust (human care) relationship.* This involves effective communication, empathy, and nonpossessive warmth.
5. *Expressing positive and negative feelings* (eg, feelings of sorrow, love, and pain), and accepting expression of those feelings from patients.
6. *Using a creative problem-solving caring process*—caring linked to the nursing process.
7. *Promoting transpersonal teaching and learning.* This factor differentiates caring from curing and shifts responsibility for wellness to the client.
8. *Providing a supportive, protective, or corrective environment.* This includes assessing the internal and external environment and the client's ability to cope with mental, physical, sociocultural, and spiritual changes; and making changes in the environment as needed.
9. *Helping with the gratification of human needs*—recognizing and attending to the physical, emotional, social, and spiritual needs of the client.
10. *Being sensitive to existential-phenomenologic-spiritual forces.* This means that you are alert to the mind-body-soul data of the immediate situation, allowing you to better understand the client's experience.

Source: Adapted from J. Watson (1988). *Nursing: Human Science and Human Care. A Theory of Nursing.* National League for Nursing Publication No. 15-2236. New York: National League for Nursing.

(1963). They described the process of nursing as a series of steps. During the 1970s, the process evolved from a three-step to a five- or six-step process (eg, Vitale, Schultz, and Nugent 1974). This text divides the planning step to create a six-step process to reflect (a) the current outcomes-driven healthcare environment and (b) the organization of the ANA *Standards of Care.*

In 1973, the ANA developed standards for evaluating the quality of care that nurses deliver. Publication of the ANA standards encouraged most states to revise their nurse practice acts to include assessment, diagnosis, planning, implementation, and evaluation as legitimate features of the nursing role. Since then, virtually all nurses have accepted the nursing process as the basis of their practice. The most recent ANA *Standards of Care* (1998) are shown in Box 1–3 on page 8. Standard II of the Canadian Nurses Association's *Definition of Nursing Practice and Standards for Nursing Practice* (1987) also requires nurses to be competent in all steps of the nursing process (see Box 1–5).

The nursing process is now taught in nearly every school of nursing. The National Council Licensure Examination for registered nurses (NCLEX, or "state board exams") integrates the phases of the nursing process into its questions. National accrediting bodies (eg, the Joint Commission on Accreditation of Healthcare Organizations and the National League for Nursing) include aspects of the nursing process in their criteria for evaluating hospitals, schools of nursing, and other healthcare agencies.

BOX 1–5

Canadian Nurses Association Standard II

1. Nurses are required to collect data in accordance with their conception of the client.
2. Nurses are required to analyse data collected in accordance with their conception of the goal of nursing, their role and the source of client difficulty.
3. Nurses are required to plan their nursing actions based upon the identified actual and potential client problems, in accordance with their conception of the focus and modes of intervention.
4. Nurses are required to perform nursing actions which implement the plan.
5. Nurses are required to evaluate all steps of the nursing process in accordance with their conceptual model for nursing.

Source: Canadian Nurses Association (1987). *A Definition of Nursing Practice and Standards for Nursing Practice.* Ottawa, ONT: CNA. Used with permission.

❑ Are all registered nurses professional nurses?
❑ Are all professional nurses registered nurses?
❑ The term "professional nurse" is used often. Who are the "nonprofessional" nurses, and what are they doing?

Purpose and Characteristics

The purpose of the nursing process is to provide a framework within which nurses can identify clients' health status and assist them in meeting their health needs. The nursing process provides a deliberate, but flexible, guide for planning, implementing, and evaluating effective, individualized nursing care. Often (but not always) the vehicle for this is a written nursing or multidisciplinary care plan. The following paragraphs describe characteristics of the nursing process and expand on its definition.

Nursing process is **dynamic and cyclic**. Nurses evaluate changing patient responses to nursing interventions in order to make necessary revisions in the plan of care. Previously completed phases (eg, assessment) are constantly reexamined for accuracy and appropriateness. Because the phases/ steps are interrelated, there is no absolute beginning or end to the process.

Nursing process is **client centered**. In the nurse-client relationship, the client's needs always take precedence. Clients are encouraged, to the extent they are able, to exercise control over their health and to make decisions about their care.

Nursing process is **planned and outcome-directed**. Interventions are carefully chosen and based on principles and research, rather than tradition (eg, "We've always done it that way"). Nursing interventions are chosen for the purpose of achieving desired patient outcomes.

Nursing process is **flexible**. It provides an organized approach to care, but it is not carried out in rigid, stepwise fashion. The nurse gives care according to a plan, but realizes that the plan will change continually.

EXAMPLE: According to the care plan, Mr. Akers was to be up in a chair for 15 minutes. However, as soon as he was out of bed he became pale and dizzy, so his nurse helped him back to bed instead of continuing toward the chair.

Nursing process is **universally applicable**. It can be used with clients of all ages, with any medical diagnosis, and at any point on the wellness-illness continuum. It is useful in any setting (eg, schools, hospitals, clinics, home health, industries) and across specialties (eg, hospice nursing, maternity nursing, surgical nursing). It is used to provide care for individuals, families, groups, and communities.

Nursing process is **patient-status oriented**. This means that care plans are organized according to statements about the patient's health status. Usually these are problem statements; however, they may also be statements describing healthy conditions or patient strengths. Of course, the nursing process cannot prevent or eliminate every patient problem (eg, chronic health problems, such as the pain and immobility associated with arthritis). When problems cannot be eliminated, the nurse provides available relief, supports the patient's strengths in coping with the problems, and helps patients to understand and find meaning in their situation.

Nursing process is a **cognitive (thinking) process**. It involves the use of intellectual skills in problem solving and decision making. Nurses use critical thinking to apply nursing knowledge systematically and logically to client data, enabling them to determine its meaning and plan appropriate care. This characteristic is discussed further in Chapter 2.

Organization: Phases of the Nursing Process

Explained very simply, the nurse using the nursing process listens to the patient's story in order to answer the following questions:

- What is the person's present health status?
- What is the person's desired health status?
- How can I help this person?
- Did it work?

Figure 1–2 shows how these questions fit with the six phases of the nursing process.

This text divides the nursing process into six phases (or steps) because it is easier to learn in smaller "chunks." However, most authors do not divide planning into two phases (their steps would be assessment, diagnosis, planning, implementation, and evaluation). This text does so in order to present planning processes gradually and in more detail. Also, a few authors still

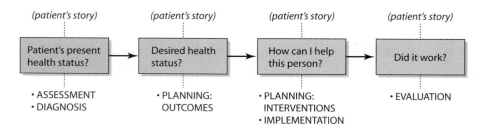

Figure 1–2
Overview of the nursing process

combine assessment and diagnosis into a single "assessment" phase (their phases are assessment, planning, intervention, and evaluation). Don't be too concerned about such inconsistencies. All such divisions are artificial anyway, because of the dynamic nature of the nursing process (see "Sequential Phases" and "Overlapping Phases" on pages 16–17).

Assessment—Getting the facts

In this phase you will collect, organize, validate, and record data about the patient's present health status. You will obtain data by examining patients, talking to them and their families, and reading charts and records. You do not draw conclusions about the data in this phase.

EXAMPLE: After Maura Greenberg's baby was born, the home health nurse performed a comprehensive assessment. She recorded on the nursing history Ms. Greenberg's statements that she is often constipated, snacks frequently, doesn't drink much, and does not take laxatives.

Diagnosis—What is the patient's present health status? What is contributing to it?

In this phase you will (1) sort, cluster, and analyze the data in order to identify the patient's present health status (actual and potential health problems and strengths); (2) write a precise statement describing the patient's present status and the factors contributing to it; (3) prioritize the diagnoses; and (4) decide which diagnoses will respond to nursing care and which must be referred to another healthcare professional.

EXAMPLE: The nurse wrote the following diagnosis on Ms. Greenberg's care plan: "Constipation related to insufficient intake of fiber and fluids."

The North American Nursing Diagnosis Association has developed a set of standardized labels for nurses to use in writing nursing diagnoses (NANDA 1999). This list is found on the inside covers of this text. It is discussed further in Chapter 6.

Planning Outcomes—What is the desired patient health status?

In this phase, you will work with the client to choose the desired outcomes. That is, you will decide exactly how you want the client's status to change and within what period of time. The outcomes chosen in this phase are the criteria you will use in the evaluation phase.

EXAMPLE: The nurse wrote the following outcomes on Ms. Greenberg's care plan:

- Will have soft, formed bowel movement at least every other day by May 15.
- Will be able to name at least six high-fiber foods before next visit on May 15.

A group of nurses in Iowa has published a standardized vocabulary and classification for describing patient outcomes thought to be sensitive to nursing interventions—the "Nursing Outcomes Classification (NOC)" (Johnson and Maas 2000). Chapter 7 discusses in more detail how nurses can use NOC in planning and evaluating care.

Planning Interventions—How can you help achieve the desired outcomes?

In this phase, you will choose interventions for promoting wellness or preventing, correcting, or relieving health problems. You will plan specific interventions for the outcomes associated with each nursing diagnosis. The end product of the planning phases is often a written care plan. However, in some cases, planning is simply the mental process of choosing what to do. You will often act without a *written* plan, but never without a plan.

EXAMPLE: The nurse wrote the following nursing orders on Ms. Greenberg's care plan:

1. Give the pamphlet "Fiber in Your Diet" to Ms. G.
2. Help Ms. G. make a meal plan using high-fiber foods.
3. Explain the relationship of fiber and fluids to bowel elimination.
4. Reassess bowel elimination status in one week (5/15).

Implementation—Doing, delegating, and documenting

In this phase, you will communicate the plan of care to other members of the healthcare team and carry out the interventions indicated on the plan or delegate them to others. The final activity in this phase is to record the care given and the client's responses.

EXAMPLE: The nurse took the pamphlet to Ms. Greenberg and talked with her about the importance of fiber and fluids and preventing constipation in the postpartum period. She recorded these interventions in the nursing progress notes.

There is also a standardized classification of nursing interventions, called the Nursing Interventions Classification (NIC) (McCloskey and Bulechek 1999). Chapters 8 and 10 describe more fully how nurses use this vocabulary to plan care and record nursing work.

Evaluation—Did it work?

In this phase, after implementing the plan, you will compare the patient's health status with the desired outcomes identified in the planning outcomes phase. You will determine which interventions were or were not helpful in achieving desired outcomes and revise the care plan as needed. The nursing process is cyclic: you will keep reexamining all the phases (assessment, diagnosis, outcomes, interventions, and implementation) to determine what is effective and what should be changed.

> EXAMPLE: On the nurse's May 15 return visit, Ms. Greenberg was able to identify high-fiber foods, but reported that she had not had a bowel movement since May 12. The nurse advised her to drink more fluids, including some prune juice, and to call her primary care provider if she did not have a bowel movement within the next 24 hours.

Table 1–3 summarizes the six phases of the nursing process.

Sequential Phases

Nursing process phases are sequential in that each step depends on the activities of preceding steps. For example:

1. *Assessment→Diagnosis.* You must have accurate data (assessment phase) in order to make the correct diagnosis (diagnosis phase).
2. *Diagnosis→Planning Outcomes.* Desired outcomes are developed directly from your diagnoses. In the preceding example of Ms. Greenberg, the diagnosis was "Constipation. . ." and an outcome was that she would have a "soft, formed bowel movement. . ."
3. *Planning Outcomes→Planning Interventions.* The desired outcomes direct your choice of interventions. You choose interventions that you expect will produce the outcomes.
4. *Planning Outcomes and Interventions→Implementation.* The plan of care guides the activities you perform during implementation.
5. *Implementation→Evaluation.* You identified the client's present health status in the diagnosis phase. You must carry out the plan (implementation) in order to produce a change in health status that you can evaluate.

Table 1–3 Phases of the Nursing Process

Phase	Activities
Assessment	Collect and organize data.
Diagnosis	Identify present health status (problems and strengths).
Planning **O**utcomes	Choose desired patient outcomes.
Planning **I**nterventions	Choose nursing interventions.
Implementation	Carry out the plan of action.
Evaluation	Determine if the plan was effective.

The phases do not always occur in the ADP$_O$P$_I$IE order; that is, you will not always complete one step before proceeding to the next. For example, nurses do not always gather a complete set of data about a patient before taking action. In an emergency, for instance, you would quickly think of an action (planning interventions) and implement it immediately (implementation) before doing formal data collection or writing a care plan. Of course, you would have had to make some observations (assessment) in order to realize that action was needed, but you would have only limited data and you probably would not have consciously formulated a problem statement. After acting, you would evaluate whether the emergency was over and then return to a more thorough and systematic collection and analysis of data. The following is another example of nonsequential phases:

EXAMPLE: The teacher brought Carlene to the school nurse's office. Carlene was crying and saying, "My stomach hurts so much!" (data). She seemed very anxious, so before attempting a complete assessment, the nurse first acted (implementation) to calm Carlene. After evaluating that Carlene was calm enough to answer questions (evaluation), the nurse proceeded with the interview and physical examination (assessment).

Overlapping Phases

This text describes the phases of the nursing process separately in order to help you learn them. However, in practice, they overlap a great deal. For example, even though the first encounter with a client usually begins with some form of data collection, assessment actually continues at each patient contact. While you are bathing a patient (implementation), you may at the same time observe the skin over his bony prominences (assessment). If you observe some redness (assessment), you may conclude that the patient has Impaired Skin Integrity (diagnosis).

The evaluation phase overlaps with all phases of the nursing process because you will constantly examine what you have done in previous phases. After performing interventions and determining their effect on client health status, you will examine the:

- *Assessment phase* to see if your data are complete and accurate.
- *Diagnosis phase* to see if the diagnoses are accurate and if any need to be added to or removed from the list.
- *Planning outcomes phase* to check whether the outcomes were appropriate/realistic.
- *Planning interventions phase* to see whether the most effective interventions were chosen.
- *Implementation phase* to determine whether the plan was actually carried out properly, and whether activities were delegated appropriately.

Relationship to Problem-Solving Processes

Problem solving is the process of identifying a problem and then planning and taking steps to resolve it. Problem solving is "the process used when a gap is perceived between an existing state (what *is* occurring) and a desired state (what *should be* occurring)" (Strader 1992, p. 228). Because the nursing process also considers wellness and strengths, it is not limited to problems. However, it is similar to the method used in solving problems of all types.

The **scientific method** is a systematic, logical approach to problem solving, based on data and hypothesis testing. The first step is to identify the problem. The next step is to define it carefully. The problem statement serves as a guide for setting criteria by which to evaluate possible solutions. Data relating specifically to the problem are then collected and solutions are generated (hypothesis formulation). After considering the consequences of each, the preferred solution is put into effect and the results are evaluated (hypothesis testing).

> EXAMPLE: Suppose you are on your way to an important job interview when your car breaks down. Your analysis of the situation is that your most important and immediate need is to get a job, not to repair the car. You have specified the exact nature of your problem: Possible loss of a job opportunity caused by being late to the interview. You have the following data: (1) it is too far to walk and (2) no one is at home to come get you. You make a quick plan. Your goal is to get there on time. You decide to walk to the nearest telephone and call a taxi for yourself and a tow truck for the car (hypothesis). The outcome of your plan is a fabulous job and a new car—you evaluate that the plan was successful.

When using the nursing process, the problem is not usually so obvious. The nurse often begins with comprehensive data collection and uses the data to identify problems or health risks. In the scientific method, the problem is identified before extensive data are collected, and the only information gathered is that which pertains to the problem. See Table 1–4, on page 19, for further comparison.

Intuition is a problem-solving approach that relies on use of one's "inner sense." Expert nurses describe instances in which they "just had a feeling" that something was wrong, even though they could not say what prompted the feeling. Although it is neither systematic nor data based, intuition is gaining credibility as a legitimate aspect of expert clinical judgment that is acquired through knowledge and experience. For example, a nurse might develop expertise in cardiovascular nursing through continuous experience with patients' responses to cardiovascular problems. The knowledge base of experienced nurses enables them to recognize patient cues and patterns and begin to make correct decisions. They are able to judge quickly which evidence is most important and act upon that limited evidence. Thus, intuition

KEY POINT
Intuition is:

- the "direct apprehension of a situation based upon a background of similar and dissimilar situations and embodied intelligence or skill" (Brenner 1984, p. 295).
- the "immediate knowing of something without the conscious use of reason" (Schraeder and Fisher 1987, p. 46).

Table 1–4   Comparison of Formal Problem Solving, the Research Process, and the Nursing Process

Research Process	Formal Problem Solving	Nursing Process
State a research question or problem	Recognize that a problem exists	Assessment: Perform comprehensive assessment (collect data)
Identify the purpose of or rationale for the study		
Review related literature	Gather information about the problem	
Formulate hypothesis and define variables	Define the exact nature of the problem	Diagnosis: Formulate the nursing diagnoses
Select method to test hypotheses	Develop solutions and decide on a plan of action	Planning: • Choose patient outcomes • Generate and choose nursing interventions and activities
Collect the data	Implement the plan of action	Implementation: Carry out the nursing interventions
Analyze the data; interpret the results	Monitor the situation over time (collect data about the effects of the plan)	
Evaluate the hypothesis	Evaluate the plan or solution to assure initial and continued effectiveness	Evaluation: Collect data about patient responses to interventions; judge whether outcomes were achieved

describes a leap (or a condensing) in the critical thinking element of considering evidence.

The danger in intuition is that sometimes the nurse's inner sense is true, but sometimes it is not. Critical thinkers realize how easy it is to confuse intuitions and prejudices. They follow their "inner sense that something is so," but only with a healthy sense of intellectual humility. Intuition is not a reliable problem-solving method for novice nurses or students because they lack the knowledge and clinical experience on which to base their judgments. Used by a novice, intuition may be little more than guessing. As a beginning practitioner, you should be cautious about flashes of intuition and discuss them with more experienced colleagues before acting on them.

In the **trial-and-error** method, you would try a number of solutions until you found one that worked. However, without considering alternatives systematically, you cannot know why one solution worked and another did not. This method is not recommended for nurses because it is inefficient and because the patient might be harmed if a solution is not appropriate.

■ QUALITIES NEEDED BY THE NURSE

The nursing process is only as good as the nurse who uses it. The following qualities and attitudes contribute to successful use of the nursing process. They are all qualities that you can improve through awareness, effort, and practice.

Cognitive (Intellectual) Skills

The nursing process is a guide to systematic thinking in nursing practice. Intellectual skills used in the nursing process are decision making, problem solving (discussed in the preceding section), and critical thinking. **Decision making** is the process of choosing the best action to take—the action most likely to produce the desired outcome. It involves deliberation, judgment, and choice. Decision making is important in the problem-solving process, but not all decisions involve problem solving (eg, you decided what to wear today). **Critical thinking** is careful, goal-oriented, purposeful thinking that involves many mental skills, such as determining which data are relevant, evaluating the credibility of sources, and making inferences. It is essential to good problem solving and decision making.

Creativity and Curiosity

Creativity and curiosity are essential to the nursing process and critical thinking. You need vision and insight to find new and better ways of doing things. Always ask yourself, "Why are we doing this? Why are we doing it *this* way?" Excellent nurses understand the rationale for every nursing activity. If they cannot find a reason for the activity or cannot show that it is having the desired effect, they work to have it discontinued.

EXAMPLE: A hospital's procedures specify the use of draw sheets. Mauricio works on a unit where most of the patients are ambulatory. One day as he was changing bed linens, he wondered, "What good is this draw sheet? We never use it for anything, and we use fitted bottom sheets." He talked to the unit manager, who changed the unit procedures, saving both money and nursing time.

Interpersonal Skills

Interpersonal skills are the activities used in person-to-person communication. In addition to verbal and written communication, they include knowledge of human behavior and social systems, as well as such nonverbal behaviors as body posture and movement, facial expression, and touch. Your success in developing a trusting relationship with patients depends on your ability to communicate—to listen and to convey compassion, interest, and information. Successful outcomes depend on successful nurse-patient relationships.

EXAMPLE: Elsa Banayos is the primary nurse for a group of patients. When she notices that the patient care assistant is not using correct body mechanics to help Mr. Davis out of bed, she draws on her interpersonal skills. She must intervene to assure the safety of both Mr. Davis and the assistant, but without embarrassing the assistant or undermining the patient's confidence in her.

Communication skills are important, but *what* you communicate is just as important. You can promote good relationships by having a positive attitude and sense of humor; by being open, honest, patient, and frank; by demonstrating humility, accountability, and reliability; by admitting when you are wrong; and by giving credit to others who deserve it.

Cultural Competence

Cultural competence means that the nurse works within the client's cultural belief system to resolve health problems. This requires the nurse to be aware of similarities and differences among cultural groups and to be culturally sensitive. Although cultural competence can be called an interpersonal skill, it also involves knowledge and attitudes.

Psychomotor Skills

Nurses use psychomotor skills, especially in the implementation phase of the nursing process when giving hands-on care. Good psychomotor skills help to gain client trust and achieve desired client outcomes.

EXAMPLE: Turning a patient smoothly minimizes pain and helps establish trust and rapport. If you are clumsy with the turning, the patient may think you are not competent and will be less likely to trust you in other situations. He may hesitate to ask you for information or help, and you may be unable to obtain important assessment data from him.

Technological Skills

Nurses work with high-technology equipment, such as heart monitors and respirators, much of which contains programmable computer chips.

EXAMPLE: In the past, nurses regulated intravenous infusions by counting drops and visualizing markings on the container. Now they must perform several steps to program a computerized pump to deliver the correct fluid rate and measure the amount infused.

Many use computers for planning and documenting patient care. For example, some nurses carry pocket-sized computers, which they use to record assessments, retrieve laboratory results, and document interventions. In addition, nurses are making on-unit use of the Internet to find information they need to choose the best nursing interventions.

KEY POINT
"**Cultural sensitivity** is the respect and appreciation of cultural behaviors based on an understanding of the other person's perspective" (Kozier et al 1995, p. 295).

KEY POINT
Examples of Psychomotor Skills

- Changing dressings
- Teaching CPR
- Giving injections
- Turning and positioning patients
- Attaching a heart monitor
- Suctioning a tracheostomy

■ NURSING PROCESS AND WELLNESS

The nursing process is not limited to use with clients who are ill. Nurses frequently work with well clients, focusing on health promotion, health protection, and disease prevention. **Health promotion** activities (eg, daily exercise) are directed toward achieving a higher level of wellness; they are not aimed at avoiding any particular disease. In health promotion, the client is seen as having more control and expertise, and the nurse serves as a facilitator (Lindsey and Hartrick 1996). **Health protection** focuses on activities that decrease environmental threats to health (eg, air pollution). **Disease prevention** involves actions that help to prevent specific health problems or diseases (eg, immunizations, prenatal care).

While most of the national health budget is spent on care and treatment of illnesses, health-promotion initiatives are receiving attention from government agencies. The US Public Health Service, in *Healthy People 2010* (2000), outlines a national strategy for improving the health of the nation during this decade. The report acknowledges that health promotion and disease prevention provide the best opportunities for preserving our healthcare resources. Following are the broad goals outlined in this report.

1. Increase the quality and years of healthy life [for Americans]
2. Eliminate health disparities [among Americans]

Consider the characteristics of the nursing process as it is applied in the following case study of a well client.

CASE STUDY A 40-year-old corporate executive has come to the company nurse for her required annual physical examination.

Assessment   The nurse takes a complete health history, which reveals no past medical problems, except that the client's father died of a heart attack at age 62. Her lab results and chest x-ray are normal. The nurse performs a complete physical examination, with normal findings, including a blood pressure of 120/74 and a pulse of 84; the client is 10 lb. overweight. The nurse asks about the client's health habits and lifestyle and discovers that: she works long hours and often takes work home; her only exercise is an occasional golf game; she eats a balanced diet, sleeps about 7 hours a day, and smokes a half-pack of cigarettes per day.

Diagnosis   If nursing were concerned only with illness, the nurse would analyze the data, diagnose that no problem exists, and conclude that no interventions are needed. However, the nurse takes a holistic perspective, rather than a disease-oriented one, and understands the importance of disease prevention and health promotion. The nurse diagnoses that the client has unmet health-promotion/disease-prevention needs.

Planning Outcomes   Using client input the nurse develops broad outcomes, that the client will (1) become aware of ways in which her lifestyle can either increase or decrease her risk of disease, and (2) experience improved health status, as evidenced by smoking cessation, beginning an exercise program, and maintaining her present weight. The nurse does not include a goal for the client to reduce her work hours, because she insists that she needs to work long hours, enjoys it, and has no interest in changing that behavior.

Planning Interventions   Based on the desired outcomes, the nurse chooses nursing interventions and writes the care plan. The nurse plans to (1) talk with the client about the effect of smoking on coronary circulation, and about the relationship of exercise and diet to weight control and a healthy heart, and (2) give the client pamphlets about basic nutrition, smoking cessation, and aerobic exercises.

Implementation   Before the client leaves, the nurse encourages her to attend the company-sponsored smoking cessation clinic. He does not refer her to a dietitian, because she seems adequately informed and motivated to avoid gaining weight.

Evaluation   The client and the nurse included in the plan that she will return in one month to be weighed, and evaluate her efforts to stop smoking and begin exercising. If desired outcomes are being achieved, the nurse plans to assess the client's stress level and coping mechanisms at the one-month follow-up, to be sure that she is still showing no effects from her strenuous work schedule. At that time, they may modify her plan of care.

■ NURSING PROCESS AND COMMUNITY HEALTH

Nursing process is not limited to caring for individual patients. Community health nurses use nursing process to focus on the health needs of groups of persons (eg, communities and systems). Parish nurses, for example, holistically address the physical, emotional, and spiritual needs of members of a church congregation (community). They provide teaching, counseling, health screening, and advocacy. Hands-on care is not their main focus (Miskelly 1995).

CASE STUDY

Parish nurse, Patti Munoz, wished to identify the parish community's health needs and priorities so that she could provide an effective health education program.

Assessment   Patti developed a survey and distributed it to church members. She collected data about their wellness behaviors and beliefs in four categories: physical, emotional/relational, spiritual, and health system relationships/knowledge base.

Diagnosis   From the data, Patti identified several groups of parishioners who were at risk. One such group consisted of adults under age 50 without regular blood pressure screening.

Planning Outcomes   For this group, Patti developed a desired outcome based on national public health standards: "Increase to at least 90 percent the proportion of adults who have had blood pressure measured within the preceding 2 years and can state whether their blood pressure was normal or high" (US Department of Health and Human Services 1990, p. 404).

Planning Interventions   To achieve this outcome, Patti planned an annual health fair. One of the activities to be included was blood pressure screening. She also planned to place related literature in the church library and write an article about heart disease prevention for the monthly newsletter.

Evaluation   A year later, after implementing her plan, Patti again surveyed the congregation regarding their health beliefs and behaviors. She discovered the desired outcome regarding blood pressure screening had been met, and decided to continue with the same interventions, except for the newsletter article, which she would not use this year.

(Case created from Miskelly, S. (1995). A parish nursing model: Applying the community health nursing process in a church community. *Journal of Community Health Nursing*, 12(1):1–14.

BOX 1–6

ANA Standard V—Ethics

The nurse's decisions and actions on behalf of patients are determined in an ethical manner.

Measurement Criteria

1. The nurse's practice is guided by the *Code for Nurses.*[1]
2. The nurse maintains patient confidentiality within legal and regulatory parameters.
3. The nurse acts as a patient advocate and assists patients in developing skills so they can advocate for themselves.
4. The nurse delivers care in a nonjudgmental and nondiscriminatory manner that is sensitive to patient diversity.
5. The nurse delivers care in a manner that preserves patient autonomy, dignity, and rights.
6. The nurse seeks available resources in formulating ethical decisions.

---

[1] American Nurses Association (1985). *Code for Nurses with Interpretive Statements.* Kansas City, MO: ANA.

Source: Reprinted with permission from American Nurses Association, *Standards of Clinical Nursing Practice.* 2nd ed. © 1998. American Nurses Publishing, American Nurses Foundation/American Nurses Association, 600 Maryland Ave. SW, Suite 100W, Washington, DC.

■ ETHICAL AND CULTURAL CONSIDERATIONS

Professional standards of practice require nurses to apply the nursing process in an ethical and culturally sensitive manner. For example, nurses are ethically responsible for evaluating the quality of the care they give and maintaining the knowledge they need to give good care. Standard V of the ANA *Standards of Professional Performance* (ANA 1998, pp. 13–14) specifically requires that nurses' decisions be made in an ethical manner and with cultural sensitivity (see Box 1–6, item 4). The other ANA professional performance standards (see Box 1–7) indirectly imply the ethical nature of nursing. Many institutions have an ethics committee for addressing ethical issues in patient care. It is important for nurses to participate in such committee work.

In addition, there are cultural variations in the ways caring is expressed and received. Nurses should try to understand how clients of different cultures view care and then work toward providing culture-specific care (Leininger 1978).

BOX 1–7

ANA Standards of Professional Performance

Standard I.   **Quality of Care.** The nurse systematically evaluates the quality and effectiveness of nursing practice.

Standard II.   **Performance Appraisal.** The nurse evaluates one's own nursing practice in relation to professional practice standards and relevant statutes and regulations.

Standard III.   **Education.** The nurse acquires and maintains current knowledge and competency in nursing practice.

Standard IV.   **Collegiality.** The nurse interacts with, and contributes to the professional development of, peers and other health care providers as colleagues.

Standard V.   **Ethics.** The nurse's decisions and actions on behalf of patients are determined in an ethical manner.

Standard VI.   **Collaboration.** The nurse collaborates with the patient, family, and other health care providers in providing patient care.

Standard VII.   **Research.** The nurse uses research findings in practice.

Standard VIII.   **Resource Utilization.** The nurse considers factors related to safety, effectiveness, and cost in planning and delivering patient care.

Source: Reprinted with permission from American Nurses Association, *Standards of Clinical Nursing Practice*. 2nd ed. © 1998. American Nurses Publishing, American Nurses Foundation/American Nurses Association, 600 Maryland Ave. SW, Suite 100W, Washington, DC.

■ SUMMARY

Nursing process

- ■ is a systematic approach to delivering holistic care to well and ill clients.
- ■ identifies the client's present health status (problems and strengths) and focuses on desired outcomes.
- ■ is used to provide care for individuals, families, and communities.
- ■ is not limited to treatment of illnesses, but is used in health promotion, health protection, and disease prevention.
- ■ benefits clients, nurses, and the nursing profession.
- ■ is organized in six interrelated phases: assessment, diagnosis, planning outcomes, planning interventions, implementation, and evaluation.
- ■ is patient-centered, flexible, dynamic, and cyclic.
- ■ requires special nursing knowledge and skills in order to be used successfully.
- ■ must be used with cultural sensitivity and in an ethical manner in order to meet standards of professional practice.

NURSING PROCESS PRACTICE

1. Think about the meanings of *caring for* and *caring about* patients. Create a short story describing a nurse who is doing each.

Caring for a patient.

Provide treatment for patient
physical

Caring about a patient.

mentaly

2. In this scenario, which of the underlined data items are appropriate concerns of the nurse and which ones are medical concerns? Brian Callaway <u>has smoked two packs of cigarettes a day for the past 30 years</u>. He has just been told that his chest x-ray shows some suspicious <u>lesions on his lung</u> and that he will need a <u>biopsy</u> to see if he has lung cancer. Mr. Callaway says <u>he coughs a lot</u> and that <u>he becomes short of breath when climbing stairs</u>. He says, "I'm scared to death I have cancer."

taking care by nurse   *by doctor*

Nursing Concerns	Medical Concerns
he coughs a lot becomes short of breath smoked two packs of	lesions on his lung biopsy

3. Match each stage of the nursing process with the examples of activities that occur in that stage.

1. _a_ Writing patient outcomes
2. _a_ Conducting a nursing interview
3. _d_ Choosing nursing interventions
4. _d_ Writing a care plan
5. _e_ Carrying out the nursing orders
6. _e_ Charting the care given to a client
7. _e_ Changing a client's dressing   I
8. _c_ Using client data to decide whether outcomes have been achieved
9. _b_ Stating the client's problem and its cause
10. _f_ Describing the client's level of wellness

a. Assessment
b. Diagnosis
c. Planning Outcomes
d. Planning Interventions
e. Implementation
f. Evaluation

4. Fill in the blanks. Use the following list to identify qualities of the nurse that are being demonstrated in each of the examples (a–e).

Cognitive skills   Psychomotor skills   Interpersonal skills
Creativity and curiosity   Technology

a. _Interperson_ The nurse sits quietly while an elderly client reminisces about old friends.

b. _techno_ The nursing student practices catheterization in the school learning lab.

c. _Creativity and curiosity_ The nursing student performs the critical thinking activities in this text.

d. __*Cognitive*__   A unit procedure book states that vital signs are to be taken every 4 hours and respirations are to be counted for one full minute. This is a unit with essentially healthy patients who have no risk for respiratory problems. After discovering that no one can provide rationale for these "routines," the unit manager specifies "routine" vital signs every 12 hours, with respirations only once a day.

e. __*physco*__   The care plan says the patient is to ambulate with help at 0900 and 2100. At 0900, Mr. Sanchez has the first visitor he has had in this three-week hospital stay. The nurse asks the patient care technician to postpone ambulation until his visitor leaves.

CRITICAL THINKING PRACTICE

Knowing yourself is an important first step in critical thinking (self-knowledge is discussed further in Chapter 2). Review the section "Qualities Needed by the Nurse" on pp. 20–21, and answer the following questions:

1. Which of the qualities/abilities best describe you?

2. How did you develop these qualities/abilities?

3. Rank the qualities from strongest to weakest.

4. Why do you think your weakest ability has not been as fully developed as the others?

5. Make a plan for strengthening your weakest qualities. What experiences will you need in order to improve them?

If you feel comfortable doing so, share your plan with a faculty adviser and ask for feedback. Otherwise, discuss it with one or two classmates. See if they agree with your self-assessment; ask for feedback about your plan.

CASE STUDY: APPLYING CRITICAL THINKING

Alma Boiko had been in an intermediate care facility since having a stroke that left her unable to care for herself. When she developed pneumonia, she was transferred to a hospital. Juan Apodaca, RN, <u>settled her comfortably in bed</u> and briefly <u>interviewed her</u> about her symptoms. He <u>obtained a temperature</u> of 101° F, pulse 120, respirations 32, and blood pressure of 100/68. Juan <u>examined Ms. Boiko's chart</u> to obtain a history of her illness and a record of her nursing care. He <u>administered oxygen by nasal cannula</u>, as ordered by the physician. When <u>performing the physical examination</u>, Juan noticed a reddened area over Ms. Boiko's coccyx.

Because she was unable to move about in bed, <u>Juan wrote a diagnosis</u> of *"Risk for Impaired Skin Integrity over coccyx related to constant pressure to bony prominences caused by inability to move about in bed."* From the list on the computer, he <u>chose an outcome</u> that the skin on Ms. Boiko's coccyx would remain intact and that the redness would be gone within 2 days. <u>He wrote nursing orders for skin care</u>, a schedule for turning Ms. Boiko every 2 hours, and orders for frequent, continued observation of her skin.

Two days later, while <u>bathing Ms. Boiko</u>, Juan <u>observed that her coccygeal area was still red</u>, a small area of skin was peeling off, and there was some serous drainage. Juan <u>concluded that the outcome had not been achieved</u>. He was sure his data were adequate, and he changed his nursing diagnosis to *"Impaired Skin Integrity over coccyx. . . ."* The other staff members assured Juan that they had carried out the 2-hour turning schedule, except for 6 hours at night when they left Ms. Boiko to sleep undisturbed. Even though turning every 2 hours while awake was a standard of care on the unit and had been adequate for other clients, Juan concluded that it was not often enough for Ms. Boiko. <u>He changed the order on the care plan</u> to read "Turn every 2 hours around the clock."

1. Label the underlined activities $A, D, P_o, P_i, I, or E,$ according to the phase of the nursing process represented by the activity.
2. List below all the client data (human responses).

3. Circle the activities that show the dynamic/cyclic nature of the nursing process.
4. List all the nursing orders that Juan wrote. Note that some are summarized here instead of being fully written out in nursing-order format.

5. Where in the case study do you see the most obvious example of overlapping nursing process phases?

6. How did the nurse demonstrate creativity?

7. Which characteristic(s) of the nursing process was/were demonstrated when Juan ordered a turning schedule that was more frequent than the unit routines?

■ SELECTED REFERENCES

American Nurses Association (1980). *Nursing: A social policy statement.* Kansas City, MO: Author.

American Nurses Association (1985). *Code for nurses with interpretive statements.* Washington, DC: Author.

American Nurses Association (1992). *House of Delegates report: 1992 convention, Las Vegas, NV.* Kansas City, MO: Author; pp. 104–120.

American Nurses Association (1995). *Nursing's policy statement.* Washington, DC: Author.

American Nurses Association (1998). *Standards of clinical nursing practice.* Washington, DC: Author.

Anderson, C. A. (1998). Nursing: A thinking profession. *Nurs Outlook.* 46:197–198.

Baggs, J. G. (1997). Collaboration between nurses and physicians: What is it? Does it exist? Why does it matter? In: J. C. McCloskey and H. K. Grace, eds. *Current Issues Nursing.* St. Louis: CV Mosby; pp. 519–524.

Benner, P. and C. Tanner (1987). How expert nurses use intuition. *Am J Nurs* 87:23–31.

Benner, P. and J. Wrubel (1989). *The primacy of caring: Stress and coping in health and illness.* Menlo Park, CA: Addison-Wesley.

Bryant, L. (1998 Winter). Scholarly dialogue: The ontology of the discipline of nursing. *Nurs Sci Quart* 11(4):145–148.

Canadian Nurses Association (1987). *A definition of nursing practice and standards for nursing practice.* Ottawa: CNA.

Hall, L. (June 1955). Quality of nursing care. *Public Health News.* Jersey State Dept of Health.

Hiraki, A. (1997). A response to Colleen Varcoe: Disparagement of the nursing process as dogma. *J Advan Nurs* 25(4):865–866.

Johnson, D. (1959). A philosophy for nursing diagnosis. *Nursing Outlook* 7:198–200.

Johnson, M. and M. Maas, eds. (2000). *Nursing Outcomes Classification (NOC)* (2nd ed.). St. Louis: CV Mosby.

Joint Commission on Accreditation of Healthcare Organizations (1992). Nursing care. *Accreditation Manual for Hospitals*: JCAHO.

Johns, C. (1996). The benefits of a reflective model of nursing. *Nursing Times* 92(27):39–41.

Johnson, J. (1994). A dialectical examination of nursing art. *Advan Nurs Sci* 17(1):1–14.

Koldjeski, D. (1993). A restructured nursing process model. *Nurse Educator* 18(4):33–38.

Kozier, B., G. Erb, K. Blais et al (1995). *Fundamentals of nursing* (5th ed.). Redwood City, CA: Addison-Wesley Nursing.

Kozier, B., G. Erb, K. Blais (1997). Chap. 4. Collaboration in health care. *Professional nursing practice: Concepts and perspectives.* Menlo Park, CA: Addison Wesley Longman, Inc.; pp. 67–85.

Leflore, E. (1998). Charting. . . in the palm of your hand. *Nursing Spectrum* (Florida ed.) 8(8):20.

Leininger, M. (1978). *Transcultural nursing: Concepts, theories, and practice.* New York: Wiley.

Lindsey, E. and G. Hartrick (1996). Health-promoting nursing practice: The demise of the nursing process? *J Adv Nurs* 23(1):106–112.

Maas, M. L. (1998). Nursing's role in interdisciplinary accountability for patient outcomes. *Outcomes Manage Nursing Prac* 2(3):92–94.

Mason, G. M. and M. Attree (1997). The relationship between research and the nursing process in clinical practice. *J Advan Nursing* 26(5):1045–1049.

McCloskey, J. and G. Bulechek (1999). *Nursing interventions classification* (3rd ed.). St. Louis: CV Mosby.

Miskelly, S. (1995). A parish nursing model: Applying the community health nursing process in a church community. *J Commun Health Nurs* 12(1):1–14.

Neuman, B. (1972). The Betty Neuman model: A total person approach to viewing patient problems. *Nurs Res* 21(3):264–269.

Neuman, B. (1980). The Betty Neuman health-care systems model: A total person approach to patient problems. In: J. Riehl and C. Roy, eds. *Conceptual models for nursing practice*. New York: Appleton-Century-Crofts.

Nightingale, F. (1969). *Notes on nursing. What it is, what it is not*. New York: Dover Publications. (Originally published in 1859)

North American Nursing Diagnosis Association (1999). *Nursing diagnoses: Definitions & Classification 1999–2000*. Philadelphia: NANDA.

O'Connell, B. (1998). The clinical application of the nursing process in selected acute care settings: A professional mirage. *Austral J Advan Nurs* 15(4):22–32.

Orem, D. (1971). *Nursing: Concepts of practice*. New York: McGraw-Hill.

Orlando, I. (1961). *The dynamic nurse-patient relationship*. New York: GP Putnam's Sons.

Parse, R. (1974). *Nursing fundamentals*. Flushing, NY: Medical Examination Publishing.

Parse, R. (1981). *Man-living-health: A theory of nursing*. New York: John Wiley & Sons.

Parse, R. (1987). *Nursing science: Major paradigms, theories, and critiques*. Philadelphia: WB Saunders.

Patterson, P. (1998). Editorial, ". . . benefits of working as a team." *OR Manager* 14(1):5.

Pavlovich-Danis, S., H. Forman et al (1998, July/August). The nurse-physician relationship. Can it be saved? *J Nurs Admin* 28(7–8):17–20.

Pender, N. J., V. H. Barkauskas, Rice, V. H. et al (1992). Health promotion and disease prevention: Toward excellence in nursing practice and education. *Nurs Outlook* 40(3):106–112.

Peplau, H. (1952). *Interpersonal relations in nursing*. New York: GP Putnam's Sons.

Reed, J. (1992). Individualized nursing care: Some implications. *J Clin Nurs* 1:7–12.

Rogers, M. (1970). *The theoretical basis of nursing*. Philadelphia: FA Davis.

Rogers, M. E. (1980). Nursing: A science of unitary man. In: J. P. Riehl and S. C. Roy, eds. *Conceptual models for nursing practice*. New York: Appleton-Century-Crofts; pp. 329–337.

Roy, C. (1970). A conceptual framework for nursing. *Nursing Outlook* 18(3):42–45.

Roy, C. (1976). *Introduction to nursing: An adaptation model*. Englewood Cliffs: NJ: Prentice Hall.

Roy, C. (1980). The Roy adaptation model. In: J. Riehl and C. Roy eds., *Conceptual models for nursing practice*. 2nd ed. New York: Appleton-Century-Crofts.

Schraeder, B., and D. Fischer (1987). Using intuitive knowledge in the neonatal intensive care nursery. *Holist Nurs Prac* 1(3):45–51.

Spitzer, A. (1998). Moving into the information era: Does the current nursing paradigm still hold? *J Advan Nurs* 28(4):786–93.

Strader, M. (1992). Critical thinking. In: E. J. Sullivan and P. J. Decker, eds. *Effective management in nursing* (3rd ed.). Redwood City, CA: Addison-Wesley Nursing.

US Dept of Health and Human Services, PHS (1990). *Healthy People 2000*. Washington, DC: US Government Printing Office.

US Dept of Health and Human Services, PHS (2000). *Healthy People 2010*. Washington, DC: US Government Printing Office.

Varcoe, C. (1996). Disparagement of the nursing process: The new dogma? *J Advan Nurs* 23: 120–125.

Vitale, B., N. Schultz, and P. Nugent (1974). *A problem-solving approach to nursing care plans: A program*. St. Louis: CV Mosby.

Walsh, M. (1997). Will critical pathways replace the nursing process? *Nurs Standard* 11(52): 39–42.

Watson, J. (1988). *Nursing: Human science and human care. A theory of nursing*. New York: National League for Nursing.

Wiedenbach, E. (1963). The helping art of nursing. *Am J Nurs* 63(11):54–57.

2
Critical Thinking

Learning Outcomes

After completing this chapter, you should be able to do the following:

- Give a definition of critical thinking.
- Explain why critical thinking is important for nurses.
- Compare and contrast five types of nursing knowledge.
- Describe some important critical thinking skills and attitudes.
- Use intellectual standards to evaluate your own thinking.
- Discuss the relationship between critical thinking and nursing process.
- List guidelines to aid in developing critical thinking.

■ WHY DO NURSES NEED TO THINK CRITICALLY?

". . . How do you choose between a butterfly or an IV intracath? [You] have to consider why you want that line in. And just learning the insertion alone is difficult. You take into consideration . . . whether it's a short-term, keep-open IV with limited medications, then the butterfly IV is more comfortable and presents less of a threat of phlebitis. Doctors vary in their preferences as well, and you have to take that into consideration. And of course, the condition of the patient and his veins makes a great deal of difference. For example, with older patients special skill is required. They look as if they are going to be so easy to get in because the veins look large, but they are so fragile. If you do not use a very, very slight tourniquet, the . . . vein will just pop open." (Benner 1984, pp. 124–125)

The preceding true exemplar, presented by an expert nurse, illustrates that nursing is both thinking and doing. Learning to be a nurse requires more than just memorizing facts. Nurses use stored-up facts along with new information to make decisions, generate new ideas, and solve problems (see Figure 2–2 on page 35). In order to transfer nursing knowledge

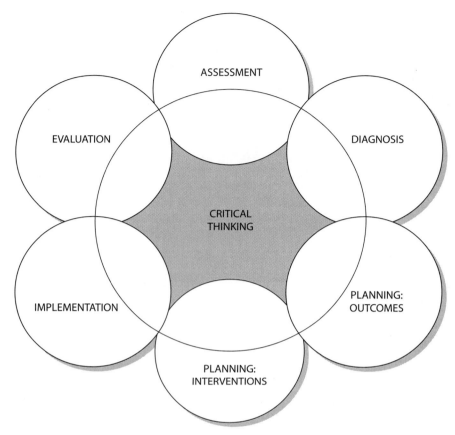

Figure 2–1
Critical Thinking and Nursing Process

into nursing practice, they must use **critical thinking**—a purposeful mental activity in which ideas are produced and evaluated and judgments are made.

Nursing Is an Applied Discipline

"Most professional practice situations are characterized by complexity, instability, uncertainty, uniqueness, and the presence of value conflicts" (Schön [1983] as cited in Gaberson and Oermann 1999, p. 4).

Nurses apply a basic core of knowledge to each new client situation. In an academic discipline (eg, mathematics), problems are well structured and the right answer can usually be found by applying the right theory or formula. In an applied discipline (eg, nursing), problems are messy and confusing. There may be insufficient or conflicting data, an unknown cause, and no single "correct" or "best" answer or solution. To manage such problems, you must know how to identify knowledge and data gaps, find and use new information, and initiate and manage change. All of these skills require critical thinking.

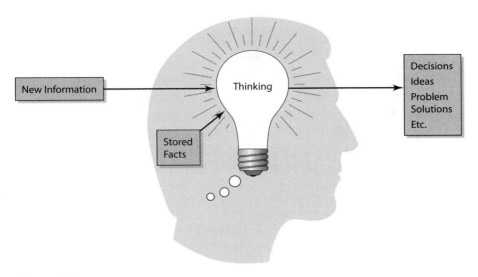

Figure 2–2
Critical Thinking

Nursing Draws on Knowledge from Other Fields

Some professionals, such as chemists and mathematicians, concentrate almost completely on the single body of knowledge that makes up their field. This is not so for nurses. Because nursing deals holistically with a wide range of human responses, nurses use information and insights from other subject areas, such as physiology and psychology, in order to understand the meaning of patient data and plan effective interventions. This, too, requires critical thinking.

Nurses Deal with Change in Stressful Environments

Nurses work in fast-paced, rapidly changing, and often hectic situations. Therefore, routine behaviors and "the usual procedure" may not be adequate for the situation at hand. For example, knowing the routine for giving 9:00 medications may not help a nurse to deal with a patient who is frightened of injections, or one who does not wish to take a medication. Treatments, medications, and technology change constantly, and a patient's condition may change from minute to minute. When anticipating or reacting to changes, nurses must base their decisions on knowledge and rational thinking in order to respond appropriately under stress.

EXAMPLE: Larry is in coronary CCU post-coronary bypass surgery and his condition begins to deteriorate. The surgeon searches for a cardiac explanation for his decline. When the nurse on the next shift makes her initial assessment, she reads [in his history] that he is a diabetic. She finds his blood sugar is 62. Interventions are implemented and he improves dramatically. (Carpenito 1999, pp. 3–4)

Nurses Make Frequent, Varied, and Important Decisions

Nurses make many decisions during a workday. These are not trivial decisions; they often involve a client's well being or even survival. Nurses use critical thinking to collect and interpret information and to make sound judgments and good decisions (eg, to decide which of their many observations to report to physicians and which to handle on their own). Although the level of decision-making may vary, all healthcare personnel need to use critical thinking.

> EXAMPLE: Part of Edna Chin's assignment as a patient care assistant is to answer patients' call lights. She has been told which patients are on bed rest and which ones need help to ambulate. She has helped Ms. Porter to the bathroom three times in the past 3 hours. Realizing that Ms. Porter usually does not void this often, Edna decides to give this information to the RN immediately instead of waiting until end-of-shift report.

■ WHAT IS CRITICAL THINKING?

By now you may be wondering, What is critical thinking? Am I doing it? How can I tell when others and I are doing it? Box 2–1, on page 37, contains questions to help you evaluate and develop your thinking.

Some Definitions of Critical Thinking

Critical thinking is both attitude and a reasoning process involving several intellectual skills. It is "the art of thinking about your thinking while you're thinking so as to make your thinking more clear, precise, accurate, relevant, consistent, and fair" (Paul 1988, pp. 2–3). Critical thinking is disciplined, self-directed, rational thinking that supports what we know and makes clear what we don't know. Some other definitions of critical thinking are found in Box 2–2 on page 38.

Characteristics of Critical Thinking

As you might expect of such a complex process, there is no single, simple definition that explains critical thinking. However, it has some characteristics that will help you to know when it is taking place.

Critical thinking is rational and reasonable. This means that the thinking is based on reasons rather than prejudice, preferences, self-interest, or

BOX 2–1

Are You a Critical Thinker?

Do you:

- Explore the thinking and assumptions that underlie your emotions and feelings?
- Base your judgments on facts and reasoning, not personal feelings, self-interest, or guesswork?
- Suspend judgment until you have all the necessary data?
- Support your views with evidence (eg, principles and research)?
- Evaluate the credibility of sources you use to justify your beliefs?
- Differentiate among facts, opinions, and inferences?
- Distinguish relevant from irrelevant data and important from trivial data?
- Ask for clarification when you don't understand?
- Use knowledge from one subject, discipline, or experience to shed light on other situations?
- Turn mistakes into learning opportunities by determining what went wrong and thinking of ways to avoid that mistake in the future?
- Fight the tendency to believe that you should have all the answers?

fears. Suppose you decide to vote for the Democratic candidate in an election because your family has always voted for Democrats. That decision is based on preference, prejudice and, possibly, self-interest. On the other hand, suppose you took time to reflect on what the candidate said about the issues in the election and based your choice on that. In that case, even though you might still vote for the Democrat, you would be thinking rationally, using facts and observations to draw your conclusions.

Critical thinking involves conceptualization. Conceptualization is the intellectual process of forming a concept. A **concept** is a mental image of reality. It is formed by generalizing an abstract idea from particular instances and it exists as a symbol (eg, a word or picture) in the mind. Concepts are ideas about events, objects, and properties as well as the relationships between them.

EXAMPLE: By experiencing headaches and minor injuries (eg, falling down when you were a child), by observing others in pain, and perhaps by reading about pain, you have an abstract idea of pain. "Pain" is not just *this* headache; it applies to many different situations.

Nursing uses concepts about **properties** (the way things are) and **processes** (the way things happen). A property concept, for example, might be about

KEY POINT
Critical thinking involves:

Rationality and reason
Reflection
Skills and attitudes
Creative thinking
Knowledge

BOX 2–2

Some Definitions of Critical Thinking

Critical thinking is:

". . . an *active, purposeful, organized cognitive process* we use to carefully examine our thinking and the thinking of others, in order to clarify and improve our understanding" (Chaffee 1994, p. 51).

"*reflective and reasonable* thinking that is focused on *deciding what to believe or do*" (Ennis 1985).

". . . a rational response to *questions* that cannot be answered definitively and *for which all the relevant information may not be available*. . . . an investigation whose *purpose is to explore* a situation, phenomenon, question, or problem to arrive at a hypothesis or conclusion about it that *integrates all available information* and that can therefore be convincingly justified" (Kurfiss 1988, p. 2).

an *attitude of inquiry* involving the use of facts, principles, theories, abstractions, deductions, interpretations, and analysis of arguments (Mathews 1979).

". . . both a *philosophical orientation* toward thinking and a cognitive process characterized by reasoned judgment and reflective thinking. Critical thinking is predicated on an intellectual disposition toward challenging accepted visions of truth and an *openness to identifying new possibilities* and explanations." (Jones and Brown 1993, p. 72)

the patient's *anxiety,* or whether there is *infection* in the patient's incision. A process concept might be about *how morphine works in the central nervous system* (Kim 1983).

Critical thinking requires reflection. Reflection means to ponder, contemplate, or deliberate something. It takes time and cannot be done during an emergency. Reflective thinking integrates past experiences into the present and explores potential alternatives. In reflection, one considers an array of possibilities and reflects on the merits of each. When reflecting, one draws "if . . . then" conclusions (eg, *if* you finish reading this chapter now, *then* you will have time to go to a movie later).

Critical thinking involves both cognitive (thinking) skills and attitudes (feelings). To think critically, you must have thinking skills as well as the motivation and desire to use them. Critical thinking skills and attitudes are discussed fully on pages 42–60.

Critical thinking involves creative thinking. Creative thinking means breaking out of established patterns of thinking and approaching situations from new directions. It results in innovative ideas and products (Reilly and Oermann 1992). Nurses use creative thinking when they encounter a new client situation or one in which traditional interventions are not effective.

> EXAMPLE: Ned, a pediatric nurse, makes a home visit to 9-year-old Pauline, who has ineffective respirations following abdominal surgery. The physician has ordered incentive spirometry breathing treatments, but Pauline is frightened by the equipment and tires quickly during the treatments. Ned offers Pauline a bottle of soap bubbles and a blowing wand, and she is delighted. Ned knows that the respiratory effort in blowing bubbles will promote alveolar expansion and suggests that Pauline blow bubbles between incentive spirometry treatments.

Creative thinking creates original ideas by establishing relationships among thoughts and concepts. It involves the ability to break up and transfer a concept to new settings or uses—in the preceding example, Ned transferred a familiar play activity to a new use: breathing treatment. Refer to Box 2–3, below, for characteristics of creative thinkers.

Critical thinking requires knowledge. Critical thinking does not occur in a vacuum. You will use it to apply a basic core of knowledge to each client situation. Your fund of knowledge affects your ability to use cognitive, interpersonal, and technical skills effectively. For example, if you did not know that normal body temperature is 98.6° F, you could not make good decisions about a client whose temperature is 102° F. The following section explains what is meant by *nursing knowledge*.

Types of Nursing Knowledge

Five "ways of knowing" make up the basic core of nursing knowledge: nursing science, nursing art, nursing ethics, personal knowledge (Carper 1978; Chinn and Kramer 1991), and practice wisdom.

BOX 2–3

Characteristics of Creative Thinkers

- Able to generate ideas rapidly
- Flexible and spontaneous; that is, they are able to discard one viewpoint for another or change directions in thinking rapidly and easily
- Able to provide original solutions to problems
- Prefer complex thought processes to simple and easily understood ones
- Independent and self-confident, even when under pressure
- Exhibit distinct individualism

Nursing Science

Scientific knowledge consists of facts, information, principles, and theories. In nursing, it includes research findings and conceptual models of nursing (eg, Roy's Adaptation model [1980]), as well as research findings and theoretical explanations from other disciplines (eg, physiology, psychology). Such knowledge is used to describe, explain, and predict. Table 2–1, below, provides examples of some subjects that make up nursing science.

Nursing Art

The **art of nursing** is the *way* in which nurses use their knowledge. Nurses express caring through their art; therefore, it must include attitudes, beliefs, and values. Scientific knowledge is acquired by scientific investigation; in contrast, art includes feelings gained by subjective experience. Scientific knowledge can be verified or explained to others, but nursing art is more difficult to describe. Sensitivity and **empathy** (the ability to imagine what another person is feeling) are important to this artistic knowing and they enable the nurse to be aware of a client's perspective and be attentive to verbal and nonverbal cues to his psychological state. This enhanced awareness makes available to the nurse a wider range of interventions.

Table 2–1   Examples of Nursing Scientific Knowledge

Subject Matter	Purpose	Example
Helping relationships, including verbal and nonverbal communication	To communicate with patients, families, and other health team members	Conveying caring and support to a patient during insertion of a urinary catheter
Effect of sociocultural and developmental factors on client behavior	To choose effective interventions and understand client behaviors	Understanding how a client's religious beliefs influence his cooperation with the treatment plan
Change theory and motivational theory	For effective team functioning	Supervising team members who are performing delegated tasks
Facts and information needed to perform technical and technologic skills	Hands-on, task-oriented skills, often involving direct contact with the client; done well, they promote patient confidence and successful nursing actions	Operating a slide projector when teaching a class about sexually transmitted diseases Keeping bed linens taut and wrinkle-free to prevent Impaired Skin Integrity

Nursing Ethics

Ethical knowledge refers to knowledge of professional standards of conduct. It is concerned with matters of obligation, or what ought to be done, and it consists of information about basic moral principles and processes for determining right and wrong actions. Nurses are accountable to clients and to each other for the ethical performance of their work. A **professional code of ethics** is a formal set of written statements reflecting the goals and values of the profession. Formal codes define professional expectations and provide a framework for making ethical decisions. Appendix A, the American Nurses Association's "Code for Nurses" (1985), is an example of a formal code of ethics for nurses.

The informal ethics of a profession are based on **conventional moral principles**—unwritten values that are widely held in a profession, expressed in practice, and enforced by rewards and sanctions (eg, the approval or disapproval of fellow professionals). The conventional moral principles of nursing are rooted in nurses' more general views of morality, their experiences, and the history of the profession.

> For each of the conventional moral principles in the margin box, write an example to illustrate how a nurse might demonstrate the principle. Compare your answers with those of a peer.

???

THINKING POINT

Personal Knowledge

Personal knowledge is concerned with knowing and actualizing one's self. It involves knowing self in relation to another human being and interacting on a person-to-person rather than a role-to-role basis. This kind of knowledge enables nurses to approach patients as people rather than objects and to establish therapeutic relationships. Highly developed self-awareness and self-knowledge, along with a good self-concept, enable you to be more attuned to your patients. The "Critical Thinking Practice" in Chapter 1 is an example of developing self-knowledge.

Practice Wisdom

Practice wisdom is acquired from intuition, tradition, authority, trial and error, and clinical experience (Ziegler et al 1986). It provides the basis for much of the nursing care that is given. As nursing develops a broader, research-based body of knowledge, nurses will come to depend less on practice wisdom. Meanwhile, you should refine and use your critical thinking skills to evaluate interventions that are based on practice wisdom and continue to seek new scientific and ethical knowledge as it becomes available.

■ CRITICAL THINKING ATTITUDES

Attitudes and character profoundly influence the ways in which people use their thinking skills. Without a critical attitude, it is easy to use thinking skills to justify prejudice, narrow-mindedness, and intellectual arrogance. Several interdependent traits of mind (attitudes) are essential to high-level critical thinking (Paul 1990). Progress with one attitude invariably leads to progress in others. For example, as you begin to fairly examine ideas or viewpoints toward which you have strong negative emotions (intellectual courage), you will become more aware of the limits of your knowledge (intellectual humility).

Independent Thinking

Critical thinkers think for themselves. They do not passively accept the beliefs of others or simply go along with the crowd. People acquire many beliefs as children because they are rewarded for them or because they do not question, not because they have rational reasons for believing. As they mature and learn, critical thinkers examine and analyze their beliefs, holding those they can rationally support and rejecting those they cannot.

Independent thinking does not mean ignoring what others think and doing whatever you please. It means that critical thinkers consider a wide range of ideas, learn from them, and then make their own judgments about them. Because they will not accept or reject a belief they do not understand, critical thinkers are not easily manipulated. Nurses must be willing to challenge orders and rituals that have no rational support.

EXAMPLE: Nurses traditionally wore white, starched caps in order to prevent hair or hair-borne contaminants from getting on patients and equipment. However, those head coverings evolved into small caps perched on the top of the head. Eventually, most nurses and institutions gave up the cap when they realized it no longer served the original purpose.

Intellectual Humility

Intellectual humility means being aware of the limits of your knowledge and realizing that the mind can be self-deceptive. Critical thinkers are not afraid to admit that they don't know. Admitting lack of knowledge or skill can enable you to grow professionally.

EXAMPLE: A nurse has just begun working on a dialysis unit. He feels insecure and unsure about how to proceed. He requests a meeting with the nurse manager to discuss his strengths and areas of inexperience and to develop a plan for gaining the needed knowledge and skills. Admitting insecurity and requesting help enables the nurse to get support and learn unit policies and procedures rapidly.

Intellectual humility also means rethinking conclusions in light of new knowledge. In the 1960s, for example, physicians and nurses believed that a client recovering from a myocardial infarction (heart attack) should stay on complete bed rest for 2 or 3 days. Research later demonstrated that this was not necessary and that using a bedpan was actually more stressful than using a bedside commode. You should assume that you may learn something new or that new evidence may be discovered that will change currently accepted knowledge.

Intellectual Courage

An attitude of courage means being willing to consider and examine fairly your own beliefs and the views of others, especially those to which you may have a strongly negative reaction. This type of courage comes from recognizing that beliefs are sometimes false or misleading and that ideas considered dangerous or absurd are sometimes rationally justified. Inevitably, after carefully examining such ideas, you will come to see some truth in those you considered wrong and some questionable elements in the ideas you so strongly believed to be true. You need courage to be true to your thinking in such cases, especially if social penalties for nonconformity are severe.

> EXAMPLE: Evelyn is a nurse in a community where there is prejudice toward homosexuality and acquired immune deficiency syndrome (AIDS). Her friends believe that the homosexual lifestyle is wrong and that AIDS is a punishment. In caring for clients with AIDS, Evelyn learns to view them as individuals rather than labeling and condemning them. Because some of her friends have difficulty accepting her view, Evelyn risks losing them. She needs courage to stand up for what she knows to be right.

New ideas may cause discomfort, and old beliefs can provide a sense of security. Therefore, a lack of courage can cause people to become resistant to change. Nurses need intellectual courage to deal with the constant changes in their practice environments.

Intellectual Empathy

Intellectual empathy is the ability to imagine yourself in the place of others in order to understand them and their actions and beliefs. It is easy to misinterpret the words or actions of a person from a different cultural, religious, or socioeconomic background, and it requires imagination to understand the feelings of a person experiencing a situation that you have not experienced yourself.

> EXAMPLE: Ginny Yamamura has cancer. Her husband does not wish her to know her diagnosis. Dave Glen, their nurse, believes that the patient has a right to know, and his first reaction is irritation toward Mr.

Yamamura. However, as he begins to reflect on what to do, Dave thinks, "I wonder why Mr. Yamamura has made that decision. What is their relationship like? What are his views about marriage, caring, and the right to know? What was his reasoning?"

Intellectual empathy also requires the ability to reconstruct the viewpoints and reasoning of others, and to reason from their viewpoints. People frequently make the mistake of believing that the way they see things is the way things really are.

???
THINKING POINT

> Abortion is a controversial issue in our society. If you are against abortion, try to argue that abortion is moral and should be legal. If you are for abortion, try to argue that abortion is immoral and should be against the law. In other words, try to take the perspective of the "other side" of the issue.

Intellectual Integrity

Intellectual integrity means being consistent in the thinking standards you apply (eg, clarity, accuracy, completeness)—holding yourself to the same rigorous standards of proof to which you hold others. By nature, people are inconsistent. For example, if people are not thinking critically, they tend to overrate their own ideas and the ideas of those who like them, and judge more harshly the ideas of those who dislike them. Knowing this, critical thinkers will question their own reasoning as quickly and thoroughly as they will challenge the reasoning of others. Critical thinkers honestly admit inconsistencies and error in their own thoughts and actions.

Intellectual Perseverance

Intellectual perseverance is a sense of the need to struggle with confusion and unsettled questions over an extended period of time to achieve understanding and insight. For nurses, this means looking for the most effective solutions to patient problems, and not settling for the easy, obvious, or routine. Perseverance enables you to sort out issues in spite of difficulties, even when others are opposed to your search. Important questions tend to be complex, confusing, and frustrating; therefore, they may require a great deal of thought and research. Critical thinkers resist the temptation to find a quick, easy answer.

Intellectual Curiosity

Intellectual curiosity is an attitude of inquiry. It means having a mind that is filled with questions: Why do we believe this? What causes that? How does that work? Does it have to be this way? Could something else work? What would happen if we did it another way? Who says this is so? Critical thinkers examine statements to see if they are true or valid rather than blindly accepting them. In response to a claim like, "Fords are better than Chevrolets," a critical thinker might ask: (1) What do you mean by "better than"? Better in what ways? and (2) What information do you have to show that this is so? Questioners tend to challenge the status quo and remove the comfort of habit, so some people see them as dangerous. But far more dangerous are individuals or disciplines who are in a "thinking rut," not even realizing that their old beliefs and practices need to be reexamined (eg, "This is how we do it here," or "Everyone knows this is the best way").

Faith in Reason

Faith in reason implies that people can and should learn to think logically for themselves, despite the natural tendencies of the mind to do otherwise. Critical thinkers believe that well-reasoned thinking leads to trustworthy conclusions. Therefore, they have confidence in the reasoning process and use logic to examine emotion-laden arguments. Critical thinkers develop skill in both inductive reasoning (forming generalizations from a set of facts or observations) and deductive reasoning (starting with a generalization and moving to specific facts or conclusions that it suggests). The confident thinker is not afraid of disagreement and, indeed, is concerned when all agree too quickly.

Fairmindedness

Fairmindedness involves making impartial judgments. It means treating all viewpoints alike, without reference to one's own feelings or vested interests, or those of one's friends, community, or nation. Fairminded thinkers understand that their personal biases or social pressures and customs could unduly affect their thinking. They actively examine their own biases and bring them to awareness each time they think or make a decision.

> EXAMPLE: A nurse spends a great deal of time trying to teach a diabetic client about his diet. The nurse is mystified when the client seems uninterested and fails to follow her advice. The nurse's egocentric tendency to assume that all clients are motivated and interested in preventive care (just because the nurse is) results in inaccurate assessment of the client's desire to learn. Both the nurse's and the client's time are wasted.

Interest in Exploring Thoughts and Feelings

Although we distinguish between thought and feeling in an effort to understand them, in reality they are inseparable. The critical thinker knows that emotions can influence thinking and that all thought creates some level of feeling. The feelings you have in response to a situation would be different if you had a different understanding of the situation.

> EXAMPLE: Todd's nursing instructor assigned him to care for a patient who required very little physical care. Todd was eager to use some of his newly learned psychomotor skills, so he was disappointed and angry. His instructor explained that this was an opportunity for Todd to concentrate on communicating with the patient and to focus on identifying and meeting *the client's* needs, rather than his own need to practice skills. As Todd's understanding (thoughts) of the situation changed, so did his feelings. He was still disappointed that he would not have a chance to give an injection, but he was no longer angry.

Nurses need to identify, examine, and control or modify feelings that interfere with good thinking. Box 2–4, on the next page, provides some suggestions for dealing with negative emotions.

■ CRITICAL THINKING SKILLS

Cognition is the act of knowing. **Thinking** is an active, organized, purposeful mental process that links ideas together by making logical connections among perceptions, beliefs, knowledge, judgments, and feelings. **Cognitive critical thinking skills** are the intellectual activities used in complex thinking processes such as critical analysis, problem solving, and decision making. For example, when solving problems (*complex process*), nurses make inferences, differentiate facts from opinions, and evaluate the credibility of information

BOX 2–4

Dealing With Negative Emotions

To deal with strong, negative emotion, take these steps:

- Limit action for awhile to avoid making hasty conclusions and impulsive decisions.
- Discuss negative feelings with a trusted peer or friend.
- Work off some of the energy generated by the emotion (eg, by walking or exercising).
- Reflect on the situation and determine whether your emotional response was appropriate.

After the strong emotion has moderated, you can then objectively move toward needed conclusions or make required decisions.

sources (*cognitive critical thinking skills*). This text addresses only those skills most important for nurses. Refer to Box 2–5, on page 48, for a list of cognitive skills covered in this section.

Although we study them separately, critical thinking skills are not used one at a time. They overlap, in that using one skill may require the use of others. For example, when *making an inference* one would need to use the skills of *identifying relevant data* and *classifying (clustering) data*.

Using Language

You use language to understand your thinking and to communicate your thoughts. Improving your use of language also improves your ability to think and make sense of things. Critical thinkers avoid general, vague, and nonspecific descriptions such as the following, given at a change-of-shift report:

Mr. Li had a *good* night.

Susan is taking fluids and *tolerating them well.*

Ms. Froelich ambulated *with no difficulty.*

KEY POINT

Make your language more precise by asking:

Who?
What?
When?
How?
Where?
Why?

Because of the vague wording, one nurse might think Mr. Li's "good night" means that he slept well. Another might think it meant he had very little pain. The nurse should have said, "Mr. Li slept from 10:00 P.M. until 6:00 A.M. and reports that he feels rested."

You should also avoid cliches (eg, "haste makes waste"), slogans (eg, "healthcare is a right"), jargon, and euphemisms. **Jargon** consists of expressions and technical terms that are understood by a particular group (eg, nurses), but not by the general public; for example, "I'm giving you some

BOX 2–5

Cognitive Critical Thinking Skills

Using Language

Using language precisely
Using critical thinking vocabulary

Perceiving

Avoiding selective perception
Recognizing differences in perception

Believing and Knowing

Distinguishing facts from interpretations
Supporting facts, opinions, beliefs, and preferences

Clarifying

Questioning to clarify meaning of words and phrases
Questioning to clarify issues, beliefs, and points of view

Comparing

Noting similarities and differences
Classifying
Comparing and contrasting ideals and actual practice
Transferring insights to new contexts

Judging/Evaluating

Providing evidence to support judgments
Developing evaluation criteria

Reasoning

Recognizing assumptions
Distinguishing between relevant and irrelevant data
Evaluating sources of information
Generating and evaluating solutions
Exploring implications, consequences, advantages/disadvantages

IV meds because of your *elevated WBC*," or "I'm going to take your *vital signs*." A **euphemism** is a supposedly more pleasant and less objectionable term that is substituted for a more direct or blunt expression. Euphemisms can be dangerous when they are used to create misperceptions. For example, an obese woman who describes herself as "pleasingly plump" may avoid dealing with the weight problem that is contributing to her diabetes and hypertension.

> What do you think about the following definitions? Are they too broad, too narrow, or just right? Explain your answer.
>
> **1.** A nurse is a professional.
> **2.** A nurse is a professional woman who works in a hospital.

???
THINKING POINT

Perceiving

Perception is the process of using the senses (sight, hearing, smell, touch, and taste) to experience the world. Perception brings sensations into your awareness; it involves three distinct activities:

- *Selecting* certain sensations to pay attention to
- *Organizing* these sensations into a design or pattern
- *Interpreting* what the design or pattern means to you

Avoiding Selective Perception

You cannot possibly attend to all the stimuli that constantly bombard you. Your mind perceives selectively—that is, you unconsciously choose what you will notice and what you will not. Selective perception may cause you to focus on things that support your own ideas and "tune out" information that does not.

> EXAMPLE: Elena believes that fat people are lazy. When an obese nurse on her unit sits to chart, Elena focuses on the fact that the nurse is sitting and thinks, "She is so lazy." Elena fails to notice the many times this nurse has offered to help her with her patients, or that the nurse often tidies the medication and supply areas. Elena perceives only evidence that supports her prejudice.

Avoid selective perception by looking for details you haven't noticed before to balance your perceptions. When you notice that you are focusing on negative details, make a conscious effort to look for positive ones and vice versa.

Recognizing Differences in Perceptions

Different points of view are often a result of different perceptions, rather than just different lines of reasoning. In the following example, two people have attended a meeting where one nurse consistently spoke in a quiet tone of voice.

> *Perception A*: "What an unassertive woman. She must lack self-esteem."
>
> *Perception B*: "How reassuring and confident she seems."

Critical thinkers do not assume that what they are perceiving is what is actually taking place, nor that what they heard is what others heard. When you notice that your perception differs from the perception of others, you should examine the way they (and you) have been selecting, organizing, and interpreting sensory information.

???

THINKING POINT

Recall an instance when you and a classmate heard a teacher's instructions differently (eg, perhaps the teacher said to wear lab coats to orientation, but you thought you were supposed to wear your full uniform). Whose perception was inaccurate, and why?

Believing and Knowing

Beliefs are interpretations, evaluations, conclusions, and predictions about the world that we take to be true. Realizing that beliefs are subject to error, critical thinkers reflect on their beliefs and revise them in light of new information and experiences.

Distinguishing Facts from Interpretations

Statements about beliefs, issues, conclusions, and claims are not statements of fact. They are interpretations. **Facts** are statements that you can verify through observation and investigation (eg, the nurse is wearing white shoes). You can check their accuracy. Statements that can be verified *in principle* are also considered facts. For example, it is a fact that arteries are less distensible than veins. Even though you cannot check it out at the moment, you *could* verify that statement if you dissected a cadaver. See Box 2–6, below, for help in distinguishing facts from interpretations.

Inferences are conclusions that are based on factual information but go beyond that information to make statements about something not presently known. (The "Critical Thinking Practice" at the end of Chapter 3 provides practice in making valid inferences.) **Judgments** are evaluations of information that reflect values or other criteria. **Opinions** are beliefs or judgments that may fit the facts or be in error. Consider the following example:

BOX 2–6

To distinguish facts from interpretations, ask the following questions:

- Is this something that I can observe directly, or would I have to interpret what I see to arrive at this conclusion?
- Could this be verified in principle? What would I need to do to verify it (eg, dissect a cadaver, weigh a patient)?
- Does this description stick to facts, or does it include reasoning and rationale?
- Is this how *anyone* would describe the situation?

EXAMPLE: Ms. Albert comes to the clinic, where the nurse weighs her. The scale indicates 250 lbs.

1. *Fact*: Ms. Albert weighs 250 lbs.
2. *Inference*: Ms. Albert consumes more calories than she needs.
3. *Judgment*: Ms. Albert is greedy or has poor self-control.
4. *Opinion*: If someone really wants to lose weight, they can do it.

Statement 1 can be verified by the scale. If the nurse had actually observed Ms. Albert's eating patterns or counted her calories, Statement 2 would also be a fact. But in this case, the nurse made an inference based on the fact of Ms. Albert's weight, together with the knowledge that excess calorie intake is the usual cause of obesity. Statement 3 is a judgment reflecting the nurse's value of self-control. For this nurse, that is a negative value judgment. However, judgments are not necessarily negative (eg, "What a pretty baby!"). Statement 4, an opinion, cannot be observed or "proven." It may or may not be in error.

Supporting Facts, Opinions, Beliefs, and Preferences

Recall that **facts** are statements that can be verified through investigation. Some statements may be made in the form of facts, but are actually incorrect. For example, if someone says, "Florence Nightingale wrote *Notes on Nursing* in 1959," it sounds as though they are stating a fact. However, Nightingale died in 1856, so that statement is actually an erroneous *belief*, not a fact. You should be able to provide support for your facts, beliefs, and opinions when others challenge them (see Table 2–2 on page 52).

A personal preference is merely a statement of something one likes or dislikes (eg, "I like strawberry ice cream better than chocolate"). You do not need to provide support for your preferences; however, when you express them in the form of opinions, you should expect others to challenge them.

Clarifying

Critical thinkers ask questions to clarify and understand complex concepts, ideas, and situations. This helps to keep them from drawing superficial, inaccurate conclusions.

Questioning to Clarify/Analyze the Meaning of Words and Phrases

If you understand a word or concept being used, you should be able to give clear, obvious, concrete examples of it. For example, if someone says, "Students are special people," you could not agree or disagree with them until you clearly understand what they meant by "students" and "special." Concrete examples of "students" might include: (1) a child in kindergarten, (2) a nursing student, or (3) a couple taking square-dancing lessons. Concrete examples of "special" might include: (1) someone who is different from the group, (2)

Table 2–2   Supporting Facts and Opinions

Guideline	Example
■ If you state a fact that is not common knowledge or that cannot be easily verified, state where you got your information.	*Common knowledge, no source needed:* "For the average person, an intramuscular injection should be given at a 90° angle." *Source of information should be given:* "The average RN is over 40 years old."
■ If you state an opinion or view with which others might disagree, include answers to questions they might ask.	"Critical thinking is important for nurses *because they work in rapidly changing environments.*"
■ If you are not sure whether a statement is a fact or an opinion, treat it and state it as an opinion.	"*In my opinion*, the ventrogluteal site is the safest one for intramuscular injections." (If you can cite references or research, you could treat this statement as a fact.)

someone you love, or (3) someone who is handicapped. See Box 2-7, on page 53 for questions to help you clarify words and phrases.

Questioning to Clarify Issues, Beliefs, and Points of View

In discussions with others, critical thinkers question and probe to gain deeper understanding. They ask questions not to embarrass others, but to learn more about what they think and to evaluate their statements for themselves. See Box 2–7, on page 53, for questions to help you clarify statements about issues, beliefs, and points of view.

Comparing

To **compare** is to examine similarities and differences among things in the same general category. For example, a nurse might compare and contrast the ways in which clients of different cultures express grief. Although each client might be from a different culture, they are all from the same general category: *people*. Making careful, systematic comparisons improves the quality of your decisions. The "Critical Thinking Practice" at the end of Chapter 5 provides practice in making comparisons.

Noting Similarities and Differences

Critical thinkers make careful, thorough observations and note significant similarities and differences, realizing that things that seem alike on the surface may be different in important ways.

EXAMPLE: A nurse is caring for two middle-aged, male clients with the same medical diagnosis: myocardial infarction (heart attack). Although

BOX 2–7

Questions for Clarifying

Questions to Clarify the Meaning of Words and Phrases

- What is a clear, concrete example of the concept *X*?
- Why is this an *X*?
- What would be an example of *X's* opposite? Or of something clearly *not X*?
- Why is this not an *X*? How is this case different from the clear-cut examples?
- What are some situations in which *X* would apply?

Questions to Clarify Statements and Conclusions

- Do I understand this issue?
- Did I state it fairly?
- How can we know whether this statement is true or false? What evidence do we need?
- Is there a clearer or more accurate way to word this statement?
- Would others accept this as a fair and accurate statement of the issue?
- What would count as evidence against this statement?
- How did you form that idea (or acquire that belief)? Have you always thought that? If not, why did you change your belief?
- Why do you believe this? What are some reasons that people believe this?
- Are there any exceptions to this view? What would someone say who disagrees with you? How would someone from a different culture see it?
- What are the consequences of this idea? What would have to be done to put this idea into action?
- What are the implications of this idea? If you believe that, wouldn't you also have to believe . . .?

these clients are similar in age and diagnosis, they are responding very differently to their disease. Mr. Jonassen is experiencing nausea, brought about by severe pain. Mr. Nguyen has no nausea and only mild pain. His main response is anxiety about being away from his business. The nurse recognizes that despite their similarities, they have very different needs.

Classifying

Classifying, or categorizing, is the process of grouping things on the basis of their similarities or common properties. For the most part, you classify things continuously and automatically as you organize and make sense of your experience. For example, the concept "thermometer" represents a type of object that nurses use to measure temperature. In order to determine whether an object is a thermometer, we focus on similarities: (1) It has a scale marked in increments, (2) It has numbers on it that represent degrees of temperature, (3) It registers temperature changes. So you would classify a variety of instruments as thermometers (eg, a mercury and glass thermometer, an electronic thermometer, a skin probe with a digital readout, a large thermometer that measures room temperature). Classifying also allows you to see how things are different—for example, to see how thermometers are different from other objects with numbers and incremental scales, such as sphygmomanometers or scales for weighing things. Chapter 4 points out some important ways in which nurses classify patient data (eg, according to nursing theories). The "Critical Thinking Practice" at the end of Chapter 6 provides practice in classifying.

Comparing and Contrasting Ideals and Actual Practice

It is important to recognize the gaps between facts and ideals. The more realistic your ideals, the more likely you are to achieve them. Unrealistic ideals, on the other hand, may lead to frustration. For example, the statement, "Nurses give holistic care," has appeared so often in the nursing literature that many take it to be a fact.

???

THINKING POINT

Think about the nurses you have observed and about your own nursing experiences.

- What, exactly, is meant by "holistic" care?
- Do nurses always, or even usually, give holistic care?
- Is holistic care really a statement of what nurses are *trying* to achieve?
- What problems do nurses have in achieving this ideal?
- Is it realistic to try to achieve this ideal?

Transferring Insights to New Contexts

By making analogies between situations, critical thinkers are able to transfer insights and information from one situation to another. An **analogy** is a special kind of comparison that points out ways in which things from different categories are similar to each other. For example, people say, "Time is money." Time and money are from completely different categories, but the analogy brings out their similarities. That is, we have only a limited amount of each, both are important, we can save or spend them both, and so on.

Critical thinkers do not compartmentalize their knowledge. They use their understanding of one subject to gain insight into other subjects. For example, to gain understanding about the present status of nurses, you could use insights from the history of nursing, the historical status of women, the sociology of oppressed groups, and the social effects of technology on the labor market and healthcare. Nurses need to connect insights from many subjects (eg, psychology, sociology, interpersonal communications, physiology, pharmacology, nutrition) in the care of each patient. As you learn a new principle, you can enrich your understanding of it by applying it to new situations. Think, "What other situation is different, but still like this one in some important ways? How would this principle work in that situation?"

Judging and Evaluating

Recall that facts are statements that can be verified, and that judgments are evaluations of facts and information that reflect certain criteria, such as our values. Facts and inferences describe what is happening, whereas judgments express your evaluation of what is happening (see "Believing and Knowing," on pages 50–51). **Opinions** are longstanding beliefs that are formed by making judgments over time, whereas a judgment can be made more or less "on the spot" and can be a one-time thing.

Providing Evidence to Support Judgments

Disagreements with others are often a result of differences in judgment rather than differences in perceptions, definition of terms, or lack of clarity. Not all judgments are equally good. Their credibility depends on the criteria used to make them and the evidence given to support the criteria. When your judgment differs from someone else's, the following is an intelligent approach to use:

1. Make explicit the criteria, standards, or values used as the basis for the judgments.
2. Try to establish the reasons that justify these criteria.

For example, a nursing instructor's judgment, "That was a good injection," is based on the criteria that: (a) sterile technique is used, (b) the needle is inserted quickly at a 90° angle, (c) the student aspirates before injecting the medication, and so forth. These criteria are justified because they can be found in current nursing literature; they are also backed by the germ theory of disease and a knowledge of anatomy.

Developing Evaluation Criteria

Evaluation, like judgment, is also the process of determining the value or worth of something. Unlike judgment, evaluation requires that you first identify the criteria or standards to be used, and then decide to what extent the thing you are examining meets those standards. Evaluation criteria should be: (a) made explicit, (b) stated clearly, and (c) applied consistently. Consider the following example:

Judgment: I really like that music.

Evaluation: I like this music because it has a beautiful melody and meaningful lyrics. The rhythm keeps the song moving along at an interesting pace.

Although the evaluation criteria are not explicit (the example does not say, "These are the criteria being used"), the evaluation statements imply that they included considerations of melody, lyrics, rhythm, and the ability of the music to capture one's attention. Undoubtedly your instructors have openly stated the criteria they use to evaluate your clinical performance. Nurses develop evaluation criteria in the form of patient outcomes, or goals, that they intend to achieve with their nursing interventions. Chapter 6 discusses outcome (evaluation criteria) development in detail. Chapter 9 discusses evaluation as it is used in the nursing process.

Reasoning

Reasoning is logical thinking that links thoughts together in meaningful ways. Reasoning is used in scientific inquiry, in examining controversial issues, and in problem solving (eg, in the nursing process). When reasons are given to provide support for a conclusion or position, it is called **argument**. Although they sometimes sound the same, arguments are different from explanations. The goal of an argument is to show *that* something is true; the goal of an **explanation** is to show *why* something is true.

EXAMPLE:
Argument: Penicillin is the drug of choice for many infections because of its low cost and low toxicity, and its effectiveness against many gram-positive bacteria.

Explanation: Penicillin is effective against a variety of gram-positive bacteria because it interferes with cell wall formation, making the bacterium susceptible to destruction by osmotic processes and autolysis.

Nurses use both inductive and deductive reasoning. **Inductive reasoning** begins with specific details and facts and uses them to arrive at conclusions and generalizations.

EXAMPLE: If you observe in a large number of cases that ice melts when it is warmed to 32° F, you will reason that all ice melts at 32° F.

EXAMPLE: A patient complains of soreness at an intravenous (IV) site. The nurse observes that the site is cool, pale, and swollen, and that the IV is not running. Having observed similar symptoms in many patients, the nurse reasons that the IV is infiltrated.

In good inductive arguments, the conclusion *probably* follows from the reasons, but one can never be absolutely certain that it will. Inductive arguments can be strong or weak, depending on the number of observations made and on the quality of the reasons given. Think about the difference in the certainty of the conclusions in the two preceding examples. When scientific induction leads to conclusions that are almost invariably true (eg, ice melts at 32° F), those conclusions can then be used as the major premises for deductive reasoning.

Deductive reasoning begins with a major theory, generalization, fact, or *major premise* that generates specific details and predictions. Reasoning is from the universal to the particular—that what is true of a class of things is true of each member of that class.

EXAMPLE:

Fact (major premise) All ice melts at 32° F.

Fact (minor premise) It is warmer than 32° F in this room.

Conclusion (correct) The ice in the patient's water pitcher will melt.

In deductive reasoning, if the facts in the premises are true, then the conclusion must be true. However, we sometimes assume that generalizations (major premises) are true when they may not be. The following is an example of wrongly assuming the truth of a major premise (the first statement).

EXAMPLE:

Fact (major premise) All infections cause fever.

Fact (minor premise) Mr. Annas's temperature is 102° F, a fever.

Conclusion (incorrect) Mr. Annas has an infection.

The major premise is incorrect in the preceding example because not all infections produce fever, although most do. In addition, factors other than infection can produce fever (eg, dehydration, heat prostration). A reasoning error can also be made if the *minor premise* (the second statement in the example) is incorrect. If Mr. Annas had a hot drink before his temperature was taken, or if the thermometer was calibrated incorrectly, the reading of 102° F would not reflect his true body temperature, and the conclusion that he has an infection would again be in error.

Recognizing Assumptions

An **assumption** is an idea or concept that you take for granted (eg, people once assumed the world was flat). Assumptions can be true or false. In the preceding example, you would incorrectly conclude that Mr. Annas has an infection if you incorrectly assumed that all infections cause fever. Of course, some assumptions are necessary for efficient performance of daily activities. For example, when you cross the street in a pedestrian crosswalk, you assume the cars will stop for you. When you take a patient's blood pressure, you assume the apparatus works properly. When you give medications, you assume the capsule marked "aspirin" is actually aspirin. These are all reasonable assumptions.

Nurses must recognize and examine their assumptions about patients and patient data. It is easy to recognize the assumptions hidden in some statements. "Have you stopped beating your wife?" assumes (a) that the person had a wife, and (b) that he has beaten his wife. A more subtle assumption is hidden in this statement about a client: "If he wanted to get well, he would keep his clinic appointments." This statement assumes that the client (a) has transportation, (b) is capable of remembering his appointment, (c) has had no emergency that prevented him from keeping his appointment, and (d) that keeping his appointments will actually help him to get well.

??? THINKING POINT

> 1. What are some assumptions nurses commonly make about patients (eg, patients are obligated to follow doctors' orders and to tell the truth when questioned about their symptoms)?
> 2. What are some assumptions you have about nurses (eg, that they know what is best for patients; that they always chart accurate data)?
>
> Compare your assumptions with another student. How are they alike or different? Are they well-founded assumptions, or are they in error?

Distinguishing Between Relevant and Irrelevant Data

When making clinical judgments, nurses sift through a great deal of data. But even data that are confirmed and verified (ie, see "facts" on page 50) are useful only if they are relevant. Critical thinkers focus on relevant facts—that is, they "stick to the point." **Relevant** statements/data are those which pertain to the issue at hand. Relevant data are facts that are important or significant. **Irrelevant** factors have nothing to do with the issue (problem, argument, and so forth), or they may be related but unimportant. The "Critical Thinking Practice" at the end of Chapter 7 will help you to differentiate between relevant and irrelevant data.

KEY POINT

Give more weight to information sources that:

- Have a good track record
- Are in a position to know
- Have a reputation for honesty
- Have a reputation for consistency
- Do not have a vested interest in the issue at hand

Evaluating Sources of Information

Critical thinkers thoughtfully examine others' statements before accepting them, and they provide credible information to support their own positions. When the source of information is something other than direct observation, they evaluate the credibility of the source. Box 2–8 provides questions to use when evaluating the credibility of sources. However, even when information is provided by a credible expert, it is often wise to seek the opinion of at least a second expert.

Generating and Evaluating Solutions

When presented with a problem, critical thinkers do not cast about wildly for solutions, nor do they accept the first solution that comes to mind. They take time to formulate problems carefully, ensuring that their problem statements are clear, accurate, and fair. They also identify and examine the causes of the

Questions for Evaluating Credibility of Information Sources

- Is this person in a position to know?
- Could the source have directly seen or heard, or did he have to reason his conclusion?
- Was the source able to make accurate observations?
- What is the person's interest in the issue? Does he have anything to gain?
- What is the person's purpose for providing the information?
- What knowledge or experience would a person need to be an expert in this area? Does this person have those credentials?
- Has this source been reliable in the past?
- Who paid for the work that went into gathering the information?

problem. As you will see in Chapter 4, nurses do these things when they make nursing diagnoses.

Because problems usually do not come with ready-made solutions, nurses need creative thinking, including flexibility and imagination, to generate and evaluate possible solutions (eg, nursing actions). For nurses, problem solving often means identifying or choosing the best nursing interventions. Chapter 7, "Planning: Interventions," addresses that in more detail. The following questions may be useful:

- Do I have all the relevant information?
- What solutions have previously been used for this problem? For similar problems?
- What makes some solutions better than others? What criteria should I use in deciding which solution is best?
- What solutions will solve the problem? What solutions will address the *cause* of the problem?
- Is this solution realistic?

Exploring Implications, Consequences, Advantages, and Disadvantages

It is certainly important to evaluate data and facts. However, when making decisions about problem solutions, policies, or actions (eg, nursing interventions), you must consider other factors as well. It is especially important to consider implications and consequences. For example, if you believe in a policy of capital punishment, the *implication* is that you believe killing is acceptable, at least in some situations. If the belief in capital punishment is actually translated into law, then one *consequence* is that some people will be killed, albeit legally. To **imply** something is to express it indirectly, suggesting it without stating it. To accept a statement is to accept its implications, or the logical connection between one statement and another (that is, if X is true, then it follows that Y must be true). Words such as *therefore, so,* and *then* point to the logical connection between two statements and may be a clue that an implication is present. For example, "*if* Madeline is a registered nurse, *then* she uses the nursing process."

Consequences are different from implications in that they are more action oriented. A **consequence** is the effect or result that is *caused* by something (that is, if one acts on X, then Y will occur). For example, "*If* a nurse gives morphine, *then* the client will experience pain relief"; or "The nurse administered morphine, *therefore* the client experienced pain relief." Refer to Box 2–9, below, for questions to help you explore possible consequences of nursing interventions. Chapter 7, "Planning: Interventions," further discusses choosing nursing interventions.

■ COMPLEX INTELLECTUAL ACTIVITIES

This chapter has presented individual critical thinking attitudes and skills one at a time to help you understand them. However, they overlap a great deal and they are not used individually or in isolation. The cognitive skills are actually used in different combinations as a part of more complex intellectual processes. For example, when nurses are solving problems (a complex activity), they use the individual skills of making inferences, differentiating facts from opinions, and evaluating the credibility of information sources.

The complex thinking processes overlap, just as the individual skills do (eg, recall from Chapter 1 that nursing process is related to problem solving and critical thinking), and even the experts do not always agree on how to define them. This section discusses the following terms and their relationship

---

BOX 2-9

Questions for Exploring Consequences

- What effect will this action probably have? (eg, what therapeutic effect will this medication have? What undesirable side effects?)
- Are there other possible actions? What would their effects be?
- Has this worked in the past? What happened?
- What are the advantages and disadvantages of this action?
- If this action is implemented, who will be affected and what will those effects be?
- Does the action (or problem solution) take into account everyone's best interests?

---

to critical thinking: critical analysis, problem solving, nursing process, clinical reasoning, decision making, clinical judgment, and reflective reasoning. Box 2–10, on page 62, provides a summary of definitions of these terms. Recall that critical thinking is careful, reflective, goal-oriented, purposeful thinking that involves a variety of mental attitudes and cognitive skills. It may be helpful to think of critical thinking as a broad umbrella for the complex thinking processes, all of which tend to be purposeful and deliberate.

Problem Solving   is the mental activity of identifying a problem (unsatisfactory state) and then planning and finding a reasonable solution to it. There are various methods of problem solving, including the *nursing process*, trial-and-error, and the scientific method. Depending on the nature of the problem, problem solving may or may not require the use of *critical thinking*. Many problems are well structured and have only a few reasonable answers, possibly only one. Such problems (eg, simple math problems such as $2 + 2 = ?$) do not require critical thinking. Problem solving requires the use of *decision making*.

Write a short paragraph describing a problem you have solved recently. Identify the problem-solving method you used.

???

THINKING POINT

Nursing Process   is a systematic, creative approach to thinking and doing that nurses use to obtain, categorize, and analyze patient data, and to plan actions to meet a patient's needs. It is a type of *problem-solving* process requiring the use of *decision-making, clinical judgment*, and a variety of *critical thinking skills*.

Decision Making   is the process of choosing the best action to take—the action most likely to produce the desired outcome. It involves deliberation, judgment, and choice. Decision making is important in the *problem-solving* process and in all phases of the *nursing process*, but not all decisions involve problem solving. For example, nurses make value decisions (eg, to keep client information confidential) and time management decisions (eg, taking clean linens to the client's room at the same time as the medication in order to save steps). Decisions must be made whenever there are mutually exclusive choices. For example, when faced with several patients' needs at one time, the nurse decides which patient to assist first. *Critical thinking* improves decision making by providing a "broader menu of options with which to analyze problems and make decisions" (Adams 1999, p. 111).

Describe a decision you made in the clinical setting that was *not* made for the purpose of solving a problem.

???

THINKING POINT

Reasoning   is logical thinking that links thoughts together in meaningful ways. Reasoning is used in scientific inquiry, in examining controversial

BOX 2–10

Complex Intellectual Processes

Critical Thinking	Goal-oriented, purposeful thinking that involves many mental attitudes and skills, such as determining which data are relevant and making inferences. Essential when a problem is ill defined and does not have a single "best" solution.
Problem Solving	The mental activity of identifying a problem (unsatisfactory state) and finding a reasonable solution to it. Requires decision making; may or may not require the use of critical thinking.
Nursing Process	A systematic, creative approach to thinking and doing that nurses use to obtain, categorize, and analyze patient data and to plan actions to meet patient needs. A type of problem-solving process requiring the use of decision-making, clinical judgment, and a variety of critical thinking skills.
Decision Making	The process of choosing the best action to take—the action most likely to produce the desired outcome. Involves deliberation, judgment, and choice. Decisions must be made whenever there are mutually exclusive choices, but not necessarily problems.
Clinical Reasoning	Reasoning is logical thinking that links thoughts together in meaningful ways. Clinical reasoning is reflective, concurrent, and creative thinking about patients and patient care—the kind of reasoning used in the nursing process.
Reflection/ Reflective Judgment	A kind of critical thinking that considers a broad array of possibilities and reflects on the merits of each in a given situation. Essential when a problem is complex and has no simple, "correct" solution.
Clinical Judgment	Judgment is the use of values or other criteria to evaluate or draw conclusions about information. Clinical judgments are conclusions and opinions about patients' health, drawn from patient data. They may or may not be made using critical thinking.
Analysis/Critical Analysis	Analysis, a critical thinking skill, is the process of breaking material down into component parts and identifying the relationships among them. Critical analysis is the questioning applied to a situation or idea to determine essential information and ideas and discard superfluous information and ideas. Critical thinking is more than just analysis.

issues, and in *problem solving*. **Clinical reasoning**, then, is reflective, concurrent, and creative thinking about patients and patient care—the kind of reasoning used in the *nursing process*.

Reflection or *Reflective Judgment*   is usually used to describe a kind of *reasoning* that considers a broad array of possibilities and reflects on the merits of each in a given situation. It is a type of *critical thinking* and is used by some experts to describe critical thinking (ie, they would say that critical thinking *is* reflective reasoning. . .). Reflection is useful in *decision making* and *problem solving*, and it is essential when the problem is complex and has no simple, "correct" solution. Nurses use reflective judgment when dealing with moral conflict and ethical problems, for example.

Clinical Judgments   are conclusions and opinions about patients' health, drawn from patient data. Clinical judgment is similar to *decision making*, in that nurses make judgments (as well as decisions) about the meaning of patient data and about nursing actions that should be taken on the patient's behalf. *Clinical judgments* are made as a part of the *nursing process*.

Judging, itself, is a *critical thinking skill*, and other thinking skills are essential for making sound judgments. However, good clinical judgments can be made without using critical thinking skills. For example, a patient might complain of a "dry mouth," and the nurse respond correctly by offering a sip of water—without thinking critically. Using *critical thinking*, the nurse would assess the oral cavity, evaluate skin turgor and temperature, evaluate input and output, review the patient's medications and treatments, and so forth. This assessment would have a goal of identifying the source of the problem (dry mouth) and planning an intervention on that basis—an intervention that could include a sip of water. *Critical thinking skills* are used to expand and "flesh out" the nursing process (Adams 1999, p. 112).

Analysis   is the cognitive process of breaking material down into component parts and identifying the relationships among them (eg, nurses use analysis to examine and interpret each piece of patient data to identify deviations from normal). **Critical analysis** is used to determine which information or ideas are essential in a situation. Analysis is used in *problem solving*, *decision making*, and *clinical judgment*. Although analysis is a critical thinking skill, *critical thinking* goes beyond analysis to focus on what to believe or what actions to take.

■ STANDARDS OF REASONING

Recall that critical thinking is, in part, "thinking about your thinking" (metacognition). You should apply a basic set of intellectual standards whenever you are checking the quality of your thinking. That is, you should check your thinking for clarity, accuracy, precision, relevance, depth, breadth, and logic. Table 2–3, on page 64, explains these intellectual standards. Subsequent

Table 2-3 Standards of Reasoning

Standard	Evaluative Questions	Examples
Clarity—A statement must be clear in order to know whether it is accurate, relevant, and so on.	■ Could you give an example? ■ Can you express that point another way?	*Unclear:* After a clinic visit, the nurse instructs a parent to call the primary care provider if the child's fever recurs. *Clearer:* The nurse instructs the parent how often to check the temperature, and the acceptable range for a child's temperature (eg, "Call if the temperature is more than 101° F.")
Accuracy—A statement can be clear but not accurate.	■ Is that really true? ■ How could you check it?	Most people weigh more than 300 lbs. (*Clearly stated, but inaccurate*)
Precision—A statement can be clear and accurate, but not precise.	■ Could you give more details? ■ Can you be more exact?	If Jack weighs 350 lbs, the statement, "Jack is overweight" is clear and accurate. A precise statement would say, "Jack is 200 lbs overweight."
Relevance—A statement can be clear, accurate, and precise, but not relevant to the issue.	■ How does that relate to the problem? ■ How does that help us understand the issue?	Students sometimes think that the amount of effort they put into a course should determine their grade. However, effort does not always measure the quality of a student's learning. When that is so, effort is not relevant to the grade.
Depth—A statement can be clear, accurate, precise, and relevant—but superficial.	■ How does the statement address the complexities of the situation? ■ Are you taking into account the problems that statement creates? ■ Does the statement deal with the most important factors?	The statement, "Just say no," which is used to discourage youthful drug use, is clear, accurate, precise, and relevant. Still, it is superficial because it does not deal with the complexities of the issue.
Breadth—A line of reasoning can meet all the other standards, but be one-sided	■ Do we need to consider another point of view? ■ Is there another way to look at this?	An argument from either a liberal or a conservative would get deeply into an issue such as the death penalty or abortion; but it would probably be narrow, presenting only one side of the question—either for or against.
Logic—Reasoning brings various thoughts together in some kind of order. When the thoughts make sense in combination, thinking is logical.	■ Does this really make sense? ■ Does the conclusion follow from what was just said (or from the data)? ■ How can both these "facts" be true?	Someone who states both, "Killing is wrong," and "We should have capital punishment" is being illogical.

Source: Adapted from R. Paul (1996)."Universal Intellectual Standards," in *Critical Thinking Workshop Handbook.* Dillon Beach, CA: Foundation for Critical Thinking. See www.criticalthinking.org.

chapters will show you how to apply these standards in each phase of the nursing process (eg, see pp. 80–81 in Chapter 3).

■ CRITICAL THINKING AND NURSING PROCESS

Critical thinking and the nursing process are interdependent, but not identical. Nurses function effectively some part of every day without thinking critically. Many decisions are based on habit, with little thinking involved; for example, selecting what clothes to wear, choosing which route to take to work, and deciding what to eat for lunch. Psychomotor skills, such as operating a familiar cardiac monitor, involve minimal thinking. But critical thinking is essential to the nursing process. Nurses use critical thinking at each stage of the process. In the following discussion, critical thinking skills are shown in italics.

Assessment is when nurses use an *attitude of inquiry* as they *use facts, principles, theories, abstractions, deductions, and interpretations* to *gather patient data and validate* what the patient says with what they observe. They must *make reliable observations* and *distinguish relevant from irrelevant data and important from unimportant data*. They also *organize* and *categorize* the relevant, important data in some useful manner, perhaps according to a theory-based nursing framework. In addition, they *identify missing information and fill in the gaps.*

> EXAMPLE: In assessing Mr. Wiley's skin, the nurse notes that it is dry, thin, and inelastic. This is relevant information that the nurse uses to diagnose Risk for Impaired Skin Integrity. The nurse also notices a 4-in. contracted scar on Mr. Wiley's lower abdomen. It is obviously an old scar and is now irrelevant to the nursing diagnosis. The nurse also notices that Mr. Wiley, age 50, is balding. This data is relevant because it pertains to the topic of skin. However, it is a normal finding, and not important in making the nursing diagnosis.

Diagnosis is when nurses *analyze* the data they have categorized to *look for patterns and relationships* among the cues and *draw conclusions* about them.

> EXAMPLE: The nurse observes that a patient is grimacing and moving about restlessly in bed. The nurse's knowledge and previous experience suggest that these symptoms mean the client is in pain. This is only an *inference* and, until verified, neither a fact nor a nursing diagnosis.

Critical thinkers are careful to *suspend judgment* when they do not have enough data. This is what nurses do when they write a "possible" rather than an "actual" nursing diagnosis. In the preceding example, there are not enough data to be sure the inference is correct. The nurse should *question the patient to validate the observations*. Even after making a valid diagnosis, a critical thinker *remains open to all possibilities*.

Planning Outcomes is when nurses *use reasonable, reflective thinking that is focused on deciding what to believe or do.* They *use knowledge* and reasoning skills (eg, *forming valid generalizations and explanations*) to *predict patient responses* and *develop evaluative criteria* (*ie, patient outcomes*). They use the outcomes developed in this stage as criteria for evaluating the client's progress and the success of the nursing actions.

Planning Interventions is when nurses *make predictions* and *form valid generalizations and explanations* when they *plan and implement creative interventions.* They *make interdisciplinary connections* when they use their knowledge of subjects such as physiology, psychology, and sociology to choose appropriate nursing actions and provide rationales for them. Finally, nurses *hypothesize* that certain nursing interventions will relieve the patient's problem or help achieve the stated health goals.

Implementation is when nurses *apply their knowledge and principles* from nursing and related courses to each specific patient-care situation. The ability to apply, not simply memorize, principles is a mark of critical thinking.

> EXAMPLE: A nursing student has learned the principles "heat is lost through evaporation" and "the normal newborn is at risk for cold stress." Although the student has never bathed a newborn and has not memorized the exact steps for doing so, she prevents cold stress by uncovering only the parts she is bathing and by drying the infant well.

Carrying out the nursing orders in the implementation phase can be compared to *hypothesis testing* in the scientific method. The nursing orders must be translated into action (or tested) in order to decide whether they were successful.

Evaluation is when nurses use *criterion-based evaluation* when they use new observations to determine whether patient goals have been met. They *analyze* outcomes to determine which nursing interventions (*hypotheses*) worked and which did not.

> EXAMPLE: When bathing a newborn, a student realizes she must evaluate the results of her actions; that is, she must determine whether she has kept the infant warm enough. The obvious criterion to use is that the infant's body temperature should be at least 98° F. Although no rule states that she should take the baby's temperature after a bath, she does so in order to evaluate whether she has achieved the goal of avoiding cold stress.

■ CRITICAL THINKING AND NURSING ETHICS

Nurses often deal with ethical questions in their work. Even beginning students encounter ethical situations in their interactions with staff, patients, faculty, and peers. Because students may feel overwhelmed and uncomfortable in their new role, it is sometimes hard for them to recognize and define the ethical issues involved. The following are some examples (Ludwick and Sedlak 1998):

- *Interactions with staff*—Students perceive nurses (and other health professionals) as experts, so it is particularly difficult when they observe nurses performing skills incorrectly, giving inappropriate care, or not paying attention when the student reports pertinent assessment findings.
- *Interactions with patients*—Students wonder, "What if I say the wrong thing? Or make a mistake?" Because of their inexperience, they may feel guilty if they do not perform perfectly 100 percent of the time. Pressure to be perfect may even tempt students to hide mistakes or falsify information.
- *Interactions with faculty*—Students rely on faculty as role models and as authority figures for handling clinical situations. Ethical questions arise when faculty ask them to do things they are afraid or unprepared to do, when a faculty member fails to use standard technique for a procedure, or when the student believes the teacher does not stand up to the staff regarding students' rights.
- *Interactions with peers*—Common questions include what to do when observing other students: violating patient confidentiality (eg, discussing patients at lunch), giving care incorrectly or incompletely (eg, failure to change linens), relying on others for information about their assigned medications, falsifying patient information, or stealing supplies. Students usually do not want to "tattle," and there are questions about when and with whom to discuss such situations.

If you encounter such situations, critical thinking can help you to: (a) think analytically and reflectively about what to do, (b) understand the basis for your decisions and the beliefs on which they are based, (c) identify your values and assumptions, and (d) examine your thinking processes for errors in reasoning (Ludwick and Sedlak 1998).

■ DEVELOPING CRITICAL THINKING

Critical thinking does not just "come naturally." By nature, people tend to believe what is easy to believe, what those around them believe, and what they are rewarded for believing. People develop and use critical thinking more or less effectively along a continuum. Some people make better evaluations than others; some believe information from nearly any source; and still others seldom believe anything without carefully evaluating the source. The following are some guidelines to enhance critical thinking (Kozier et al 2000):

- **Perform a self-assessment**. Determine which critical thinking attitudes (see p. 37) you already have and which need to be cultivated. Reflect on situations where you made decisions that you later regretted, and analyze the thinking processes or attitudes that you used. This could also be done with a trusted colleague or as a group.

- **Tolerate dissonance and ambiguity**. For example, to develop fair-mindedness, you could practice being open to other viewpoints by deliberately seeking out information that is in opposition to your views. As another example, you could practice suspending judgment (or tolerating ambiguity). If an issue is complex, it may not be resolved quickly and neatly. For a while, you might need to say, "I don't know," and be comfortable with that answer until more is known.
- **Seek situations where good thinking is practiced**. Attend conferences in clinical or educational settings that support open examination of all sides of issues and respect opposing viewpoints.
- **Create environments that support critical thinking**. Nurses in leadership positions must be particularly aware of the climate for thinking that they establish. They should create a stimulating environment that encourages differences of opinion and fair examination of ideas and options. As leaders, nurses should encourage colleagues to examine evidence carefully before they come to conclusions and to avoid "group think," the tendency to defer unthinkingly to the will of the group.
- **Practice critical thinking**. Everyone can achieve at least some level of critical thinking skill. Although critical thinking is not easy, with practice you can develop a critical attitude and good thinking skills. You are taking the first steps on the path to critical thinking when you realize that understanding is more important than memorizing, and when you trust your own ability to make sense of information and principles. The application and critical thinking exercises in this book help you to practice critical thinking. A "Critical Thinking Practice" exercise at the end of every chapter explains a particular critical thinking skill and asks you to apply it. As you develop habits of critical thinking, you will find that your thinking is no longer limited by the influences of your unexamined beliefs, feelings, and values. This will help you in your efforts to bring about good outcomes for your clients.

■ SUMMARY

Nurses:

- must be critical thinkers because of the nature of their work.
- use critical thinking skills in each step of the nursing process.
- use five types of knowledge: nursing science, nursing art, nursing ethics, personal knowledge, and practice wisdom.

Critical thinking:

- involves both attitudes (feelings) and cognitive thinking skills.
- is rational and reasonable.
- involves creative thinking.
- involves cognitive skills, such as using language, perceiving, believing and knowing, clarifying, comparing, judging and evaluating, and reasoning.

- includes complex intellectual activities, such as problem solving, clinical reasoning, reflective judgment, clinical judgment, and critical analysis.
- can be improved with practice.

Critical thinkers:

- consider issues before forming an opinion.
- believe in their ability to think things through and make decisions.
- apply knowledge and principles to specific situations.
- think for themselves and are not easily manipulated.
- are aware of the limits of their knowledge.
- have an attitude of inquiry.

Nursing Process Practice

To answer items 1 through 4, refer to situations a–d in the box on page 70:

1. Which situation is the best example of an attitude of intellectual humility?_____
   Explain your answer.

2. Which situation is the best example of an attitude of independent thinking?_____
   Explain your answer.

3. In the four situations (a–d), underline all nursing activities that represent *clinical judgment.*

4. This chapter gave reasons to support the belief that nurses need to be critical thinkers; they are listed below. Fill in the blanks with the letter (a, b, c, d) of the situation that best matches each reason. Compare your answers with a classmate. Explain the choices you made.

   _____ Nursing is an applied discipline.
   _____ Nursing draws on knowledge from other subjects and fields.
   _____ Nurses deal with change in stressful environments.
   _____ Nurses make frequent, varied, and important decisions in their work.

   a. Sally Sims works in a critical care unit. Today she performed neurological checks on her patient every hour. When her client stopped breathing she helped resuscitate him and put him on a ventilator. He has three different intravenous (IV) solutions running. Sally also attended a required inservice meeting to learn how to use a new IV pump. When she returned to the unit, she learned that her client had orders to receive a new, experimental medication and now needed neurological checks every 15 minutes.

b. Patrick Patel is taking a psychology course because he wants to better understand his patients. Today at work, he looked up a new medication on the Internet. He also reviewed the inflammatory process in a physiology text.

c. Recalling that a local lack of nutrients and oxygen results in tissue damage, Roberto Saldona turns his immobile patient at least every 2 hours to prevent pressure sores.

d. Today Samantha Wiles chose to use a smaller-than-usual needle to inject a client with frail tissues and little muscle mass. She decided to let a patient's family stay past visiting hours because the patient needed their support. When another patient had symptoms of low blood glucose, she decided to give him some juice and wait to see how he responded before calling the physician.

5. Look at each of the responses to the following case. Which nurse(s) demonstrated critical thinking? Circle the correct nurse(s): A, B, C, or D.

CASE: The night nurse has just given this shift report: "Mr. Stewart doesn't look very good to me. He said he felt 'sick' when I took his vital signs at 0600. Probably he just needs some orange juice." The day nurse has floated to a new unit and does not know any of her patients today. She also knows from the shift report that Mr. Stewart is 80 years old, has diabetes, and had vital signs within normal limits at 0600.

Nurse A, realizing that the regular staff probably knew the patients better than she did, followed the night nurse's advice and gave Mr. Stewart some orange juice right away, before making rounds on her other patients. After making rounds she returned to see if he was feeling better.

Nurse B, realizing that she was not an expert on diabetes, immediately called Mr. Stewart's physician and relayed the night report so that she could get orders about how to proceed.

Nurse C went to Mr. Stewart's room immediately after report, took his vital signs, listened to his heart and lungs, and asked him to describe how he was feeling. Unable to recall the symptoms of low blood glucose, she looked them up in a nursing text before giving Mr. Stewart the orange juice. Her plan was to call the physician if Mr. Stewart's condition did not improve within the hour.

Nurse D gave Mr. Stewart the orange juice immediately. She then charted that Mr. Stewart had a hypoglycemic reaction (low blood glucose) and initiated a care plan for that problem, including nursing orders to give orange juice as needed and to reassess the patient within 30 minutes.

6. In the preceding situations, for each nurse who did not use critical thinking, explain what the nurse did wrong. In your explanations, use the information from "Definitions of Critical Thinking" and "Characteristics of Critical Thinking" on pp. 36–39.

7. Fill in the blanks. Which kind of thinking does each of the following situations demonstrate?

Reflective thinking   Creative thinking
Rational/reasonable thinking   Conceptualizing

a. _creative_____ Mr. Adams is having difficulty understanding the calorie content of different foods, so his nurse thinks of an entirely new way to present the information to him.

b. _Rational_____ The nurse determines that a client is too weak to sit at the lavatory and assigns an aide to bathe him.

c. _Reflective_____ Before surgery, Ms. Morris's nurse notices that her facial expression is tense and her hands are trembling. The nurse analyzes the relationship between these cues and recognizes that the client is anxious.

d. _Conceptu_____ The nurse notices that Ms. Ginsburg has been left alone in the corridor to wait for surgery. She imagines how lonely the client must feel and she is reminded of the time her mother was in the hospital. She pats Ms. Ginsburg's hand as she walks by to another client's room.

8. Enter the letter for the kind of knowledge demonstrated by the following examples:

(S) Scientific, (E) Ethical, (P) Practice Wisdom
(A) Nursing Art, (SK) Self-Knowledge

a. _A_ The nurse is having lunch with colleagues who are discussing her client's personal life. One of them says, "I heard she made all that money in real estate. Is that true?" The nurse replies, "I can't discuss personal information about her, especially where it could be overheard."

b. _E_ Mr. Castaneda is reading his wife's chart, which was accidentally left at her bedside. The nurse says, "I'm sorry, Mr. Castaneda, but I must have Ms. Castaneda's permission in order to give you information that is in the chart."

c. _____ After reading several research reports, the head of the newborn nursery discontinued the requirement that parents must wear special gowns when holding the infants.

d. _____ The nurses on a surgical floor urge patients to ambulate to help promote the return of peristalsis after surgery. No one can say exactly how it helps, but they all remember patients who passed flatus after ambulating (and some who did not).

Critical Thinking Practice: Using Language

Review pp. 47–48, "Using Language."

A. Using Language Precisely

First reactions are usually fairly general, as in the statements below. One way to make your language more precise is to follow-up your first reactions by restating them with "because," and then give your reasons for the general conclusion you drew.

a. Mr. Li had a good night *because*: (1) he only woke up once in 8 hours and (2) he did not need any pain medication).
b. Susan is taking fluids and *tolerating them well.*
c. Ms. Froelich ambulated *with no difficulty.*

1. For the preceding statements, "b" and "c," add "because" and write reasons that might have caused the nurse to make the general statement. Statement "a" has been done for you.

2. In the following admission note, underline the words that are vague or imprecise.
"2 P.M. Elderly patient admitted to Room 212 in a moderate amount of distress. States that if he becomes terminally ill he does not want any heroic measures or treatments."

3. Rewrite the admission note as though you were the client being admitted. Remove all vague or ambiguous terms by answering the questions: Who? What? Where? When? How? and Why? Supply any information you need to make the terms specific (eg, although you don't know the patient's age, write in "80-year-old" for "elderly."

B. Jargon, Cliches, and Euphemisms

Underline any jargon, clichés, and euphemisms in the following statements. Write (J), (C), or (E) to identify the words you underline as jargon, cliché, or euphemism. Rewrite the statements, as needed, to create a more honest version of each thought.

1. Your husband is rather stocky, so this low-calorie diet is important.

2. Have you been living alone since your husband passed away?
   Are you alone after your husband die ?
3. Now that he is middle-aged, he is overweight and his waistline is much larger.
   Now that he is in 40's
4. I'm a little full-figured. Can you find me a larger hospital gown?
   enough with this
5. If your child's ear infections become more frequent, we should consider tubes.
   too bad

6. Mrs. Adams, I'll need to check your tummy every 15 minutes for the first hour after you have your blessed event.

    Stomak

7. Do you need to go to the little girls' room?

    chil's

8. I know you're having a hard time, Mr. Jones. Just remember, it's always darkest just before dawn.

    You feel bad before you feel good.

9. We need to get you ambulating today.

10. The I & O shows 350 cc voided and 500 cc residual obtained by cath.

11. Healthcare is a right.

    care for your heath is a right

12. Lab will be here soon to do a stick for your gases and lytes.

    workers who is working in the lab

13. I'll take your vital signs and then we'll take you for your ECG.

Case Study: Applying Critical Thinking

Mrs. Lutz is a 78-year-old woman who has undergone radiation therapy and three surgeries for cancer. She is not progressing well, cannot eat, and is losing weight. The physician has decided to place a subclavian catheter in order to administer total parenteral nutrition. The nurse takes the informed consent form to Mrs. Lutz for her signature and explains to her that "the doctor will place a small tube in your vein, about here, so we can give you more nutrients and help you regain your strength and heal." Mrs. Lutz says, "I'm so tired of all this pain. I'm not sure I want anything else done, and I surely don't want to be hurt again."

1. What factors does the nurse need to assess that might affect Mrs. Lutz's *ability* to consent?

2. Before Mrs. Lutz signs the consent form, how can the nurse be certain that her consent was truly "informed"? (Informed consent means that the client has been informed about and understands the treatment, including its risks and benefits.)

    The nurse replies to Mrs. Lutz: "Now, now, your doctor has ordered this to make you well. Don't worry, we'll make sure you don't feel a thing. Your doctor will be here soon and he will expect this permit to be signed. Won't you please sign it now?"

3. Evaluate the nurse's approach to Mrs. Lutz in regard to this invasive procedure. (What do you think about it, and why?)

4. Which phase of the nursing process is the nurse using in Items 1 and 2?

5. In Items 1 and 2, which standard(s) of reasoning is involved (see Table 2–3, on page 64).

■ SELECTED REFERENCES

Alfaro-LeFevre, R. (1998). Improving your ability to think critically. *Nursing Spectrum* (Illinois ed.) 11(4):14–16.

Adams, B. L. (1999). Nursing education for critical thinking: An integrative review. *J Nurs Edu* 38(3):111–119.

American Nurses Association (1985). *Code for nurses with interpretive statements*. Washington, DC: ANA.

Benner, P. (1984). *From novice to expert*. Menlo Park, Calif.: Addison-Wesley Publishing Co.

Carpenito, L. J. (1999). Editorial. *Nurs Forum* 34(2):3–4.

Carper, B. (1978). Fundamental patterns of knowing in nursing. *Adv Nurs Sci 1(October): 13–23*.

Chinn, P. and M. Kramer (1991). *Theory and nursing*. St. Louis: Mosby Year Book.

Dexter, P., M. Applegate, et al (1997 [May-June]). A proposed framework for teaching and evaluating critical thinking in nursing. *J Prof Nurs* 13(3):160–167.

Foundation for Critical Thinking (1996). *Critical thinking workshop handbook*. Rohnert Park, CA: Foundation for Critical Thinking.

Gaberson, K. B. and M. H. Oermann (1999). *Clinical teaching strategies in nursing*. New York: Springer.

Green, C. (2000). *Critical thinking in nursing. Case studies across the curriculum*. Upper Saddle River, NJ: Prentice Hall Health.

Jameton, A. (1984). *Nursing practice. The ethical issues*. Englewood Cliffs, NJ: Prentice-Hall.

Kennison, M. and J. Brace (1997). Critical thinking. Digging deeper for creative solutions. *Nursing* 27(9):52–54.

Kim, H. (1983). *The nature of theoretical thinking in nursing*. Norwalk, CT: Appleton-Century-Crofts.

Kozier, B., G. Erb, A. Berman et al (2000). *Fundamentals of nursing: Concepts, process, and practice*. Upper Saddle River, NJ: Prentice-Hall.

Lauri, S. and S. Salantera (1998). Decision-making models in different fields of nursing. *Res Nurs Health* 21(5):443–452.

Lenburg, C. B. (1997). Confusing facets of critical thinking. *Tennessee Nurse* 60(5):11–13.

Ludwick, R. and C. A. Sedlak (1998 [Fall]). Ethical perspectives. Ethical issues and critical thinking: Students' stories. *Nursing Connections* 11(3):12–18.

Paul, R. (1988). *What, then, is critical thinking?* The Eighth Annual and Sixth International Conference on Critical Thinking and Educational Reform. Rohnert Park, CA: The Center for Critical Thinking and Moral Critique, Sonoma State University.

Paul, R. (1990). *Critical thinking*. Rohnert Park, CA: The Center for Critical Thinking and Moral Critique, Sonoma State University.

Reilly, D. E. and M. H. Oermann (1992). *Clinical teaching in nursing education*. New York: National League for Nursing.

Roy, C. (1980). *The Roy adaptation model. Conceptual models for nursing practice*. J. Riehl and C. Roy, eds. New York: Appleton-Century-Crofts.

Taylor, C. (1997). Problem solving in clinical nursing practice. *J Advan Nurs* 26(2):329–336.

Trauner, L. (1998). It is time to move from the nursing process to critical thinking. [Letter] *JAORN* 67(1):18.

Ziegler, S., B. Vaughan-Wrobel, and J. Erlen (1986). *Nursing process, nursing diagnosis, nursing knowledge: Avenues to autonomy*. Norwalk, CT, Appleton-Century-Crofts.

3

Assessment

Learning Outcomes

On completing this chapter, you should be able to do the following:

- Relate assessment to the other phases of the nursing process.
- Differentiate between subjective and objective data.
- Compare initial and ongoing assessment.
- Describe effective interview techniques.
- State the contents of an initial comprehensive nursing assessment.
- Use a nursing framework to structure and record data collection.
- Give examples of a "special purpose" assessment.
- Describe the nursing assessments pertinent to healthy clients.
- Explain why and how data should be validated.
- Apply critical thinking standards to your assessment activities.
- Explain the need for honesty and confidentiality when collecting data.

■ ASSESSMENT: THE FIRST PHASE OF THE NURSING PROCESS

Assessment, the first phase in the nursing process, is the systematic gathering of relevant and important patient data. **Data** are information or facts about the patient. Nurses use data to: (1) identify health problems, (2) plan nursing care, and (3) evaluate patient outcomes. During the assessment phase, the nurse collects, validates, records, and organizes data into predetermined categories (see Box 3–1 on page 77, and Figure 3–1 on p. 76).

Standards of Practice American Nurses Association and Canadian Nurses Association practice standards outline nurses' accountability for assessment. Adhering to the standards in Box 3–2 on page 78 will help you to collect data in a professional manner. Keep these standards of practice in mind as you work through this chapter.

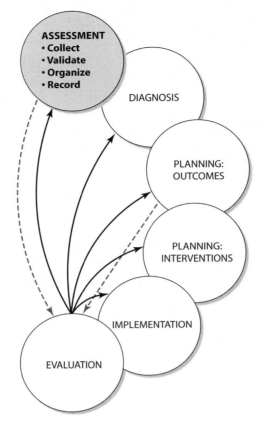

Figure 3–1
The Assessment Phase

Purpose of Nursing Assessment

The purpose of nursing assessment is to get a total picture of the patient and how he can be helped. This requires data about patient, family, and community patterns of health and illness, deviations from normal, strengths, coping abilities, and risk factors for health problems. The nursing assessment focuses on patient responses—unlike the medical assessment, which focuses on disease processes and pathology. The nurse may gather data about a medical diagnosis, but this is not the focus of the assessment. For example, when admitting a patient to the hospital for surgery, the nurse is interested in the disease symptoms and the nature of the surgery, but focuses primarily on how the symptoms affect the patient's ability to care for himself, what he expects from the surgery, how his recovery period will affect his life, and what his main concerns are at this time.

BOX 3-1

Overview of Assessment Phase

1. Collect data
   Interview
   Observation
   Physical examination
2. Validate data with client and significant others
   Compare subjective with objective data
   Validate conflicting data
3. Organize and record data
   Initial assessment: Use printed form (admission database)
   Ongoing assessment: Use nursing model to organize; record on care plan or nursing progress notes
   Special purpose assessments: Perform as needed

Relationship to Other Phases of the Nursing Process

Recall from Chapter 1 that even though the steps of the nursing process are discussed separately to help you understand them, they are actually interrelated and overlapping. This is especially true of the assessment phase. Assessment data must be accurate and complete because they form the basis for the decisions made in the remaining steps of the nursing process. The usefulness and validity of the nursing diagnoses depend greatly on thorough, accurate data collection. In the planning phase, the nurse uses patient data to decide which goals are realistic and which nursing orders will be most effective.

In effect, assessment is a continuous process carried out during all phases of the nursing process. For example you may begin to formulate a tentative problem in your mind (diagnosis phase) while still collecting data. Assessment overlaps with implementation and evaluation in that you will continue to collect patient data while carrying out these steps.

> **KEY POINT**
>
> **Assessment** is the systematic gathering of relevant and important patient information for use in identifying health status and planning and evaluating nursing care.

EXAMPLE: As the nurse is bathing a patient (implementation), she is observing his skin condition and joint mobility. After the nursing orders have been carried out, during the evaluation phase, the nurse collects data to determine patient progress toward goal achievement (eg, she observes the skin to see if turning and positioning the patient have prevented pressure sores).

Critical Thinking in Assessment

Assessment is more than just writing information on an assessment form. You will need critical thinking skills and a good knowledge base to decide

Standards of Practice

American Nurses Association Standard I: Assessment. The nurse collects patient health data.

Measurement Criteria

1. Data collection involves the patient, family, and other healthcare providers as appropriate.
2. The priority of data collection activities is determined by the client's immediate condition or needs.
3. Pertinent data are collected using appropriate assessment techniques and instruments.
4. Relevant data are documented in a retrievable form.
5. The data collection process is systematic and ongoing.

Source: Reprinted with permission from American Nurses Association, *Standards of Clinical Nursing Practice*, 2nd ed, © 1998, American Nurses Publishing, American Nurses Foundation/American Nurses Association, 600 Maryland Ave., SW, Suite 100 W, Washington, DC 20024-2571.

Canadian Nurses Association Standard II. Nursing practice requires the effective use of the nursing process.

Collection of Data

1. Nurses are required to collect data in accordance with their conception of the client. The nurse in any practice setting:
    1.1 systematically and continuously collects data, utilizing knowledge from nursing and related fields, that are consistent with the conception of the client
    1.2 systematically and continuously collects data that are consistent with the goals of nursing and related disciplines
    1.3 determines the client's expectations for care
    1.4 uses all appropriate sources for data collection including: client, physician, family, relevant others, records, the nurse's own knowledge and experience
    1.5 employs various techniques in data collection including: interview, consultation, physical examination, observation, measurement
    1.6 treats data with regard for the confidentiality of those concerned
    1.7 makes available relevant data to appropriate persons with the client's permission

Source: Reprinted with permission from the Canadian Nurses Association. From *Standards for Nursing Practice* (1987). 2nd ed. Ottawa, Ontario: CNA.

which assessments to make, how much information you need, and where and how to get that information. When performing assessments, you will apply principles and theories about basic human needs, anatomy and physiology, disease processes, human growth and development, human behavior, socioeconomic patterns and trends, and various cultures and religions.

You must make reliable observations, distinguish relevant and important data from irrelevant and unimportant data, and recognize when information is missing. All of this requires critical thinking, as does organizing and categorizing data in a useful manner. To check the quality of your thinking in the assessment phase, review the standards of reasoning in Table 2–3, on page 64, and ask yourself the questions in Table 3–1, on pp. 80–81.

> Think about measurement Criteria 1–5 in Box 3–2 (ANA Standard I). Which of the standards of reasoning (in Table 3–1) are implied by each criterion? For example, Criterion 1 implies *breadth* because it helps assure that the data include more than one perspective. What other standards are implied by Criterion 1? By the other criteria?

Reflective Practice

Recall from Chapter 2 that critical thinking requires reflection. In the assessment phase, the core question for reflection is: What information do I need to care for this person, family, or community? This will require you to reflect more deeply, asking such questions as:

- Who is this person?
- What is this person's story (eg, what health event caused the person to seek care)?
- How has this person's life been changed by this illness/event?
- Who and what are this person's supports?
- How is this person feeling?

■ COLLECTING DATA

Data collection is the process of gathering information about client, family, or community health status. This section will help you develop your data-collection skills.

Subjective and Objective Data

Subjective data are sometimes called *covert data* or *symptoms*; objective data are sometimes called *overt data* or *signs*. Both types of data are needed for a thorough assessment.

Subjective data are not measurable or observable. They can be obtained only from what the client tells you. Subjective data include the client's thoughts, beliefs, feelings, sensations, and perceptions of self and health (eg,

Table 3–1   Assessment: Think About Your Thinking

Standard of Reasoning	Questions to Ask Yourself	Discussion/Examples
Clarity—A statement must be clear in order to know whether it is accurate, relevant, and so on.	■ Did the patient express herself clearly in the interview? ■ Are the data the recorded clearly?	*Unclear*: "Patient states he has been sick for a long time." *Clearer*: Nurse should ask for and record more details: How does patient describe "sick," and exactly how long is "a long time"?
Accuracy—A statement can be clear, but not accurate.	■ Are my measurements correct? ■ Is there reason to believe that the patient gave me incorrect information? ■ Did I validate data when necessary (eg, compare subjective and objective data)?	■ *Example*: If the blood pressure was difficult to hear, you would ask another nurse to check it. Also, data may be inaccurate if instruments need to be calibrated (eg, meters for checking blood glucose, heart monitors). ■ *Example*: A patient may not feel comfortable enough to be frank with the nurse, may be embarrassed if family members are present, or have mental deficits.
Precision—A statement can be both clear and accurate, but not precise.	■ What details can I provide to make these data more exact? ■ Would someone else know exactly what I mean by this?	*Imprecise*: "Patient states he has a headache." *More precise*: "Patient states he has a mild, throbbing pain in his left temple, which began about an hour ago."
Relevance—A statement can be clear, accurate, and precise, but not relevant to the issue.	■ Do I have data that relate to this nursing diagnosis or problem? ■ Do I have data about factors that are contributing to the problem?	In the admission (comprehensive) assessment, almost anything may be relevant. Focus assessments are more selective (eg, to evaluate the status of a decubitus ulcer, the appearance of the ulcer is relevant; you also need data about the patient's mobility and nutrition; it is irrelevant that the patient is coughing).

Table 3–1 Assessment: Think About Your Thinking (continued)

Standard of Reasoning	Questions to Ask Yourself	Discussion/Examples
Depth—A statement can be clear, accurate, precise, and relevant—but superficial.	■ Did I cover all areas on the assessment form? ■ Are there any other data that would shed some light on the problem? ■ In the interview, did I follow up on patient leads with probing questions?	*Example:* A nurse was to obtain a patient's signature on a surgery consent form. She first checked the patient's chart and noted that she had a designated power of attorney for her healthcare. This alerted the nurse that she needed more data in order to determine whether the patient was actually competent to sign the form.
Breadth—A line of reasoning can meet all the other standards, but be one-sided	■ Did I get data about patient and family concerns, as well as my own? ■ Did I see only what I expected to see?	*Example:* A nurse who expects patients to be anxious preoperatively might be inclined to "see" signs of anxiety: to see normal moving about as "restlessness."
Logic—Reasoning brings various thoughts together in some kind of order. When the thoughts make sense in combination, thinking is logical.	■ Do these data make sense? ■ How can both of these "facts" be true?	See "Validating the Data" on pp. 100–101.
Significance—Related to relevance. What is *most* important?	■ Which of the facts are most important? ■ Are there abnormal findings that I need to report to someone immediately?	As a student, you should report abnormal data to your instructor or an experienced nurse as soon as possible. Be prepared in advance; know the "norms" for relevant data.

Source: Based on R. Paul (1996) *Critical thinking workshop handbook.* Dillon Beach, CA: Foundation for Critical Thinking. See www.Criticalthinking.org.

pain, dizziness, nausea, sadness, happiness). Although you will usually obtain subjective data from the client, data from significant others and other health professionals may also be subjective if they consist of opinion and perception rather than fact. You may not always be able to obtain subjective data. Some clients, such as infants, unconscious people, or the cognitively impaired, may not be able to provide subjective data, or their data may be unreliable. See Table 3–2 for approaches to use when it is difficult to obtain subjective data.

Table 3–2 Nursing Actions to Use When It Is Difficult to Obtain Subjective Data

Contributing Factor	Symptoms	Nursing Activities
Language barrier (eg, not fluent in English)	Unable to communicate information clearly	Use simple, clear language; obtain an interpreter.
Severe illness or pain	Short responses; patient's main concern is to obtain relief; impatient with "questioning."	Provide needed intervention (eg, give pain medication) before interviewing. Ask closed questions; obtain only essential data. Ask family or friends.
Anxiety	Rapid, incoherent speech; distorted or inaccurate information	Speak slowly and quietly to the person. Emphasize that you need accurate information to give appropriate help.
Fear of incapacitating effects of illness	Denying certain symptoms or deliberately giving misleading facts	Explore discrepancies between client statements and physical findings or data from other sources (see "Validating Data" pp. 100–101).
Limited mental capacity	May give inaccurate, unreliable information	Encourage client to provide as much information as possible; then use secondary sources to fill in gaps and validate data.
Previous negative experience with health-care professionals; lack of trust	Reluctant to provide data. Believes, "It won't help me anyway. It didn't do any good before."	Acknowledge previous experience and the imperfection of health professionals. Request another chance to help. Demonstrate competence. Convey respect for client's thoughts and feelings.

Source: Adapted from Kozier et al (1995) *Fundamentals of Nursing*. 5th ed. Redwood City, CA: Addison-Wesley Nursing.

Objective data can be detected by someone other than the client. You will usually obtain it by observing and examining the client. Examples of objective data include: pulse rate, skin color, urine output, and results of diagnostic tests or x-rays.

When used in the nursing process, the terms *subjective* and *objective* have the special meanings described above. *Subjective* does not suggest biased information or personal interpretation of meaning, as it does in common use; and *objective* does not necessarily carry the common meaning of *impartial*. See Table 3–3 for examples of subjective and objective data.

Primary and Secondary Data Sources

Data sources fall into two broad categories: *primary* and *secondary*. You should use the most reliable source of data, whether it is the patient or a significant other, and you should indicate the source on the patient's record. The client is the **primary data** source; all other data sources are secondary. Both primary and secondary source data can be subjective or objective; that is, it can be obtained from what the client tells you or by observation and examination. **Secondary data** are obtained from sources other than the client (eg, other people, client records).

Significant others, such as family or friends, are especially valuable sources when the client is a child or has difficulty communicating. When possible, you should get the client's consent before collecting data from significant others.

Other healthcare providers, such as the physician, social worker, and respiratory therapist, can provide information about the areas of client functioning with which they are involved. Sharing information among disciplines is especially important when the client is being transferred from one institution to another (eg, from a nursing home to a hospital) or discharged from the institution for follow-up care at home.

The client's written record from present and past hospitalizations is a secondary source. The client's record should be reviewed early in the data-collection process to help you plan the initial nursing assessment and to confirm the other data.

Table 3–3   Examples of Subjective and Objective Data

	Subjective	Objective
Description	*Covert data; symptoms.* What the patient says. Can be perceived and verified only by the patient.	*Overt data; signs.* Can be observed by others or measured against a standard.
Examples	Itching Pain Anxiety "I'm afraid." "I feel weak all over."	Pulse rate 100 bpm Blood pressure 120/80 mm Hg Skin pale and cool to touch Urine output 350 mL X-ray results Skin turgor Posture

Information from nursing and other literature is especially important for students and beginning practitioners. For example, if you have never cared for a client with trigeminal neuralgia, you should read a textbook in order to know what signs and symptoms to expect. The literature also provides helpful information about developmental norms, cultural differences, and spiritual practices to use as a guide during data collection. Table 3–4 provides examples of primary and secondary data sources.

Initial Versus Ongoing Assessment

Assessment begins with the nurse's first contact with the client and continues throughout all subsequent encounters. Initial and ongoing assessment differs in purpose and, usually, in scope.

The **initial assessment** is made during the first nurse-client encounter and is usually comprehensive, consisting of all subjective and objective data pertinent to the client's health status. When the initial assessment is performed on the client's arrival at a healthcare agency, it is called the **admission assessment**. Each client should have an initial assessment to determine the need for care and further assessment.

Ongoing assessment consists of data gathered after the database is completed—ideally, during every nurse-patient interaction. These data are used to identify new problems and to evaluate the status of problems that have already been identified. See Table 3–5 on page 85 for a summary comparison of initial and ongoing assessment.

Table 3–4   Examples of Primary and Secondary Data Sources

	Primary	Secondary
Description	Subjective or objective data obtained directly from the patient.	Information about the patient obtained from family and friends, verbal reports from other healthcare professionals, information from patient records.
Examples	Itching Patient statement of pain Patient statement of anxiety Pulse rate Skin color Posture	Statements from records (eg, x-ray results; nurse's note that "Client refused dinner.") Verbal report from caregivers (eg, "Needed pain medication at 8 AM") Family statement, "He has been in pain all day."

Table 3–5 Initial Versus Ongoing Assessment

Initial	Ongoing
Admission assessment	Focus assessment
Database assessment	Focuses on specific problems, activities,
Comprehensive assessment	or behaviors
Can include focus assessment	Focuses on identified problems (can also
Data are used to make initial	be used to identify new problems)
problem list	Data are used to evaluate outcomes
	achievement and problem resolution

Comprehensive Versus Focus Assessment

A **comprehensive assessment** provides an overall picture of the client's health status. The nurse obtains data about all the client's body systems and functional abilities, without necessarily having a particular health problem in mind. It usually follows the agency's printed assessment form (eg, Figure 3–2 on pp. 86–87).

Information obtained from the comprehensive assessment makes up the **nursing database**. In fact, the initial (admission) assessment is also called "database assessment." Figure 3–3 on p. 88 illustrates the place of the database in the assessment phase. The complete database consists of the nursing history and physical examination, as well as data from the patient's records, consultations and, sometimes, a review of the literature. Figure 3–2, on pp. 86–87, is an example of a nursing database, as is Appendix B.

In a **focus assessment**, the nurse gathers data about an actual, potential, or possible problem that has been identified (Alfaro-Le Fevre 1998). The assessment focuses on a specific topic or particular area of the body instead of the client's overall health status. Data from focus assessments are used to evaluate the status of existing problems and to identify new problems.

EXAMPLE: *Evaluation of an existing problem.* The care plan for Hassim Asad included the problem of Fluid Volume Deficit. When performing ongoing assessment during Mr. Asad's bath, the nurse noted that his oral mucous membranes were moist and that he had good skin turgor—signs that his fluid volume problem was resolving.

EXAMPLE: *Identification of a new problem.* During his bath, Mr. Asad mentioned that his head was beginning to hurt. He had not mentioned headaches before. The nurse took his blood pressure and questioned him about the nature and onset of the pain. Mr. Asad's blood pressure was elevated, and his vision was blurred. The nurse elevated the head of the bed, relieving his pain somewhat, and notified the physician of this new development.

A focus assessment is not limited to ongoing data collection; it can also be used in the initial assessment when the client reports a symptom or other

ADMISSION DATA

Date 4-16-00   Time 3:15 p.m. Primary Language English
Arrived Via: ☐ Wheelchair ☐ Stretcher ☑ Ambulatory
From: ☐ Admitting ☐ ER ☑ Home ☐ Nursing Home ☐ Other
Admitting M.D. R. Katz   Time Notified 5 p.m.

ORIENTATION TO UNIT

	YES	NO		YES	NO
Arm Band Correct	☒	☐	Visiting Hours	☒	☐
Allergy Band	☒	☐	Smoking Policy	☒	☐
Telephone	☒	☐	TV, Lights, Bed Controls,		
Electical Policy	☒	☐	Call Lights, Side Rails	☒	☐
Educational Mat'l	☒	☐	Nurses Station	☒	☐
(TV Brochure)	☒	☐			

Family M.D. R. Katz
Weight 125 lb   Height 5ft. 2in.   BP:R — L 122/80
Temp. 103 F   Pulse 92. weak   Resp. 28. shallow
Source Providing Information ☑ Patient ☐ Other
Unable to Obtain History ☐
Reason for Admission (Onset, Duration, Pt.'s Perception) "Chest
cold" X2 weeks S.O.B. on exertion. "Lung pain,
fever," "Dr. says I have pneumonia."

ALLERGIES & REACTIONS

Drugs Penicillin
Food/Other
Signs & Symptoms rash, nausea
Blood Reaction ☐ Yes ☑ No   Dyes/Shellfish ☐ Yes ☑ No

MEDICATIONS

Current Meds	Dose/Freq.	Last Dose
Synthroid	0.1 mg. daily	4-16, 8 a.m.

Disposition of Meds: ☒ Home ☐ Pharmacy ☐ Safe*At Bedside

MEDICAL HISTORY

☑ No Major Problems   ☐ Gastro
☐ Cardiac   ☐ Arthritis
☐ Hyper/Hypotension   ☐ Stroke
☐ Diabetes   ☐ Seizures
☐ Cancer   ☐ Glaucoma
☐ Respiratory   ☑ Other Childbirth-1992

Surgery/Procedures	Date
Appendectomy	1978
Partial thyroidectomy	1991

SPECIAL ASSISTIVE DEVICES

☐ Wheelchair ☐ Contacts ☐ Venous ☐ Dentures
☐ Braces ☐ Hearing Aid Access ☐ Partial
☐ Cane/Crutches ☐ Prosthesis Device ☐ Upper
☐ Walker ☐ Glasses ☐ Epidural ☐ Lower
                              Catheter
☐ Other None

VALUABLES

Patient informed Hospital not responsible for personal belongings.
Valuables Disposition: ☐ Patient ☐ Safe ☐ Given to
Patient/SO Signature None

PSYCHOSOCIAL HISTORY

Recent Stress None
Coping Mechanism Not assessed because of fatigue
Support System Husband, co-workers, friends
Calm: ☑ Yes ☐ No
Anxious: ☐ Yes ☐ No Facial muscles tense; trembling
Religion Catholic, Would want last rites
Tobacco Use: ☐ Yes ☑ No
Alcohol Use: ☐ Yes ☑ No
Drug Use: ☐ Yes ☑ No

NEUROLOGICAL

Oriented: ☑ Person ☑ Place ☑ Time ☐ Confused ☐ Sedated
          ☐ Alert ☐ Restless ☑ Lethargic ☐ Comatose
Pupils: ☑ Equal ☐ Unequal ☑ Reactive ☐ Sluggish
          ☐ Other 3mm
Extremity Strength: ☑ Equal ☐ Unequal
Speech: ☑ Clear ☐ Slurred ☐ Other

MUSCULO-SKELETAL

Normal ROM of Extremities ☑ Yes ☐ No
☑ Weakness ☐ Paralysis ☐ Contractures ☐ Joint Swelling ☑ Pain
☐ Other related to fatigue   when coughing

RESPIRATORY

Pattern: ☐ Even ☐ Uneven ☑ Shallow ☑ Dyspnea
          ☑ Other diminished breath sounds
Breathing Sounds: ☐ Clear ☑ Other inspiratory crackles
Secretions: ☐ None ☑ Other pink, thick sputum
Cough: ☐ None ☑ Productive ☐ Nonproductive

CARDIOVASCULAR

Pulses: Apical Rate 92-W ☑ Reg. ☐ Irregular ☐ Pacemaker
          S = Strong W = Weak A = Absent D = Doppler
Radial R 92   L —   Pedal R —   L —
Edema: ☑ Absent ☐ Present ☐ Site
Perfusion: ☐ Warm ☐ Dry ☑ Diaphoretic ☐ Cool ☐ (Hot)

GASTROINTESTINAL

Oral Mucosa ☐ Normal ☑ Other pale and dry
Bowel Sounds: ☑ Normal ☐ Other Abd. soft
Wt. Change: ☐ ☑ N/V Stool Frequency/Character 1/day;soft
Last B/M 4-15-00 ☐ Ostomy (type)
Equip.

GENITOURINARY

Urine: Last Voided This morning
☐ Normal ☐ Anuria ☐ Hematuria ☐ Dysuria ☐ Incontinent
☒ Other decreased amount & frequency since
☐ Catheter (type)   Other
LMP 4-1-00   ☐ Vaginal/Penile Discharge
Other

SELF-CARE

Need Assist with: ☐ Ambulating ☐ Elimination
                  ☐ Meals ☒ Hygiene ☐ Dressing
                  while fatigued

☀ **NORTH BROWARD HOSPITAL DISTRICT**
NURSING ADMINISTRATION ASSESSMENT

Figure 3–2

Assessment for Luisa Sanchez (*Source*: Nursing assessment tool courtesy of Broward General Medical Center, Broward County, Florida. Reprinted with permission.)

General Appearance: ☑ Well Nourished ☐ Emaciated ☐ Other_____

Appetite: ☐ Good ☐ Fair ☑ Poor -x2 Days

Diet _Liquid_   Meal Pattern _3/day_

☐ Feeds Self ☐ Assist ☐ Total Feed

SKIN ASSESSMENT

Color: ☐ Normal ☐ Flushed ☑ Pale ☐ Dusky ☐ Cyanotic ☐ Jaundiced ☑ Other _Cheeks flushed, hot_

General Description _Surgical scars: RLQ abdomen; anterior neck_

Note Cultures Obtained _____

PRESSURE SORE "AT RISK" SCREENING CRITERIA

OVERALL SKIN CONDITION
Grade
- 0 Turgor (elasticity adequate, skin warm and moist)
- ☑1 Poor turgor, skin cold & dry
- 2 Areas mottled, red or denuded
- 3 Existing skin ulcer/lesions

BOWEL AND BLADDER CONTROL
Grade
- ☑0 Always able to ask for bedpan
- 1 Incontinence of urine
- 2 Incontinence of feces
- 3 Totally incontinent Confined to bed

REHABILITATIVE STATE
Grade
- 0 Fully ambulatory
- ☑1 Ambulated with assistance
- 2 Chair to bed ambulation only
- 3 Confined to bed
- 4 Immobile in bed

NUTRITIONAL STATE
Grade
- 0 Eats all
- ☑1 Eats very little
- 2 Refuses food often
- 3 Tube feeding
- 4 Intravenous feeding

MENTAL STATE
Grade
- ☑0 Alert and clear
- 1 Confused
- 2 Disoriented/Senile
- 3 Stuporous
- 4 Unconscious

CHRONIC DISEASE STATUS
(i.e. copd, ascvd. Peripheral Vascular Disease, Diabetes, or Renal Deficits, Cancer, Motor or Sensory Deficits, Elderly, Other)
Grade
- ☑0 Absent
- 1 One Present
- 2 Two Present
- 3 Three or more Present

TOTAL_____ Refer to Skin Care Protocol

FALLS SCREENING

If one or more of the following are checked, institute fall precautions/plan of care
☐ History of Falls ☐ Unsteady Gait ☐ Confusion/Disorientation ☐ Dizziness

If two or more of the following are checked institute fall precautions/plan of care
☐ Age over 80
☐ Impaired vision
☐ Multiple
☐ Utilizes cane, walker, w/c
☐ Impaired hearing
☐ Multiple diagnoses
☐ Sleeplessness
☐ Urgency/frequency in elimination
☐ Medication/Sedative/ Diuretic, etc.
☐ Inability to understand or follow directions

NURSE SIGNATURE/TITLE	DATE	TIME
Mary Medina, RN	4-16-00	3:30 pm
NURSE SIGNATURE/TITLE	DATE	TIME

---

1. What do you know about your present illness? _"Dr. says I have pneumonia." "I will have an I.V."_
2. What information do you want or need about your illness?
3. Would you like family/SO involved in your care? _Husband Michael_
4. How long do you expect to be in the hospital? _"1-2 days"_
5. What concerns do you have about leaving the hospital?

CHECK APPROPRIATE BOX

Will patient need post discharge assistance with ADLs/physical functioning? ☐ Yes ☑ No ☐ Unknown

Does patient have family capable of and willing to provide assistance post discharge?
☑ Yes ☐ No ☐ Unknown ☐ No family

Is assistance needed beyond that which family can provide?
☐ Yes ☑ No ☐ Unknown

Previous admission in the last six months?
☐ Yes ☑ No ☐ Unknown

Patient lives with _Husband and 1 child_

Planned discharge to _Home_

Comments: _Fatigue and anxiety may have interfered with learning. Re-teach anything covered at admission, later._

Social Services Notified ☐ Yes ☑ No

NARRATIVE NOTES

S—c/o sharp chest pain when coughing and dyspnea on exertion. States unable to carry out regular daily exercise for past week. Coughing relieved "if I sit up and sit still." Nausea associated with coughing. Having occasional "chills." Occasionally becomes frightened, stating, "I can't breathe." Well groomed but "too tired to put on make-up."

O—Chest expansion < 3 cm, no nasal flaring or use of accessory muscles. Breath sounds and insp. crackles in ® upper and lower chest.

Assesses own supports as "good" (eg, relationship c̄ husband). Is "worried" about daughter. States husband will be out of town until tomorrow. Left 3-year-old daughter with neighbor. Concerned too about her work (is attorney). "I'll never get caught up." Had water at noon—no food today. Informed of need to save urine for 24 hr. specimen. IV D₅W LR 1000 mL started in ® arm, 100 mL/hr. Slow capillary refill. Keeping head of bed↑ to facilitate breathing.

Figure 3–2
Continued

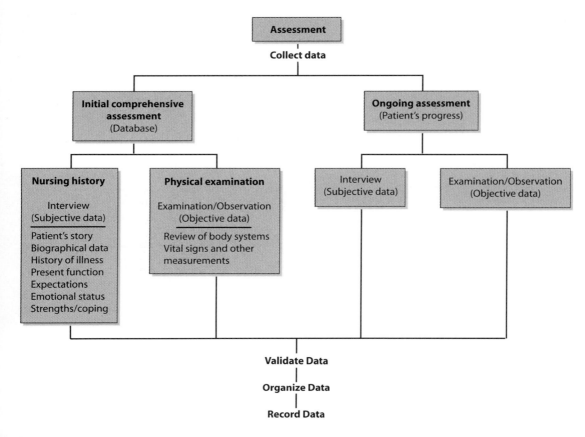

Figure 3–3
Overview of Assessment

unusual findings. Any symptom or difficulty the client reports should be expanded on by asking further questions about it (eg, When did it begin? What makes it worse? What relieves it?). When a client needs repeated in-depth assessment of a particular problem area, most agencies have special assessment forms for recording the ongoing focus assessment (eg, a flow sheet for hourly neurologic assessments).

Use of Computers in Assessment

Many healthcare agencies use computerized information systems to facilitate data collection. In some automated assessment systems, patients respond directly to interview questions on the computer screen. In other systems, the nurse interviews the patient and enters the data into a bedside terminal. Nurses may also use bedside terminals to prompt them through a systematic and complete physical examination of a patient. And finally, nurses use computers to record the interview and examination data. Figure 3–4 is an example of a computer screen showing a portion of a flowsheet on which nurses record their ongoing assessments at a bedside computer.

In addition, a variety of monitors can be programmed to make continuous or periodic patient assessments. Examples are digital thermometers, digital scales, pulse oximeters, electrocardiogram/telemetry/hemodynamic monitors, apnea monitors, fetal heart monitors, and blood glucose analyzers. Most of these instruments keep a record of the most recent values. Some can transmit their data to a more sophisticated computer or print out a paper record. Some have digital displays that "talk" to the user, giving instructions or results. Most have alarms to indicate either that the instrument is malfunctioning or that the assessed value is outside predetermined parameters. These devices, with their tiny but powerful computer chips, make it possible to extend the nurse's observations and provide valid and reliable data (Kozier et al 2000).

Data-Collection Methods

Three methods of collecting data are used in both comprehensive and focus nursing assessments: observation, physical examination, and interview.

Observation

Observation is the conscious, deliberate use of the physical senses to gather data from the patient and the environment. It occurs whenever the nurse is in contact with the client or support persons. Examples of data observed through use of the senses are found in Table 3–6 on page 91. Nursing observations must be systematic so that no significant data are missed. At each patient contact, try to develop a sequence of observation, such as the following:

1. As you enter the room, observe the patient for signs of *distress* (eg, pallor, labored breathing, behaviors indicating pain or emotional distress).
2. Scan for *safety* hazards (eg, Are the side rails up? Are there spills on the floor?)
3. Look at the *equipment* (eg, urinary catheter bag, intravenous [IV] pumps, oxygen, monitors). Is the equipment working? Do any of the alarms or screens indicate a need for immediate attention? Is the IV running? Is the urinary catheter draining?
4. Scan the room. Who is there (*people*) and how do they interact with the patient?
5. Observe the patient more closely for data such as skin temperature, breath sounds, drainage odors, condition of dressings, condition of bed linens, and need for repositioning.

			10/12 08:00	12:00	16:00	20:00	10/13 00:00	04:00	08:00	12:00
NEURO	Behavior		Anxious	Cooperat	Restless	Calm	Sleeping	Anxious	Calm	Cooperat
	Level of Consciousness	Orientation	x3 P-P-T	No Change	No Change	x3 P-P-T	Reorients	x3 P-P-T	x3 P-P-T	No Change
		LOC	Alert	No Change	No Change	Alert		Alert	Alert	No Change
	Mentation		Normal	No Change	No Change	Normal	Normal	Normal	Normal	No Change
	Speech		Clear	No Change	No Change	Clear	Clear	Clear	Clear	No Change
	Movement	RA	Normal	No Change	No Change	Normal	No Change	No Change	Normal	No Change
		LA	Normal	No Change	No Change	Normal	No Change	No Change	Normal	No Change
		RL	Normal	No Change	No Change	Normal	No Change	No Change	Normal	No Change
		LL	Normal	No Change	No Change	Normal	No Change	No Change	Normal	No Change
	Pupil Size(mm)/Reaction	R	5 Brisk	4 Brisk	4 Brisk	4 Brisk	3 Brisk	4 Brisk	5 Brisk	4 Brisk
		L	5 Brisk	4 Brisk	4 Brisk	4 Brisk	3 Brisk	4 Brisk	5 Brisk	4 Brisk
CV	Heart Sounds		Murmur	No Change	No Change	Murmur	No Change	No Change	Murmur	No Change
			Irregular	No Change	No Change	Irregular	No Change	No Change	Regular	No Change
	Edema Assessment	Edema	Dependent	No Change	No Change	Dependent	No Change	Dependent	Dependent	No Change
		Type	2+Pitting			1+Pitting		2+Pitting	1+Pitting	
		Location	BilAnkles			BilAnkles		BilAnkles	BilAnkles	
	Femoral	R	PalpStrng			PalpStrng			PalpStrng	
		L	PalpStrng			PalpStrng			PalpStrng	
	Popliteal	R	PalpWeak			PalpWeak			PalpWeak	
		L	PalpWeak			PalpWeak			PalpWeak	
	Posterior Tibialis	R	PalpWeak	No Change	No Change	PalpWeak	No Change	No Change	PalpWeak	No Change
		L	PalpWeak	No Change	No Change	PalpWeak	No Change	No Change	PalpWeak	No Change
	Dorsalis Pedis	R	PalpWeak	No Change	No Change	PalpWeak	No Change	No Change	PalpWeak	No Change
		L	PalpWeak	No Change	No Change	PalpWeak	No Change	No Change	PalpWeak	No Change
RESP	Breath Sounds	R	Decreased Clear	FineRales	InspWheez ExpWheez	FineRales	FineRales ExpWheez	No Change	Crackles	Crackles ExpWheez
		L	Decreased Clear	FineRales	InspWheez ExpWheez	FineRales	FineRales ExpWheez	No Change	Crackles	Crackles ExpWheez
				R>L					bases	
GI	Abdomen		Rounded NonTender	No Change	No Change	Soft NonTender	No Change	No Change	Rounded NonTender	No Change
	Bowel Sounds	R	Present	No Change	No Change	Present	No Change	No Change	Hypo	Present
		L	Present	No Change	No Change	Present	No Change	No Change	Hypo	Present
			Present	No Change	No Change	Present	No Change	No Change	Hypo	Present
		Flatus	Present			Present			Hypo	Present
GU	Urine	Route	Foley	No Change	Foley	Foley	No Change	Foley	Foley	Foley
		Color	Yellow	No Change	Amber	Yellow	No Change	Amber	Amber	Yellow
		Character	No Change	No Change	Sediment	Sediment	No Change	Cloudy	Cloudy	Sediment
SKIN	Skin Vitals	Color	Pale	No Change	Pale	Pale Pink	No Change	Pale Pink	Pale Pink	No Change
		Temp	Warm	No Change	Cool	Warm	No Change	Cool	Warm	No Change
		Moisture	Dry	No Change	Clammy	Dry	No Change	Dry	Dry	No Change
		Cap Refill	< 3 sec	No Change	< 3 sec	< 3 sec	No Change	< 3 sec	< 3 sec	No Change
		Nailbeds	Pink	No Change	Dusky	Pink	No Change	Pink	Pink	No Change
		Turgor	Elastic	No Change	Elastic	Elastic	No Change	Elastic	Elastic	No Change

Figure 3–4

Computer Screen-portion of Assessment Flowsheet. (*Source:* Courtesy of Shore Memorial Hospital, Somers Point, NJ.)

Physical Examination

The **nursing physical examination** is a systematic assessment of all body systems. It is concerned with identifying strengths and deficits in the client's functional abilities, rather than identifying pathology. Physical examination provides objective data that can be used to validate the subjective data obtained in the interview or to clarify the effect of the patient's disease on her ability to function. Data from the initial physical examination serve as a baseline for comparing the client's later responses to nursing and medical interventions.

One approach is to proceed from *head to toe*. In this case, the head and neck would be examined first, and then the shoulders, chest (including heart and lungs), and back. Another approach is to examine each of the *body systems* in a predetermined order; for example, respiratory, neurologic, cardiovascular, musculoskeletal, and so on. Whatever approach you choose, the examination should follow the same order each time to prevent omission of data.

You will use the techniques of inspection, auscultation, palpation, and percussion when performing a physical examination. Refer to a text on the fundamentals of nursing or physical assessment for in-depth discussion of these techniques and other aspects of the physical examination.

Inspection is done visually, either with the naked eye or with instruments such as an otoscope, which is used in examining the ears. Abdominal distention and skin pallor are examples of data found on inspection.

Auscultation uses the nurse's hearing. Using *direct* auscultation with the unaided ear the nurse can hear sounds such as the client's coughing. A stethoscope is used for *indirect* auscultation to amplify the sounds made within the client's body, such as crackles and wheezes in the lungs.

Percussion is the striking of a body surface, usually with the tip of the finger, to elicit sound or vibration. Different sounds are produced, depending on whether the finger strikes over a solid, fluid-filled, or air-filled area. It is useful, for instance, in determining whether a patient's abdomen is distended with air or fluid.

Palpation uses the sense of touch. The finger pads are usually used because they are the most sensitive to tactile stimulation. The nurse uses palpation, for example, to check for bladder distention and to obtain the patient's pulse rate and strength.

Interview

A **nursing interview** is purposeful, structured communication in which the nurse questions a patient to obtain subjective data. An admission interview is formal and planned. During ongoing assessment, interviews may be informal, brief, narrowly focused interactions between nurse and patient, but they are still purposeful, structured communication.

KEY POINT

Examination Examples

- Taking a patient's pulse
- Weighing a patient
- Listening to heart sounds
- Palpating the abdomen
- Auscultating bowel sounds

Table 3–6 Examples of Observation Data

Sense	Examples of Data Obtained
Touch	Pulse rate and rhythm; lesions (eg, masses, nodules); firmness of uterine fundus in postpartum woman; skin temperature
Vision	General appearance (eg, estimate of height and weight, posture, grooming), skin color, facial expression, body movements, personal articles in room (eg, religious books, icons, beads, family pictures), equipment (eg, intravenous pump, electrocardiogram monitor)
Smell	Body, breath, or urine odors; wound secretions
Hearing	Blood pressure, breath sounds, bowel sounds, heart sounds, spoken words (eg, to indicate thoughts, feelings, ability to communicate, and orientation)

Purpose of the Interview   During the initial assessment, the main purpose of the interview is to obtain subjective data for the nursing history. The **nursing history** contains data about the effects of the illness on the patient's daily functioning and ability to cope. It considers the whole person, including data about all the patient's basic needs, not just the biological ones. The specific content of a nursing history varies in different settings, but usually includes the general content areas shown in Box 3–3, on page 93.

At the time of the initial interview, the nurse usually also orients the patient to the room and provides some information about the hospital stay (eg, how to call for help, where to put belongings). Although the focus is on obtaining data, the nurse should provide enough teaching and counseling to relieve some of the patient's anxieties. This is important because impressions gained in the initial interview form the basis for the beginning of the nurse-patient relationship.

Preparing for the Interview   As a rule, you should begin by reviewing the chart, so you will know who the patient is and what you want to accomplish. This will prevent you from covering topics already assessed by someone else, which can be tiring and annoying for patients. Be careful, though, not to form preconceived ideas about the client. Failure to approach the client with an open mind can cause you to miss some data. After forming goals for the interview, think of some initial leading questions. Schedule a time when you will be free from interruptions—not too close to mealtime, treatment time, or visiting hours. Provide privacy, wait until visitors are gone, or ask them to leave the room. Be sure the patient is comfortable: ask if he is thirsty or needs to use the bathroom. Consider the patient's emotional state as well. If he is very anxious or frightened, you may need to relieve his anxiety before proceeding with the interview.

Types of Interviews   There are two basic types of interview: directive and nondirective. A **directive interview** is highly structured. The nurse controls the subject matter and asks questions in order to obtain specific information. This is an efficient way to obtain factual, easily categorized information, such as age, sex, and analysis of symptoms.

During a **nondirective interview** the nurse allows the patient to control the purpose, subject matter, and pacing. The nurse clarifies, summarizes, and uses open-ended questions and comments to encourage communication. Nondirective interviewing is time-consuming and can result in a great deal of irrelevant data; however, it is useful in helping a patient to express feelings, promoting communication, and building rapport.

Kinds of Interview Questions   Questions are classified as closed or open-ended (see Table 3–7 for examples). **Open-ended questions**, associated with the nondirective interview, invite patients to discover and explore (elaborate, clarify, or illustrate) their thoughts and feelings. An open-ended question may specify the topic of discussion, but it is broad and requires elaboration from the patient.

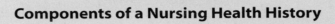
BOX 3-3

Components of a Nursing Health History

Component	Example or Explanation
Biographical information	Age, sex, marital status
Chief complaint or reason for visit	Specifically, what initiated the patient to seek help (eg, chest pain, weight loss, check-up)
History of present illness	Includes usual health status, chronology of the illness, and effect of the illness on the client's daily life
Past health status	Previous hospitalizations or surgeries, childhood diseases
Review of systems and their effect on client's functioning	Subjective data regarding body systems such as respiratory system (cough, shortness of breath, etc). Difficulties with activities such as dressing, grooming, eating, and elimination
Social and family history	Family relationships, friendships; ethnic affiliation; occupational history; economic status; home and neighborhood conditions; exposure to toxic materials
Lifestyle, including usual habits and patterns of daily living	Personal habits such as alcohol and tobacco use; usual diet; sleep/rest patterns; exercise
Spiritual well-being	Client's source of strength or hope
Psychological data	Major stressors; usual coping pattern; available supports; communication style; self-concept
Client's perception of health status and illness	Does the client realize the implications of the illness (eg, does he think his arthritis can be cured)?
Client's expectations of caregivers	What the client thinks will be done for him. What he wants the nurses to do to help

Table 3–7. Closed and Open-Ended Questions

Closed Questions	Open-Ended Questions
When was the accident?	Tell me about your accident.
Are you in pain?	Describe your pain to me.
Was this a planned pregnancy?	What were your thoughts/feelings when you found out you were pregnant?

Closed questions, used in the directive interview, generally require only "yes," "no," or short factual answers giving specific information. Thus the amount of information gained is limited. Closed questions often begin with "when," "where," "who," "what," "do (did, does)," "is (are, was)" and sometimes "how." Closed questions are especially effective in emergency situations or when a patient is highly stressed, anxious, or has difficulty communicating.

The nursing interview requires a combination of directive and nondirective techniques. Use closed questioning to obtain the more specific information on the nursing history (eg, biographical information, previous surgeries, childhood diseases). Then use broad statements to guide the patient to talk about other topics, such as sleep patterns, pain, and usual routines; finally, follow up or clarify those responses with specific, closed questions.

EXAMPLE:

(Closed question)	*Nurse:*	How many times have you been pregnant?
	Patient:	Four.
(Closed question)	*Nurse:*	Were there any problems with your other deliveries?
	Patient:	Yes, with my last one.
(Open-ended question, directing topic)	*Nurse:*	What happened?
	Patient:	I was in labor a long time, and then something happened to the baby's heart rate. They did an emergency cesarean section.
(Open-ended question)	*Nurse:*	What plans have you made for this delivery?

The last, broad question elicits information about a topic of the nurse's choice. A more directive, closed question along the same lines would be, "Do you plan to have a cesarean birth again this time?" If the nurse wanted to explore the patient's feelings, she might have said, "What are your concerns for *this* delivery?"

Table 3–8 on pages 96–97, lists some common interviewing problems, along with some suggestions for handling them. Along with Box 3–4 on pages 98–99, these suggestions should help you improve the quality of your interviews.

Active Listening   When first learning to interview, students tend to focus on what questions to ask and how to phrase them. However, the most important communication strategy is active listening. Most people think they are listening, but often they are focusing on preparing a response to what they are hearing, rather than trying to understand what they are hearing. Active, empathic listening is done with ears, eyes, and heart (Straka 1997). It means being attentive to the patient's verbal and nonverbal messages, listening for feelings, and conveying acceptance, respect, and trust. The following acronym will help you to remember behaviors of active listening (Townsend 1996):

S   Sit or stand facing the patient to indicate that you are interested in what he is saying.
O   Open posture: arms and legs uncrossed.
L   Lean forward toward the patient.
E   Establish and maintain eye contact.
R   Relax to convey a sense of connection with the patient. (p. 104)

---

1. Observe a conversation between peers or family members. What nonverbal behaviors did you see? Did the speakers (a) put words in each other's mouth? (b) interrupt? (c) make value judgments or give advice?
2. Recall a recent conversation between a nurse and a patient. Did the nurse do a, b, or c? Did the nurse make eye contact? Use silence as a technique?

???
THINKING POINT

Interviewing Older Adults   Interview techniques in this chapter focus on patients with normal cognitive and communication abilities. However, some patients, such as the elderly, require special communication techniques. Older adults make up an ever-growing proportion of the US population, and most nurses will care for at least some of these patients. In addition to the general interview guidelines in Box 3–4, consider the following when interviewing older adults:

1. *Proceed slowly.* Speak slowly and clearly, giving the client plenty of time to form an answer.
2. *Check for sensory deficits at the beginning of the interview.* Don't wait until you come to that area of the assessment form. Until you have checked the patient's hearing, look at him as you speak, to allow for lip reading.
3. *Don't assume all elderly people are deaf or unable to understand your meaning.* The fact that you need to speak slowly does not mean that you need to speak loudly.

Table 3–8 Common Interviewing Problems

Source of Problem	Explanation	Suggested Nursing Actions
Interviewer's own discomfort	■ You may feel you are imposing on the patient, perhaps because you do not clearly know how the information will be used. (Especially true for students.) ■ You may feel uncomfortable asking personal questions of a stranger.	■ Do your "homework." Be sure you understand the purpose of the interview; explain it to the patient during the introduction phase. ■ Remember that nurses are concerned with the whole person and that data are needed in order to give comprehensive care. Early in the interview, tell the patient to respond only as he feels comfortable. Remember that patients can choose what they wish to tell you, so they have some power to preserve their own privacy. Remind yourself that patients are usually at ease if you are at ease. Also, it may be that the patient has felt the need to talk about the subject, did not know how to bring it up, and is relieved that you have done so.
	■ Knowing that patients may respond to some questions with tears or anger, you may be afraid to ask such questions.	■ It may be hard to accept another's expressions of feelings, but it is important that you learn to do so. Avoiding potentially upsetting topics can leave large gaps in the database. Remember that the patient usually feels better after expressing emotions—even though you may be uncomfortable.
Interviewer's curiosity	■ There is a fine line between interest and curiosity. Patients appreciate interest, but resent curiosity. This may cause them to be less inclined to talk to you.	■ Don't become too emeshed in the details of the patient's story. Focus on getting the information you need for planning care.
Patient's family and visitors inhibit responses	■ The client may be embarrassed to discuss personal information in front of others, or it may be information clients do not wish others to know (eg, a wife may not want her husband to know that she was treated for a sexually transmitted disease before they were married).	■ Unless the visitor is an important source of information (eg, when the patient is a small child), ask the visitor to step out for a few minutes or postpone the interview until the visitor leaves.

(continues)

Table 3–8   Common Interviewing Problems *(continued)*

Source of Problem	Explanation	Suggested Nursing Actions
Patient's family and visitors inhibit responses *(Cont'd)*	■ Spouses often answer the questions you address to patients.	■ Thank the spouse for the information, but remind him or her that it is important for you to get the information from the patient's perspective.
Nurse is not culturally sensitive	■ There are cultural variations in communication (eg, in some cultures social courtesies must be established before personal topics are discussed).	■ Be aware of differences in the meaning of phenomena such as touch, facial expressiveness, use of silence, and need for physical space. For example: ■ In some cultures, strangers do not make direct eye contact. ■ As a rule, men of all cultures require more space than women.

4. *Be aware that appropriate affect and articulate speech do not always go together*. Likewise, inappropriate affect and incoherent speech do not necessarily indicate lack of understanding. A patient may speak coherently and make sense as she tells you about her loss of appetite, and then begin crying for no apparent reason. Nevertheless, the information about her appetite may be credible. Another patient may laugh appropriately at something funny, and yet be unable to speak clearly or find the words to express what he means.

5. *Rely more than usual on body language*. Be aware of nonverbal communication, such as quivering of the lips, tears in the eyes, or movements of the hands and feet. As noted above, some older patients have difficulty finding the words to express their ideas and feelings.

6. *Be alert for intermittent confusion*. Some older clients are confused at one time and not another. A client may be giving you credible information and then, as the interview progresses, begin to lose track of the topic or introduce irrelevant material. When the patient seems confused, use focus assessment to determine his mental status. If you conclude that his answers are unreliable, you can finish the interview later when he is no longer confused.

7. *When possible try to get data directly from the client*. Some clients are reluctant to answer questions. Also, families are sometimes very protective of clients, and tend to answer for them. Explain to them that it is important for you to hear what the client has to say.

These suggestions apply in some degree to people of all ages, but they are especially important in meeting the challenges that occur when the aging process is superimposed on a disease process.

BOX 3–4

Guide for Interviewing

1. **Prepare for the interview**
   - **Read the chart.** Think of some initial questions.
   - **Provide privacy.** Ask visitors to leave; pull the bed curtain.
   - **Don't rush.** Schedule a block of time for the interview.
   - **Reduce distractions** (eg, turn off the television).
   - **Make the client comfortable** (eg, offer bedpan, drink of water).
2. **Set the stage**
   - **Call the patient by name.** Ask what name the patient prefers you to use.
   - **Introduce yourself**, including your position and the purpose of the interview.
   - **SOLER** (see page 95)
   - **Set a time limit** at the beginning of the interview.
3. **Obtain the data**
   - **Start with the client's main complaint** ("Why are you here?").
   - **Ask about non-threatening subjects and symptoms.** Introduce personal or threatening material later in the interview when you are both more at ease.
   - **Don't mechanically "fill out the form."** Follow patient leads for expanding on or introducing a new topic.
4. **Use good communication techniques**
   - **Say "I," not "we"** ("We need some information from you"). "We" indicates lack of personal involvement and creates psychological distance between you and the patient.
   - **Don't use endearing names**, such as "grandma, dear, sweetie." Many people feel belittled by this.
   - **Use language the patient can understand.** Many patients do not know the meaning of "void" or "vital signs." Check the patient's understanding of a word by saying, for example, "Explain what happens when you have *diarrhea*."
   - **Don't "talk down" to the patient** (eg, "I need to feel your tummy.")
   - **Don't ask too many questions**—you may seem curious rather than concerned. Instead, use neutral statements and reflection to obtain information (eg, instead of, "Where do you work?" say, "Tell me about your job.")
   - **Use an appropriate balance of closed and open-ended questions**.
   - **Avoid asking "why" questions** (eg, "Why have you been unable to stop smoking?"). For many people, "why" connotes disapproval and may provoke a defensive response.

BOX 3-4

Guide for Interviewing (*continued*)

- **Don't put words in the patient's mouth**. Avoid leading questions such as, "Are you worried about your surgery tomorrow?"
- **Don't give advice**.
- **Encourage the patient to continue** by nodding or saying, "Um-hm," "Yes. . .," or "Go on."
- **Don't interrupt**. If the patient is rambling, allow him to finish a sentence and then try to redirect the conversation by saying something like, "You hadn't finished telling me about. . . ."
- **Use and accept silence**. Give the patient time to search for and organize thoughts.
- **Validate your understanding** of the content and feeling of the patient's message. Summarize the meaning of what you have heard and ask for feedback (eg, "Did I understand you to say. . ." or "I hear you saying. . . Do I have it right?").

Cognitive Deficits   In addition to the normal changes of aging, many older people have mild to severe problems with memory and at least one other ability (eg, judgment, thinking, language, or coordination). This is referred to as **dementia**. Nearly 50% of people older than age 85 are affected by Alzheimer's disease, a type of dementia. People with dementia have difficulty speaking and comprehending. Consult gerontology journals and texts for help in communicating with patients affected by dementia, because the techniques vary from those discussed in this chapter. The following are a few examples of such variations (Zimmerman, 1998):

- Repeat the words *exactly* if the patient does not respond to your comment or question. Usually when someone does not understand, you would try a new word, hoping it will be in their vocabulary. For patients with dementia, giving new information only adds to their confusion.
- Use simple, short sentences containing a single item or thought. Ask, "Where does it hurt?", not "What does it feel like and when did it start?"
- Do not use vague comments such as "Um-hmm" and "I see" to show attentive listening; the patient will not be able to interpret them. Echo the patient's comment and bluntly state your response: "You are thirsty. I will bring you a drink."
- Understand that the patient's reality is confused and he cannot behave differently. This is easy to forget, because when the patient is smiling and conversing superficially, he may seem competent.

■ VALIDATING THE DATA

Validation is the act of "double-checking" or verifying data. Critical thinkers validate data in order to:

- Ensure that assessment information is complete, accurate, and factual
- Eliminate their own errors, biases, and misperceptions of the data
- Avoid jumping to faulty conclusions about the data

To collect data accurately, you must be aware of your own biases, values, and beliefs, and be able to separate fact from interpretation and assumption. The unthinking acceptance of assumptions is called **premature closure**. For example, a nurse seeing a man holding his arm to his chest might assume that he is experiencing chest pain, when in fact he has a painful hand. To avoid premature closure the nurse should ask the man why he is holding his arm to his chest. His response may validate the nurse's assumption (of chest pain) or prompt further questioning. Not all data require validation though. For example, data such as height, weight, birth date, and most laboratory studies can be accepted as factual. As a rule, you should validate data when:

1. *Subjective and objective data (or interview and physical examination data) do not agree.*

    EXAMPLE: Ms. Dolan states she has never had high blood pressure. However, the nurse obtains a reading of 190/100 mm Hg.

2. *The client's statements differ at different times in the assessment.*

    EXAMPLE: A labor patient initially stated that this was her first pregnancy. Later, when the nurse asked about prior hospitalizations, she said, "Once, in 1994, to have my appendix removed; and in 1998 when I had a miscarriage." The nurse realized that a miscarriage is counted as a pregnancy, making this the patient's second pregnancy.

CRITICAL THINKING QUESTIONS: JARGON

Imagine you are a patient, and the nurse says to you: "Lab will be here STAT to do a stick for gases, lytes, and enzymes. Then you'll go down for a CAT scan and an ECG. Meanwhile, I need to take your vitals. Also, do you take any OTC meds?"

- ❏ Would you understand what the nurse means?
- ❏ How would patients feel about these statements?
- ❏ Which terms are jargon that should be clarified?

3. *The data seem extremely abnormal.*

EXAMPLE: The client has a resting pulse of 50 bpm and a blood pressure of 190/100 mm Hg.

4. *Factors are present that interfere with accurate measurement.*

EXAMPLE: A crying infant will have a higher than normal respiratory rate and should be quieted in order for assessment data to be correct.

Table 3–9 contains suggestions for ways to validate data:

■ ORGANIZING DATA

ANA Standard I and CNA Standard II require that data collection be systematic (see Box 3–2 on page 78). This means that in addition to collecting and validating data, nurses organize related cues into predetermined categories.

Table 3–9   Suggestions for Validating Data

Nursing Activities	Examples
Clarify vague or ambiguous statements by asking the patient more questions.	*Client*: "My son has been acting strange this week." *Nurse*: "What, exactly, did your son do when he started 'acting strange'?"
Always compare subjective and objective data to verify the patient's statements with your observations.	■ Compare pain behaviors to the patient's statements about the pain. ■ Take the patient's temperature when he complains of "feeling hot."
Recheck your measurement to be sure it is accurate.	Take the blood pressure a second time in the opposite arm.
Ensure that your measuring device is working correctly or use a different piece of equipment.	■ Calibrate the glucose monitor. ■ Take the patient's temperature with two different thermometers. ■ Palpate the pulse rate and compare with electronic monitor reading.
Ask someone else to verify your findings.	Ask a more experienced nurse to listen to the patient's lungs. Ask a nursing assistant to retake the blood pressure.
Use references (eg, journals, the Internet, textbooks) to explain findings.	When the nurse discovered tiny purple swollen areas under an elderly client's tongue, she considered it abnormal. When she consulted a text about physical changes of aging, she discovered that such varicosities are common among the elderly.

Most healthcare agencies have standardized forms for the comprehensive nursing assessment (eg, Figure 3–2). Such forms help to assure that no data are missed. They are also efficient, enabling you to organize data at the same time you collect and record it. For ongoing and focus assessment, you will not always have a data-collection form, so you will need to organize (cluster) the data *after* you collect it. Chapter 4 explains data clustering more fully. The content of assessment forms (tools) is determined by:

1. the requirements of government agencies (eg, Medicare), insurance companies, and accrediting agencies, such as the Community Health Accreditation Program (CHAP).
2. the type of patients seen on the unit or the agency (eg, nurses working in a hospital maternity unit need different information about their patients than do nurses working in a long-term care facility).

Regardless of the content of the form, the agency determines the framework that will be used to organize the information. A **framework** is, very simply, a way of looking at something.

EXAMPLE: A patient is trembling. A nurse using a psychological framework might conclude the patient is frightened; a nurse using a biological framework might conclude that the patient is cold.

Some frameworks focus on body systems, some on human needs, adaptive responses, self-care abilities, and so on. A framework indicates which data are significant and guides the nurse in selecting which patient characteristics to observe. A framework groups related data, helping the nurse to find the patterns necessary for identifying client strengths, problems, and risk factors.

Nursing Models

A **nursing model (theoretical framework)** is a set of interrelated concepts that represents a particular way of thinking about nursing, clients, health, and the environment. Such models are also called *theories, frameworks,* or *conceptual frameworks.* Those terms differ in meaning, depending on the extent to which the set of concepts has been used and tested in practice, and on the level of detail and organization of the concepts. For the purposes of this chapter, you do not need to know whether a theorist's ideas are a framework, a model, or a theory. Any level of organized concepts can be used to guide data collection.

A nursing model tells you what to assess and why. The major concepts of the framework provide the categories for collecting and organizing data. Whereas a medical, or body systems, model provides data that are useful for medical diagnoses and treatments, a nursing model will produce data that are useful in planning nursing care. The following are some examples:

Gordon's Functional Health Patterns Framework directs nurses to collect data about common patterns of behavior that contribute to health, quality of life, and achievement of human potential (Gordon 1994, p. 69). Using this framework, you would note emerging patterns and determine whether the client's functioning in each of the patterns is functional or dysfunctional (see Table 3–10, on pp. 104–105, and Appendix B).

Orem's Self-Care Model focuses on the patient's abilities to perform self-care to maintain life, health, and well being. Using this framework, you would identify self-care deficits that require nursing intervention (Orem 1991) (see Table 3–11 on page 105).

Roy's Adaptation Model describes patients as biopsychosocial beings, constantly adapting to external and internal demands. Using this model, you would note patterns indicating the client's inability to adapt in one of four modes: physiological, self-concept, social role, and interdependence (see Table 3–12 on page 106).

The North American Nursing Diagnosis Association's Taxonomy II adopted at NANDA's 14th biennial conference (2000) provides a framework for assessing and diagnosing. Strictly speaking, though, it is not a nursing theory. It classifies data and nursing diagnoses into 13 domains. See Table 3–13 on pp. 107–108.

Nonnursing Models

Frameworks from other disciplines may also be helpful for clustering data. **Maslow's Hierarchy of Needs** organizes data according to basic human needs that are common to all people. This model theorizes that a person's basic needs (eg, physiological) must be met before their higher needs (eg, self-esteem). See Table 3–14, on page 109, for examples.

A **body systems (medical) model** is useful for identifying data that may indicate a medical problem. Most assessment forms have at least a section that is organized by body systems (see Box 3–5 on p. 109). A form that combines body systems with other models (eg, Maslow's Hierarchy of Needs or a nursing model) provides a holistic approach that enables the nurse to identify both medical and nursing problems.

No matter which model you use, it is important to use it consistently in order to become familiar with it. Even if you do not use a form to collect data, you will still classify related cues according to your framework. Remember that a framework gives you a special way to view the patient, helps you to make thorough, systematic assessments, and makes the data more meaningful.

Does your school provide a nursing assessment form for you to use in clinical? What model(s) does it use to organize data? What are the major categories? How is it different from the forms used by the nurses on your clinical unit?

???

THINKING POINT

Table 3–10   Using Gordon's 11 Functional Health Patterns to Organize Data

Functional Health Pattern	Describes	Examples
Health Perception/ Health Management	Client's perception of health and well-being and how health is managed.	Compliance with medication regimen; use of health-promotion activities, such as regular exercise, annual check-ups.
Nutritional/ Metabolic	Pattern of food and fluid intake relative to metabolic need indicators of local nutrient supply.	Condition of skin, teeth, hair, nails, mucous membranes; height and weight, fluid and electrolyte balance.
Elimination	Patterns of excretory function (bowel, bladder, and skin); includes client's perception of "normal" function.	Frequency of bowel movements, voiding pattern, pain on urination, appearance of urine and stool.
Activity/Exercise	Patterns of exercise, activity, leisure, and recreation.	Exercise, hobbies; may include cardiovascular and respiratory status, mobility, and activities of daily living.
Cognitive/ Perceptual	Sensory-perceptual and cognitive patterns.	Vision, hearing, taste, touch, smell, pain perception and management; cognitive functions such as language, memory, and decision making.
Sleep/Rest	Patterns of sleep, rest, and relaxation.	Client's perception of quality and quantity of sleep and energy, use of sleep aids, routines client uses.
Self-Perception/ Self-Concept	Client's self-concept pattern and perceptions of self, emotional patterns.	Body comfort, body image, feeling state, attitudes about self, perception of abilities, objective data such as body posture, eye contact, voice tone.
Role/Relationship	Client's pattern of role engagements and relationships.	Perception of current major roles and responsibilities (eg, father, husband, salesman); satisfaction with family, work, or social relationships.

(continues)

**Table 3–10   Using Gordon's 11 Functional Health Patterns
to Organize Data** *(continued)*

Functional Health Pattern	Describes	Examples
Sexual/ Reproductive	Patterns of satisfaction and dissatisfaction with sexuality; reproductive pattern and stage.	Histories of pregnancy and childbirth; difficulties with sexual functioning; satisfaction with sexual relationship.
Coping/Stress Tolerance	General coping pattern and effectiveness of the pattern in terms of stress tolerance.	Client's usual manner of handling stress, available support systems, perceived ability to control or manage situations.
Value-Belief	Patterns of values, beliefs (including spiritual), and goals that guide client's choices or decisions.	Religious affiliation, what client perceives as important in life, value/belief conflicts related to health, special religious practices.

Source: Adapted with permission from Gordon (1994). *Nursing diagnosis: Process and application*. 3rd ed. St. Louis: CV Mosby, p. 70.

■ RECORDING DATA

ANA Standard I (see Box 3–2 on page 78) requires that assessment data be accessible, communicated, and *recorded*. The nursing database becomes a part of the client's permanent record. Therefore, you should record the assessment in ink on the form provided by the agency, on the same day the

Table 3–11   Using Orem's Self-Care Model to Organize Data

Group data into the following categories of "universal self-care requisites."

1. The maintenance of a sufficient intake of air
2. The maintenance of a sufficient intake of water
3. The maintenance of a sufficient intake of food
4. The provision of care associated with elimination processes and excrements
5. The maintenance of a balance between activity and rest
6. The maintenance of a balance between time alone and time with others
7. The prevention of hazards to human life, human functioning, and human well-being
8. The promotion of human functioning and development within social groups in accord with human potential, known human limitations, and human desire to be normal (as determined by science, culture, and social values).

Source: Adapted from Orem (1991) *Nursing: Concepts of practice*. 4th ed. St. Louis: Mosby-Year Book, p. 126.

Table 3–12   Using Roy's Adaptation Model to Organize Data

Categories (Adaptive Modes)	Explanation
Physiological needs Activity and rest Nutrition Elimination Fluid and electrolytes Oxygenation Protection Regulation: temperature Regulation: the senses Regulation: endocrine system	Balance must be maintained in each of the sub-categories.
Self-concept Physical Self Personal Self	Adaptation means developing a positive self-concept, including the physical self, moral-ethical self, and self-ideal. Includes self-esteem and psychological integrity.
Role Function	Ability to function in various roles, such as parent, spouse, worker, and so on.
Interdependence	Achieving balance between dependence and in-dependence.

Source: Roy and Andrews (1991) *The Roy adaptation model: The definitive statement*. Norwalk, CT: Appleton & Lange, pp. 15–17.

client is admitted. Write neatly and legibly, using only the abbreviations approved by the agency. Do not try to write everything the client says word for word, because this is likely to interfere with the communication between you and the client.

Record subjective data in the client's own words when possible, using quotation marks. Alternatively, you may paraphrase or summarize what the client says and omit the quotation marks. Be sure to record the data, not what you think they mean. Record **cues** (what the client tells you and what you see, hear, feel, smell, and measure) not **inferences** (your judgment or interpretation of what the cues mean). Table 3–15 on page 110 compares cues with conclusions (inferences).

Avoid vague generalities such as *good, normal, adequate,* or *tolerated well.* These words mean different things to different people. Suppose a nurse writes, "Vision adequate." Does this mean the client can read newsprint without eyeglasses? Or when she is wearing glasses? Or that she can see well enough to ambulate without assistance? It would be better to record "Able to read newsprint at 24 in. while wearing glasses."

Table 3-13   Using NANDA Taxonomy II to Organize Data

Domains	Definitions	Classes
Domain 1. **Health Promotion**	The awareness of wellbeing or normality of function and the strategies used to maintain control of and enhance that wellbeing or normality of function	1. Health awareness 2. Health management
Domain 2. **Nutrition**	The activities of taking in, assimilating, and using nutrients for the purposes of tissue maintenance, tissue repair, and the production of energy to support life processes for absorption and assimilation	1. Ingestion 2. Digestion 3. Absorption 4. Metabolism 5. Hydration
Domain 3. **Elimination**	Secretion and excretion of waste products from the body	1. Urinary 2. Bowel 3. Skin 4. Lung
Domain 4. **Activity/Rest**	The production, conservation, expenditure, or balance of energy resources	1. Sleep/rest 2. Activity-Exercise 3. Energy balance 4. Cardiovascular/ Pulmonary responses
Domain 5. **Perception/ Cognition**	The human information processing system including attention, orientation, sensation, perception, cognition, and communication	1. Attention 2. Orientation 3. Sensation/Perception 4. Cognition 5. Communication
Domain 6. **Self-Perception**	Awareness about self	1. Self-Concept 2. Self-Esteem 3. Body image
Domain 7. **Role Relationships**	The positive and negative or associations between persons or groups of persons and the means by which those connections are demonstrated	1. Caregiving roles 2. Family relationships 3. Role performance
Domain 8. **Sexuality**	Sexual identity, sexual function, and reproduction	1. Sexual identity 2. Sexual function 3. Reproduction
Domain 9. **Coping/Stress Tolerance**	Contending with life events/life processes	1. Post-Trauma responses 2. Coping 3. Neurobehavioral stress

(continues)

Table 3–13   Using NANDA Taxonomy II to Organize Data *(continued)*

Domains	Definitions	Classes
Domain 10. **Life Principles**	Beliefs and values underlying conduct, thought and behavior about acts, customs, or institutions viewed as being true or having intrinsic worth	1. Values 2. Beliefs 3. Values/Belief congruence
Domain 11. **Safety/ Protection**	Freedom from danger, physical injury or immune system damage, preservation from loss, and protection of safety and security	1. Infection 2. Physical injury 3. Violence 4. Environmental hazards 5. Immune response 6. Thermoregulation
Domain 12. **Comfort**	Sense of mental, physical, or social well being or ease	1. Physical comfort 2. Environmental comfort 3. Social comfort
Domain 13. **Growth/ Development**	Age appropriate increases in physical dimensions, organ systems, and/or attainment of developmental milestones	1. Growth 2. Development
Domain 14. **Other**	This category is for diagnoses that do not fit in any of the other domains.	

Source: Adapted from materials handed out at the 14th Biennial Conference on Nursing Diagnosis, North American Nursing Diagnosis Association, April 5–8, 2000, Orlando, FL.

???

THINKING POINT

Scenario: You are making a focus assessment for Sleep Pattern Disturbance. Your patient says, "Well, of course, I'm tired! I didn't sleep a bit last night. My roommate snores like a freight train, and the night nurse was in here making noise all night long. If she'd get organized, she wouldn't have to disturb us so much." (1) In this case, what do you think of your text's directions to "record subjective data in the client's own words"? (2) What would you write when recording these data? Why?

■ SPECIAL PURPOSE ASSESSMENTS

You may wish to perform an in-depth assessment of certain areas of a client's functioning. Most agencies have developed forms for special assessments. For example, you may gather in-depth data about a client's nutritional status, using a form provided by your school. Or you may use a special form to

Table 3–14 Using Maslow's Basic Human Needs to Organize Data

Data Categories (Needs)	Examples of Data
Physiological (Basic survival needs)	Oxygen, nutrition, fluids, body temperature regulation, warmth, elimination, shelter, sex
Safety and Security (Need to be safe and comfortable)	Physical safety (infection, falls, drug side effects); psychological security (knowledge of procedures, bedtime rituals, usual routines, fear of isolation dependence needs); pain
Love and Belonging (Need for love and affection)	Information about family and significant others, social supports
Esteem and Self-Esteem (Need to feel good about self)	Changes in body image (eg, puberty, surgery); changes in self-concept (eg, ability to perform usual role in family); pride in capabilities
Self-Actualization (Need to achieve one's maximum potential; need for growth and change)	Extent to which goals are being achieved, autonomy, motivation, problem-solving abilities, ability to give and accept help, feelings about accomplishments, roles

Source: Adapted from Maslow (1970) *Motivation and Personality*. 2nd ed. New York: Harper & Row.

monitor the level of consciousness, pupil reaction, and limb movement of a comatose patient. This section discusses functional, home health, cultural, spiritual, wellness, family, and community assessments.

Home Care and Functional Assessment

Reimbursement and accrediting agencies mandate patient education and discharge planning to aid patients in the transition from acute care to self-care. Data about the patient's knowledge and self-care abilities enable the nurse to

---

BOX 3–5

Body Systems Model

Integumentary	Musculoskeletal
Respiratory	Gastrointestinal
Cardiovascular	Genitourinary
Nervous	Reproductive
Endocrine	Immune

Table 3–15   Comparison of Data and Conclusions (Cues and Inferences)

| Cues (Data) | | Inferences (Conclusions) |
Subjective	Objective	
"My back really hurts." (Paraphrase: Patient states his back hurts.)	Lying rigidly in bed. Facial grimacing observed.	Patient is in pain.
"My armband to too tight and my arm is really sore." (Paraphrase: Patient says his armband is too tight and his arm is sore.)	Left arm is hot, red, and swollen in a 4" × 4" area around IV insertion site.	Left arm is infected at IV site.
"I'm not sure I should have this surgery. It might not even help, and it is very dangerous. I guess I'm scared."	Tearful. Facial muscles tense. Pulse rate 100 bpm. Hands trembling.	Patient is afraid of having surgery.

Remember: You should record cues, not inferences.

develop an individualized teaching plan. However, nurses have less time than ever to focus on the patient as an individual. One way to overcome this obstacle is to have the patient complete a self-assessment checklist. One such tool assesses patients' self-care abilities. For each of the following abilities, patients check responses to indicate what information they have, their perceptions and feelings about it, and what they actually do (Johannsen 1992).

- Seeking and securing medical assistance
- Understanding and attending to the effects of illness
- Effectively carrying out the therapeutic regimen
- Regulating discomfort/harmful effects of the regimen
- Living with the illness in a style conducive to health
- Modifying self-concept

Accreditation and managed care companies also require outcomes data from home care agencies. For example, Medicare is piloting the Outcomes Assessment Information System (OASIS). Box 3–6 provides examples of the data included in a comprehensive home health care assessment (ie, environment, family, psychosocial, education, physiologic, functional). Functional assessment data are important because they are part of the OASIS data and because they help the nurse determine a client's rehabilitative prognosis. Three functional assessment tools—PULSES, the Barthel Index, and the Functional Independence Measure—are summarized in Table 3–16 on p. 112. These tools measure only "basic" activities of daily living. They

BOX 3–6

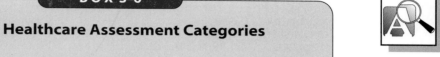

Home Healthcare Assessment Categories

Category	Examples of Data
Environment	Appearance of house, location of bathroom, location of cooking area, water source, type of bed and couch, pets
Family	Significant other/spouse, number of children, flexibility of family roles (eg, child care, cooking), availability of day care, stress reactions of family unit, able to verbalize appropriate coping mechanisms
Psychosocial	Social groups (eg, exercise group), church groups, level of education/ability to understand, anxiety associated with condition, availability of neighbors
Education Needed	Use of any medical equipment (eg, IVs), treatments (eg, special exercises, dressing changes, medications), limitations (eg, avoid lifting), signs and symptoms of complications of disease, safety in the home
Physiologic	Depends on the purpose of the home visit. For example, it might be a prenatal assessment, an assessment of wound healing, or a nutritional assessment for an elderly person
Functional (Self-Care)	Activities of daily living (eg, bathing, dressing, hygiene) and instrumental activities of daily living (eg, cooking, cleaning, shopping)

Source: Adapted from Kodakek, M., and M. Boland (1998). Assessing the high-risk pregnant woman at home. *Home Healthcare Nurse* 16(3):162.

do not measure "instrumental" activities of daily living, such as cooking, driving, and shopping. Therefore, a high score indicates that a patient should not require attendant care, but not necessarily that the patient can live alone (Neal 1998).

Cultural Assessment

Because nurses are expected to provide individualized care, they must understand how clients' cultural beliefs and practices can affect their health and

Table 3–16 Functional (Self-Care) Assessment Tools

Instrument	Description	Categories Assessed
PULSES (Moskowitz and McCann 1957)	Expands functional assessment to include the client's physical condition and support system. The patient is scored 1 to 4 on each item, with 1 representing independence.	**P**hysical condition **U**pper limb functions **L**ower limb functions **S**ensory components **E**xcretory functions **S**upport factors
Barthel Index (Mahoney and Barthel 1965)	Assesses independence with basic activities of daily living (ADL). The patient is scored "independent" or "with help" on each category.	Feeding Moving from wheelchair to bed and return Performing personal toilet (eg, wash face, shave) Getting on and off toilet Bathing Walking on level surface Propelling wheelchair Going up and down stairs Dressing and undressing Bowel continence Bladder control
Functional Independence Measure	Measures basic ADL in a bit more detail than the Barthel Index and has been used primarily with children (Neal 1998).	Self-care Sphincter control Mobility Locomotion Communication Social cognition (eg, problem solving)

illness (ANA, 1991a, p. 1). **Cultural sensitivity** begins in the first phase of the nursing process, when the nurse obtains culturally specific information for the client health history. **Cultural competence** requires knowledge of the values, beliefs, and practices of various cultures, along with an attitude of awareness, openness, and sensitivity. Figure 3–5, on page 113, is a heritage assessment that analyzes the degree to which a person identifies with the dominant culture and with a traditional culture (Spector 1994). You may wish to use this tool with clients or as a self-assessment to discuss with your peers. The remainder of this section provides an overview of phenomena that must be assessed in order to provide culturally competent nursing care (Kozier et al 2000; McNeal 1998).

Ethnicity/Race/Cultural Affiliation The four federally defined ethnic minorities of color are African Americans, Asian Americans and Pacific Islanders, Hispanic Americans, and American Indians and Alaska Natives.

Heritage Assessment

I. Demographic Data

1. Location _____
2. (a) Age _____
   (b) Date of Birth _____
   (c) Place of Birth _____
3. Sex
   (1) Female   (2) Male
4. What is the highest grade completed in school? _____
5. Are you
   (1) Married   (2) Widowed
   (3) Divorced   (4) Separated
   (5) Never married

II. Heritage Assessment: Your Ethnic, Cultural, and Religious Background

1. Where was your mother born?
   _____

2. Where was your father born?
   _____

3. Where were your grandparents born?:
   a. Your mother's mother?
      _____

   b. Your mother's father?
      _____

   c. Your father's mother?
      _____

   d. Your father's father?
      _____

4. How many brothers do you have?_____ sisters?_____

5. In what setting did you grow up?
   Urban   Rural   Suburban

6. In what country did your parents grow up?
   Father _____
   Mother _____

7. How old were you when you came to the United States?

8. How old were your parents when they came to the U.S.?
   Mother _____
   Father _____

9. When you were growing up, who lived with you? _____
   _____

10. Have you maintained contact with:
    a. Aunts, uncles, cousins   Yes   No
    b. Brothers and sisters?   Yes   No
    c. Parents?   Yes   No
    d. Your own children?   Yes   No

11. Did most of your aunts, uncles, cousins live near to your home?
    Yes   No

12. Approximately how often did you visit your family members who lived outside of your home?
    (1) Daily (2) Weekly (3) Monthly
    (4) Once a year or less (5) Never

13. Was your original family name changed?
    Yes   No

14. What is your religious preference?
    (1) Catholic   (2) Jewish
    (3) Protestant   (4) Denomination
    (5) Other   (6) None

15. Is your spouse the same religion as you?
    Yes   No

16. Is your spouse the same ethnic background as you?
    Yes   No

17. What kind of school did you go to?
    (1) Public   (2) Private
    (3) Religious

18. As an adult, do you live in a neighborhood where the neighbors are the same religion and ethnic background as yourself?
    Yes   No

19. Do you belong to a religious institution?
    Yes   No

20. Would you describe yourself as an active member?
    Yes   No

21. How often do you attend your religious institution?
    (1) More than once a week
    (2) Weekly   (3) Monthly
    (4) Special holidays only (5) Never

22. Do you practice your religion in your home?
    Yes   No
    (if yes, please specify)
    (1) Praying   (2) Bible reading
    (3) Diet
    (4) Celebrating religious holidays

23. Do you prepare foods of your ethnic background?
    Yes   No

24. Do you participate in ethnic activities?
    Yes   No
    (if yes, please specify)
    (1) Singing
    (2) Holiday celebrations
    (3) Dancing   (4) Festivals
    (5) Costumes   (6) Other

25. Are your friends from the same religious background as you?
    Yes   No

26. Are your friends from the same ethnic background as you?
    Yes   No

27. What is your native language?
    _____

28. Do you speak this language?
    (1) Prefer   (2) Occasionally
    (3) Rarely

29. Do you read your native language?
    Yes   No

III. Beliefs and Practices Regarding Personal Health and Illness

(Note: Use a separate sheet of paper for long answer questions.)

1. How do you describe "health"?

2. How do you rate your health?
   (1) Excellent   (2) Good
   (3) Fair   (4) Poor

3. How do you describe "illness"?

4. What do you believe causes illness?
   (1) Poor eating habits?   Yes   No
   (2) Incorrect food combinations?   Yes   No
   (3) Viruses, bacteria, "germs?"   Yes   No
   (4) God's punishment for sin?   Yes   No
   (5) The "Evil Eye?"   Yes   No
   (6) Other people's hexes or spells? Yes   No
   (7) Witchcraft?   Yes   No
   (8) Changes in environment, i.e., cold/hot weather? Yes   No
   (9) Exposure to drafts   Yes   No
   (10) Overwork?   Yes   No
   (11) Underwork?   Yes   No
   (12) Grief and loss?   Yes   No
   (13) Other

5. What did your mother do to keep you from getting sick?

6. How do you keep yourself from getting sick?

7. What home remedies did your mother use to treat illness?

8. What home remedies do you use?

9. Describe in 200–300 words an incident in your nursing practice when cultural differences (religious, ethnic, or lay nursing) caused a problem for you.

Figure 3–5

Heritage Assessment. (*Source*: Courtesy of Rachel E. Spector, PhD, RN, CTN, FAAN. Reprinted with permission.)

This is important information because of biological variations, such as lactose intolerance, and susceptibility to specific disease process, such as sickle cell anemia or Tay Sachs disease. Be aware that skin color is not necessarily an indicator of either race or culture. Do not assume ethnic or racial affiliation; allow patients to self-report these data. You might ask an open-ended question such as: "I want to learn about your cultural heritage. Can you tell me about your cultural group?"

Birthplace and Place of Residence   Patients who have lived in this society only a short time may not have assimilated Western healthcare practices. This information may provide an idea of the degree to which the patient may be able to adhere to a prescribed regimen. Part II of Figure 3–5 covers this category thoroughly.

KEY POINT

Assess for Communication:

Native language
Regional dialect
Different meanings
   for same word
Speech volume
Emotional tone
Nonverbal behavior

Communication Abilities   Gestures, touch, eye contact, and body language are culturally related (eg, some Asian Americans may avoid direct eye contact as a show of respect). Determine which nonverbal cues given by the client or the nurse facilitate or hinder communication. Assess the client's language fluency and obtain an interpreter if needed. Be aware that from the client's point of view, if the interpreter is too young, of the wrong sex, or of a different sociocultural background, the client may not wish to share personal information.

Food Sanctions or Restrictions   Food choice and selection have more than just nutritional value and may be closely related to religious practices and health beliefs. Ask, "What kind of foods do you eat to maintain health? What foods do you eat during illness? Do they require special preparation?" Ask about religious restrictions on eating (eg, is the client required to fast or to avoid certain foods?). Consult a nutritionist as needed for making culturally acceptable food substitutions.

Religious and Spiritual Beliefs and Practices   The nurse should facilitate patients' observance of spiritual beliefs. Some cultures rely on spiritual healers; others may require presence of a religious representative during delivery of healthcare; still others sanction the use of mood-altering substances during ceremonies. For more information, refer to Figure 3–5 on p. 113, and "Spiritual Assessment," on pp. 115–116.

Health Beliefs, Theories of Illness, Folk Practices   Western health practices are based on the *scientific perspective* (all diseases have a measurable cause and effect). The *holistic model* of illness emphasizes a balance between mind-body-spirit and the universe (eg, "hot-cold theory," "Yin-Yang theory"). The *magicoreligious model* holds that the supernatural forces of good and evil cause disruptions in health. People often hold a combination of these beliefs. Part III of Figure 3–5, on page 113, provides questions for assessing health beliefs. In addition, ask, "What are you considering now, and how can we help?"

Family and Support System   In some families, decisions are made by one dominant authority; in others, decisions are made by the collective community and the patient must abide by them. Ask questions such as: "Who are the members of your family? What family duties do women and men usually perform in your culture? Whom do you consult when making healthcare decisions (eg, family member, cultural or religious leader)? Who will be able to help you during and after treatment?"

Space Orientation   The relationship between one's body and objects and persons in the environment is learned. People in Western societies tend to be more territorial (eg, "You are in my space"). The patient may withdraw if the nurse is perceived as being too close (eg, to assess the lungs, a nurse needs to move into the patient's intimate space).

Time Orientation   Time may have a different meaning and value to people of different cultures. Time orientation also refers to the person's focus on the past, the present, or the future. Most cultures combine all three orientations, but one is more likely to dominate. Healthcare workers tend to value time and an orientation toward the future (eg, medication schedules, appointment times).

Pain Responses   There are both cultural and individual differences in pain perception and responses. In some cultures, pain may be considered a punishment for bad deeds, so the patient is expected to tolerate pain without complaint. In other cultures, tolerance of pain suggests strength and endurance; in still others the expression of pain elicits attention and sympathy.

Spiritual Assessment

A holistic assessment includes information about the client's spiritual well-being. For healthy clients, the spiritual dimension is important to overall well-being. For those who are ill, spirituality can be either a source of support or difficulty. Nurses usually elicit spiritual data as a part of the general history. It is best to do the spiritual assessment at the end of the interview, once you have developed a relationship with the client. The following questions may be helpful when working with clients who indicate a religious affiliation:

- Please tell me about any particular religious practices that are important to you.
- Has being here (or being ill) interfered with your religious practices?
- Do you feel that your faith is helpful to you? In what ways is it important to you right now?
- How can I help you carry out your faith? For example, would you like me to read your prayer book to you?
- Would you like a visit from your spiritual counselor, minister, or the hospital chaplain?

KEY POINT

Cultural Assessments:

Ethnicity/race/ cultural affiliation
Birthplace and place of residence
Communication
Food sanctions and restrictions
Religious beliefs and practices
Health beliefs
Folk practices
Family and social organization
Space orientation
Time orientation
Pain responses
Environmental control

Nurses sometimes hesitate to ask questions about spirituality because they are afraid they may impose their own ideas of spirituality on the patient or because they fear that using "religious language" would alienate a client who does not express his spirituality in such language (eg, "Do you pray regularly?" or "Are you saved?"). It may help to think of spirituality in a broad sense, not as limited to religion. The following are some questions and observations that may help you to assess the client's spiritual status without asking direct, spiritual questions (Cathell 1991; Stoll 1979):

1. *The patient's concept of "God."* Most people are religious in the sense that they need something to give meaning to their life. For some, "God" is the religious meaning of God; for some it is their work; for others it is their lifestyle, their children, and so on. Listen to what the patient says about how he spends his time and energy. Observe the books at his bedside and the programs he watches on television. Does the patient's life have meaning, value, and purpose? Does he seem to be at peace with himself?

2. *The patient's source of hope and strength.* This might be God in the traditional sense, a family member, or the client's "inner source" of strength. Notice who the client talks about most often; or ask, "Who is important to you?", "Where do you go to feel loved and understood?" or "What helps you when you feel afraid or in need of special help?"

3. *The significance of religious practice and rituals.* In addition to asking specific questions, notice whether the client seems to be praying when you enter the room, before meals, or during procedures. Observe whether he is visited by a clergy member. Look for such items as religious literature, pictures, rosaries, church bulletins, and religious get-well cards at the bedside. These provide clues to the kind of spiritual support that are meaningful to the client.

4. *The patient's thoughts about the relationship between spiritual beliefs and his state of health.* Is the client questioning the meaning of his illness: "Why did God let this happen to me?" Some people believe illness is a punishment for some wrong they have done. Others may see illness as a test of their faith. Still others may see their faith as therapy for their illness: "If I have faith, I will get well." You might ask questions such as, "What has bothered you most about being sick?" or "What is most frightening or meaningful about your illness?"

5. *The patient's fear of alienation, loneliness, or solitude.* This can take many forms. Instead of appearing lonely, patients may use distancing behaviors such as joking. Some patients are overly sophisticated about their illness. They talk about it in terms of lab values, pathophysiology, and medications, but do not say how they feel about it or what it means in their life. Other clients may pace the halls, have sleep disturbances, or seem angry, apathetic, or preoccupied.

KEY POINT

Be aware of spiritual needs:

Look for visual cues (eg, Bible, prayer beads)

Listen for verbal cues (eg, refers to God or church)

Assess for spiritual distress (eg, crying, anger, wishing to die)

Wellness Assessment

A thorough assessment of the client's health status is basic to health promotion. **Health promotion** is more than avoidance or prevention of disease. It includes activities undertaken for the purpose of improving well-being and achieving a higher level of health (eg, stress management and physical fitness). See Table 3–17 for a summary of the components of a wellness assessment (Pender 1996, pp. 117–135).

Health promotion assumes that people can identify their own health needs. In this framework, assessment involves active listening and a dialogue between the nurse and the client. The nurse and client collaborate to achieve a deeper understanding of the client's health experiences. The nurse may ask questions in order to make the client more aware of factors that may be influencing his condition, and the client asks questions of the nurse (Lindsey and Hartrick 1996). This type of assessment promotes mutual input into decision making and planning to improve the client's health (Pender 1996, p. 116).

Family Assessment

Nurses assess the health of individuals, families, and communities. When a family is the client, the nurse determines the health status of the family and its individual members, as well as the level of the family's functioning, interaction patterns, and strengths and weaknesses. Even if the client is an individual, data about the family enable the nurse to reflect more holistically on the client's story. Nurses assess families in a variety of settings (eg, mental health clinics, schools, community health, home care, inpatient maternity units). Box 3–7, pp. 122–123, provides a guide for making family assessments.

Community Assessment

Community assessment is not limited to public health nurses. Acute care nurses use knowledge of community resources to make referrals and coordinate clients' transition from hospital to home care. Clients also benefit if their home care nurse is aware of groups and services available for continuing support.

> EXAMPLE: An elderly woman has fallen and has a lacerated foot that is healing slowly. A nurse visits her daily to make dressing changes. Because she is diabetic and has poor circulation, the client needs to be treated by wound care specialists. However, she is not able to drive. Is there a wound care clinic in the community? Are there transportation services that she could use?

A community assessment answers these kinds of questions. In addition, the data can be analyzed to determine the overall health status of a particular group (eg, pregnant adolescents, home health clients with diabetes) or community (eg, a neighborhood, the city government, the American Diabetes Association). Major

Table 3–17   Components of a Wellness Assessment

Assessment Categories	Explanation and Examples
Physical Fitness Evaluation	Because of sedentary lifestyles, this is a critical component. Includes cardiovascular tolerance (eg, step test), general appearance, muscle strength (eg, sit-ups), joint flexibility, body proportions, percent of body fat.
Nutritional Assessment	Poor eating habits and dietary risk factors are widespread in all socioeconomic groups. Includes muscle mass, 24-hour recall of food intake, knowledge of nutrition, effect of sociocultural beliefs on diet, use of the Food Guide Pyramid and Recommended Daily Allowances of essential nutrients, comparison of weight to body build and height.
Health Risk Appraisal	Assessment of a client's risk of disease or injury over the next 10 years by comparing the client's characteristics with those of corresponding age, sex, and racial group. A **risk factor** is anything that increases a person's chance of acquiring a specific disease, such as cancer (eg, exposure to the sun is a risk factor for skin cancer). Risk factors may be categorized according to age, genetic factors, biologic characteristics, personal health habits, lifestyle, and environment. Many health risk tools are available. They commonly assess five categories of risk: cardiovascular disease, cancer, automobile accidents, suicide, and diabetes.
Lifestyle Assessment	Categories generally assessed are physical activity; nutritional practices, stress management, safety practices, healthcare practices (eg, last Pap smear, last chest x-ray), and such habits as smoking, alcohol consumption, and drug use. Figure 3–6, on pp. 120–121, is an example of a lifestyle assessment.
Health Beliefs	Healthcare beliefs provide an indication of how much the person believes he/she can influence or control health through personal behaviors (eg, breast self-examination). Assess clients' beliefs about such things as exercise benefits and barriers, social support for exercise, the definition of health, and health locus of control (ie, whether the person, chance, or powerful others influences the person's health).
Life Stress Review	People who have a high level of stress are more prone to illness and less able to cope with illness. Various tools have been developed that assign numerical values to recent life events (eg, divorce, pregnancy, retirement). High scores are associated with an increased likelihood of illness.
Social Support Systems Review	Social support is the subjective feeling of belonging and being accepted; being valued for oneself. The *natural support system* is the family; this is usually the primary support group. *Peer support systems* are people who function informally to meet the needs of others (eg, a group of widows and widowers).

(continues)

Table 3–17   Components of a Wellness Assessment *(continued)*

Assessment Categories	Explanation and Examples
Social Support Systems Review *(continued)*	*Organized religious support systems* (eg, churches) provide support through shared values. *Professional supports* consist of helping professionals with a specific set of skills and services (eg, financial counselor, bereavement counselor). *Organized support systems not directed by health professionals* include voluntary service groups and mutual help groups, such as Alcoholics Anonymous.
Spiritual Health Assessment	Because spiritual beliefs affect the client's interpretation of life events, they are a critical component of health assessment. Spiritual assessment goes beyond religious affiliation to explore feelings about the meaning of life, love, hope, forgiveness, life after death, and connectedness. Refer to "Spiritual Assessment," on pages 115–116.

Sources: Edleman, C. L. and C. L. Mandle, eds (1998), *Health promotion through the life span,* 4th ed. (St. Louis: Mosby); Kozier, B. et al, *Fundamentals of nursing: Concepts, process, and practice.* 6th ed. (Upper Saddle River, NJ: Prentice Hall Health, pp. 128–131); Murray, R. B. and J. P. Zentner (1997), *Health assessment and promotion strategies through the life span,* 6th ed. (Stamford, CT: Appleton & Lange); Pender, N. J. (1996), *Health promotion in nursing practice,* 3rd ed. (Stamford, CT: Appleton & Lange, pp. 116–135); Pinnell, N. and M. de Meneses (1986), *The nursing process: Theory, application, and related processes* (Norwalk, CT: Appleton & Lange, pp. 89–90).

aspects of a community assessment are shown in Box 3–8 on p. 124. The best way to assess a community is to live in it. However, the nurse can gather data while traveling through the community and observing the surroundings (eg, types of buildings, condition of roads, people walking about), and by networking with other professionals who live or work there (Lindell 1997).

■ ETHICAL AND LEGAL CONSIDERATIONS

As in all aspects of care, nurses must be aware of their ethical responsibilities when assessing clients. According to the ANA "Code for Nurses" (1985),

> the nurse provides services with respect for human dignity and the uniqueness of the client. . . . The nurse safeguards the client's right to privacy by judiciously protecting information of a confidential nature.

Issues of honesty and confidentiality are frequently encountered during assessment.

Honesty

The principle of **veracity** (honesty) holds that we should tell the truth and not lie. In assessing patients, this means that you should be honest about how you will use the data: to plan the patient's care, for research, for a student

All of us want good health. But many of us do not know how to be as healthy as possible. Health experts now describe *lifestyle* as one of the most important factors affecting health. In fact, it is estimated that as many as seven of the ten leading causes of death could be reduced through common-sense changes in lifestyle. That's what this brief test, developed by the Public Health Service, is all about. Its purpose is simply to tell you how well you are doing to stay healthy. The behaviors covered in the test are recommended for most Americans. Some of them may not apply to persons with certain chronic diseases or handicaps, or to pregnant women. Such persons may require special instructions from their physicians.

Cigarette Smoking

If you <u>never smoke</u>, enter a score of 10 for this section and go to the next section on *Alcohol and Drugs*.

	Almost Always	Sometimes	Almost Never
1. I avoid smoking cigarettes.	2	1	0
2. I smoke only low tar and nicotine cigarettes *or* I smoke a pipe or cigars.	2	1	0

Smoking Score: _____

Alcohol and Drugs

	Almost Always	Sometimes	Almost Never
1. I avoid drinking alcoholic beverages *or* I drink no more than 1 or 2 drinks a day.	4	1	0
2. I avoid using alcohol or other drugs (especially illegal drugs) as a way of handling stressful situations or the problems in my life.	2	1	0
3. I am careful not to drink alcohol when taking certain medicines (for example, medicine for sleeping, pain, colds, and allergies), or when pregnant.	2	1	0
4. I read and follow the label directions when using prescribed and over-the-counter drugs.	2	1	0

Alcohol and Drugs Score: _____

Eating Habits

	Almost Always	Sometimes	Almost Never
1. I eat a variety of foods each day, such as fruits and vegetables, whole grain breads and cereals, lean meats, dairy products, dry peas and beans, and nuts and seeds.	4	1	0
2. I limit the amount of fat, saturated fat, and cholesterol I eat (including fat on meats, eggs, butter, cream, shortenings, and organ meats such as liver).	2	1	0
3. I limit the amount of salt I eat by cooking with only small amounts, not adding salt at the table, and avoiding salty snacks.	2	1	0
4. I avoid eating too much sugar (especially frequent snacks of sticky candy or soft drinks).	2	1	0

Eating Habits Score: _____

Exercise/Fitness

	Almost Always	Sometimes	Almost Never
1. I maintain a desired weight, avoiding overweight and underweight.	3	1	0
2. I do vigorous exercises for 15–30 minutes at least 3 times a week (examples include running, swimming, brisk walking).	3	1	0
3. I do exercises that enhance my muscle tone for 15–30 minutes at least 3 times a week (examples include yoga and calisthenics).	2	1	0
4. I use part of my leisure time participating in individual, family, or team activities that increase my level of fitness (such as gardening, bowling, golf, and baseball).	2	1	0

Exercise/Fitness Score: _____

Stress Control

	Almost Always	Sometimes	Almost Never
1. I have a job or do other work that I enjoy.	2	1	0
2. I find it easy to relax and express my feelings freely.	2	1	0
3. I recognize early, and prepare for, events or situations likely to be stressful for me.	2	1	0
4. I have close friends, relatives, or others whom I can talk to about personal matters and call on for help when needed.	2	1	0
5. I participate in group activities (such as church and community organizations) or hobbies that I enjoy.	2	1	0

Stress Control Score: _____

Safety

	Almost Always	Sometimes	Almost Never
1. I wear a seat belt while riding in a car.	2	1	0
2. I avoid driving while under the influence of alcohol and other drugs.	2	1	0
3. I obey traffic rules and the speed limit when driving.	2	1	0
4. I am careful when using potentially harmful products or substances (such as household cleaners, poisons, and electrical devices).	2	1	0
5. I avoid smoking in bed.	2	1	0

Safety Score: _____

(continues)

Figure 3–6

Healthstyle: A Self Test. (*Source*: Courtesy of National Health Information Clearinghouse, Washington, DC.)

What Your Scores Mean to YOU

Scores of 9 and 10

Excellent! Your answers show that you are aware of the importance of this area to your health. More important, you are putting your knowledge to work for you by practicing good health habits. As long as you continue to do so, this area should not pose a serious health risk. It's likely that you are setting an example for your family and friends to follow. Since you got a very high test score on this part of the test, you may want to consider other areas where your scores indicate room for improvement.

Scores of 6 to 8

Your health practices in this area are good, but there is room for improvement. Look again at the items you answered with a "Sometimes" or "Almost Never." What changes can you make to improve your score? Even a small change can often help you achieve better health.

Scores of 3 to 5

Your health risks are showing! Would you like more information about the risks you are facing and about why it is important for you to change these behaviors. Perhaps you need help in deciding how to successfully make the changes you desire. In either case, help is available.

Scores of 0 to 2

Obviously, you were concerned enough about your health to take the test, but your answers show that you may be taking serious and unnecessary risks with your health. Perhaps you are not aware of the risks and what to do about them. You can easily get the information and help you need to improve, if you wish. The next step is up to you.

Figure 3–6
Continued.

paper, and so forth. When you introduce yourself to the patient, tell him what to expect from the interview and how the information will be used.

Truthfulness also affects the patient's autonomy. The moral principle of **autonomy** holds that a person has the right to be independent and to decide for himself what is to happen to him. If the patient does not know how the data will be used, he cannot make a truly informed choice about whether to participate in the interview and thereby loses some of his autonomy.

Confidentiality

Treat assessment data as confidential. Failure to do so robs the patient of his autonomy, because it removes his control over how data are used and shared. Among other things, confidentiality means that assessment notes should be kept in the patient's chart, not lying about where others can read them. It also means that you should not use the patient's name on any written learning assignments; and you should not talk about patient data at the desk, in the halls, or in the lunchroom, where casual observers might overhear.

A client may tell you something in confidence that you feel you must tell in order to protect her; for example, a client might tell you of her plans for suicide. If you believe you cannot keep the information confidential, then you are obligated (by the principle of veracity) to tell the client that, in her best interest, you must share the information with other caregivers. A similar situation arises when a client tells you something that you feel you must

BOX 3–7

Family Assessment Guide

Family Structure

- Family type: traditional, nuclear, blended, extended, single-parent, or other
- Age, sex, and number of family members

Lifestyle

- Level of knowledge of sexual and marital roles (eg, teenage pregnancy and marriage)
- Child, spouse, or elder abuse
- Chemical dependency, including alcohol and nicotine
- Safety of the home environment

Psychosocial Factors

- Adequacy of income
- Adequacy of child care when both parents work
- Availability of support persons (eg, friends, church groups)
- Work or social pressures that create stress

Developmental Factors

- Older adults, especially if living alone
- Adolescent parents
- Families with new babies

Family Roles

- Persons working outside the home; type of work; satisfaction with work
- Divison of household responsibilities; family members' satisfaction with this arrangement
- Person who makes the major decisions; person making day-to-day decisions
- Who is the most significant family member in each person's life?

Communication and Interaction

- Openness and honesty in communication among family members
- Ways of demonstrating love, sorrow, anger, and other feelings
- Degree of emotional support given to each other
- Methods of handling conflict and stressful situations among family members

(continues)

BOX 3-7

Family Assessment Guide (continued)

Physical Health

- Current health status of each member
- Ways the family obtains health services
- Preventive measures (eg, immunizations, dental hygiene, visual examinations)
- Genetic predisposition to disease (eg, cardiovascular disease, diabetes)
- Health practices (eg, foods eaten, bedtime, exercise)

Family Values

- Views about importance of education, teachers, and school
- Cultural affiliation and degree to which cultural practices are followed
- Religious orientation; degree of importance in family life
- Use of leisure time and whether shared or individual
- Extent to which health is valued (eg, preventive care, exercise, diet)

reveal in order to protect someone else. There is no rule about when to tell and when not to tell. You will, each time, have to balance the need to preserve autonomy against the need to protect the client or others.

In both instances, it is better from an ethical standpoint to stop the client from telling you something you cannot keep confidential. Of course this is not always possible, but often you can pick up clues from the client that she is about to disclose this kind of information. If you do, you might say something like, "This sounds like something I may not be able to keep confidential. Are you *sure* you want to go on with it?"

Malpractice Suits

Monitoring is frequent, ongoing assessment often done at specified intervals. It is focused assessment; for example, you might monitor the reflexes of a patient receiving magnesium sulfate, or the fluid intake and output of a patient with burns. Monitoring is sometimes ordered by the physician, but some monitoring can also be ordered by a nurse (eg, monitoring the mental status of a patient who has had episodes of disorientation and confusion). Failure to monitor is a common cause of malpractice suits. If a physician orders frequent monitoring for a patient, be sure to do the following:

1. Have the physician specify the frequency or follow the frequency specified in your agency's policies and protocols.

BOX 3-8

Major Aspects of a Community Assessment

Category	Examples
Physical Environment	Geographic size, types of housing, density, crime rate
Education	School lunch programs, parental involvement in schools, health services handled by the schools
Safety and Transportation	Police, fire, ambulance, and sanitation services; public transportation, air quality
Politics and Government	Type of government; influential people and organizations, recent election issues
Health and Social Services	Hospitals, clinics, home care, long-term care, accessibility of health care services
Communication	Newspapers, radio stations, postal services
Economics	Major employers in the community, income levels, employment rate
Recreation	Number and types of churches, playgrounds, parks, sports facilities, and theaters

Source: Adapted from Anderson, E. and J. McFarlane (1996). *Community as partner: Theory and practice in nursing*, 2nd ed. Philadelphia: Lippincott-Raven, p. 178.

---

2. Perform the monitoring as specified.
3. Thoroughly document the monitoring (and all interventions)

> EXAMPLE: (Actual case) An infant was admitted to a hospital for heart surgery. After surgery, a nurse allegedly failed to monitor the infant's urinary output and delayed obtaining blood gas analysis, which were ordered by the physician. The infant's injuries resulted in cerebral palsy, and the case was settled for $2.2 million (Eskreis 1998, p. 38).

An unreasonable delay in a comprehensive admission assessment could also create a risk for malpractice because the patient might be harmed by a delay in treatment. If you are unable to perform a timely admission assessment, inform your supervisor. When you have time, document your conversation and request in writing that your unit be given additional staff. As soon as possible, assess the patient fully.

■ SUMMARY

Assessment

- is the collection, validation, organization, and recording of data using interview, observation, and examination.
- requires critical thinking skills, a good knowledge base, and an awareness of ethical issues.
- uses directive and nondirective interviewing techniques, adapting to the special needs of the client.
- may be comprehensive or focused.
- may involve various conceptual frameworks to collect and organize data.
- may include in-depth assessment for special purposes (eg, wellness, spiritual, and cultural assessment).
- may be performed for individuals, families, or communities.
- should consider the moral issues of honesty and confidentiality.
- should meet professional and legal standards.

ASSESSMENT THINKING QUICK-CHECK

- ❑ Are the data accurate?
- ❑ Is anything missing?

Nursing Process Practice

1. Listed below are data-collection practices observed on various nursing units. You are the quality-control nurse. Place a check mark beside the practices that meet ANA Standard I. For those you do not check, explain which criterion of the standard they violate.

   a. _____ Admission data are recorded on a printed form in predetermined categories.

   b. _____ There is an admission assessment in the chart. The nursing progress notes on two different days list care given to the patient, but no assessment data about the patient.

   c. _____ The nurses record the comprehensive assessment in paragraph form on the nursing progress notes; they do not all record the data in the same order.

   d. _____ Each patient's chart contains a nursing history and physical examination. A divider with a tab makes these easy to locate.

   e. _____ The comprehensive database contains only primary source objective data (no subjective data).

f. _____ For a woman in labor, the fetal heart rate and the woman's vital signs are automatically transmitted from an electronic monitor to a computer. The nurse records subjective data and nursing activities/observations on a keypad at the bedside. The notes are automatically and continuously printed out on the monitor strip as it comes out of the machine.

2. Place a _C_ beside the cues. Place an _I_ beside the inferences.

   a. _____ The client's blood pressure is 140/80 mm Hg.

   b. _____ The client states he is in pain.

   c. _____ The client is afraid.

   d. _____ The client is depressed.

   e. _____ The client's wife says he forgets to take his pills.

   f. _____ The incision is draining pink fluid.

   g. _____ The incision is infected.

   h. _____ There is no wound care clinic closer than 150 miles.

   i. _____ The client and his wife are not speaking to each other.

   j. _____ The couple needs marital counseling.

3. Classify the data below by placing the letters in the appropriate columns. Note that most letters will be placed in _two_ columns (subjective/objective and primary/secondary). The first one is done for you.

Subjective Data	Objective Data	Primary Source	Secondary Source
	a		a

a. You read in the chart that the client's blood pressure is 140/80 mm Hg.

b. The client's wife says he doesn't sleep well.

c. You observe that the client is pale.

d. The aide tells you the client is pale.

e. You palpate the client's pulse. It is 84 bpm.

f. Mrs. Jones says, "I can't sleep."

g. The nursing progress notes say, "Client is breathing rapidly."

h. The night nurse reports the client's temperature is 98.6° F.

i. The client is coughing.

j. Client states he is cold.

k. The client is walking with a limp.

l. Urine output measured at 100 mL.

m. You feel the dressing. It is dry.

n. Client says she cannot void.

o. You auscultate wheezes in the patient's lungs.

p. The anesthetist tells you the pulse is weak and thready.

q. You palpate a weak, thready pulse.

r. The patient tells you his leg hurts.

s. Driving through a town, you smell an odor of sulphur in the air.

4. Suppose your instructor gives you the following patient assignment for the next day.

You are to perform the admission assessment, including interview and physical examination, on Melissa Bourque, who is being admitted for cosmetic surgery. Patient is a 45-year-old woman. Her preoperative lab work has been done and will be on the chart, along with her medical records from the physician's office.

Will you read Ms. Bourque's chart before interviewing her? Why or why not?

5. Indicate whether the *nurse* (you) obtained the data by interview (*I*), observation (*O*), or physical examination (*E*).

a. _____ You read in the chart that the client's blood pressure is 140/80 mm Hg.

b. _____ Client's wife says he doesn't sleep well.

c. _____ You see that the client is pale.

d. _____ You feel the dressing. It is dry.

e. _____ You count the client's pulse at 84 bpm.

f. _____ You hear the client cough.

g. _____ Client states he is cold.

h. _____ Urine output is measured at 100 mL.

i. _____ Client says she cannot void.

j. _____ You auscultate wheezes in the client's lungs.

k. _____ Anesthetist tells you the pulse is weak and thready.

6. Identify the type of question: *C* = Closed, *O* = Open-ended.

a. _____ Would you like a backrub?

b. _____ Where would you like me to begin?

c. _____ Did you sleep well?

d. _____ How did you sleep?

e. _____ What do you think kept you from sleeping well?

f. _____ Are you hearing voices?

g. _____ Tell me about the voices.

h. _____ Are you worried about the operation?

i. _____ How do you feel now?

j. _____ Tell me about the delivery.

7. The client says, "I have this pain in my stomach." Write examples of questions the nurse could ask to find out more about it.

a. A closed question:

b. An open-ended question:

8. You need to perform the database assessment for Stella Contini. You have read her chart and know that she is 50 years old, unmarried, and has no children. She has severe arthritis in several joints and is being admitted for a total knee replacement. Her mother and sister are at the bedside. Ms. Contini has a roommate in the adjoining bed.

   a. To *prepare* for the interview, what do you need to do?

   b. There is a section on the assessment form labeled "Reason for Hospitalization." What would you say to Ms. Contini to elicit this information?

   c. There is a section on the form labeled "Usual sexual functioning" and another labeled "Changes in sexual functioning since illness." Would you ask these questions? Why or why not?

9. Place a check mark beside the data that should be validated.

   a. _____ The patient tells you he is not anxious about the barium enema. He is lying quietly in bed with no obvious muscle tension. His hands are still. His skin is warm and dry.

   b. _____ The patient says, "On a scale of 1 to 10, the pain is a 10. The worst I can imagine." Less than 5 minutes ago, you observed the patient talking on the telephone in a normal tone of voice.

   c. _____ The patient says he smokes two packs of cigarettes a day. You observe that his teeth and fingers are brown-stained.

   d. _____ The client tells you on admission that she lives alone. In a later conversation, she refers to her roommate.

e. _____ The data were obtained early in the interview, and then the client became confused and began to ramble incoherently.

f. _____ The mother says her little boy "eats like a horse." You observe that the child is thin and small for his age.

g. _____ A client tells you that there is no Alcoholics Anonymous group in the county.

10. Write the correct word in the blank: Is the situation a question of *honesty, or confidentiality,* or *neither*?

a. _____ The nurse asks the patient whether he prefers a bedbath or a whirlpool bath.

b. _____ Before beginning the interview, the nurse tells the patient she needs the information to help plan his care.

c. _____ Nora Morenz is collecting data about pain relief measures for a research project. Because it does not change the patients' care and because they are not mentioned by name, she decides not to tell them she is collecting data for research.

d. _____ A patient's wife overhears the staff discussing information about her husband in the lunchroom.

e. _____ The client tells the nurse she has a knife hidden in the room and that "Someone is going to be sorry." The nurse looks for the knife, but cannot find it. She tells the client, "I am afraid for you and for the other patients. I'm sorry, but I will have to share what you've told me with the rest of the staff."

11. You are caring for Mr. Abbott while his nurse has gone to lunch. When you go in to take his noon vital signs, he tells you that he is feeling better since having his pain pill, but that he now feels a little nauseated. Will you chart the vital signs and the subjective data, or will you report it to Mr. Abbot's nurse? Why?

12. Refer to the data in Question 3. Classify the data into the following categories from NANDA Taxonomy II (see Table 3–13 on pp. 107–108)

Health Promotion	
Nutrition	
Elimination	
Activity/Rest	
Perception/Cognition	
Self-perception	
Role Relationships	
Sexuality	
Coping/Stress Tolerance	
Life Principles	
Safety/Protection	
Comfort	
Growth/Development	
Other	

13. Compare home health assessment in Box 3–6 on page 111, with the family assessment in Box 3–7 on pp. 122–123.

   a. How are they alike?

   b. How are they different?

Critical Thinking Practice: Believing and Knowing

Part I: Differentiating Facts from Interpretations

Review pages 50–52 in Chapter 2. Nurses must know whether they are charting and reporting facts or interpretations. A fact can be verified by investigation, often by observation. Inferences, judgments, and opinions are interpretations of facts.

Learning the Skill

Determine whether the following statements are facts or interpretations.

   a. A break in the skin can be a portal of entry for pathogens.
   Step 1. Can the statement be verified by investigation or observation? (yes or no)
   Step 2. If yes, it is a fact.
   Step 3. If it is a fact, how could you verify the information or check its accuracy?

   b. Nurses who wear caps are more professional than those who don't.
   Step 1. Can the statement be verified by investigation or observation? (yes or no)
   Step 2. If yes, it is a fact.
   Step 3. If it is a fact, how could you verify the information or check its accuracy? If it is
   not a fact, what other facts, observations, or values might have formed the basis
   for the interpretation?

   c. Patient vomited 100 mL green-tinged fluid.

   d. Patient feels nauseated.

   e. Patient was tearful during the interview.

   f. Client is confused.

   g. Patient tolerated clear liquids well.

h. Ms. Benitez is very fearful of this surgery.

i. Patient's abdomen is distended.

Applying the Skill

Determine whether the following statements are facts or interpretations (fill in the blanks). If it is a fact, list ways you could verify the information or check its accuracy. If the statement is an interpretation, (1) what facts, observations, or values might have formed the basis for the interpretation? and (2) Is the statement a belief, opinion, preference, inference, or judgment?

j. _____ No-smoking policies are a good idea because they help prevent fires.

k. _____ Diaper rash is caused by skin bacteria reacting with urea in the urine.

l. _____ If a baby has diaper rash, it is because his parents do not change him often enough.

m. _____ In order to meet ANA Standards of Practice, nursing assessments must be systematic, timely, and retrievable.

n. _____ Good nursing assessments are systematic, timely, and retrievable.

o. _____ "Mrs. Brady complained about the food." (A statement by the nurse giving you the shift-change report.)

p. _____ "I don't want my lunch. I hate cabbage!" (A statement to you by Mrs. Brady.)

q. _____ A patient says, "This illness is a punishment from God."

r. _____ The nurse replies to the patient in "q": "Oh, that can't be true; you're a good Christian."

s. _____ The patient replies to the nurse in "r": "The Bible says that we will be punished for our sins."

t. _____ The nurse replies to the patient in "s": "Well, the Bible *is* the word of God."

Part II: Making Inferences

Review Table 2–2 and pages 50–52 in Chapter 2. We think some things are true because we have direct evidence. For instance, you might see your dog standing outside the door. You know the dog is there because you can see her. We also believe that things are true even when we do not have such clear evidence. Suppose you are in your house and you hear a scratching noise coming from the front door. Again, you might believe that your dog is standing at the door, but this time the evidence is different. You don't actually see your dog, but the sound you hear makes you think she is at the door. This is the best explanation you can think of for the noise. That is the process of *making an inference*. An inference is something we believe to be true based on consideration of the evidence (or facts).

You can never be sure of the truth of an inference. Obviously, some inferences are supported by more evidence than others. If, in addition to hearing scratching, you also hear your dog's chain rattling and hear her barking, you would be very sure that she is outside the door. On the other hand, if all you heard was some scratching, you would be less sure about your inference. It could be that some other animal, perhaps a cat or a raccoon, was scratching.

Sometimes we become so accustomed to making a particular inference that we do not even realize we are inferring. If every time you hear scratching at the door you go and find your dog, then you assume that scratching always means your dog is out there. You have tested your inference so many times that it seems more like a fact. Many of the so-called "facts" of science are really inferences that we make so often that we do not stop to consider that they are not actually "proven" facts. It is important to remember that patient problems are really inferences from evidence; in most cases, they have not been observed directly.

Learning the Skill

Practice thinking about inferences by answering the following questions.

1. While sitting in a sunlit room, you notice that the direct sunlight has stopped coming through the window. List several things that might be causing this (these are things you might infer).

2. A few minutes after the sunlight stops, you observe through the window that drops of water are falling from the sky. Does this provide any additional evidence for one of the inferences you listed in Question 1? Explain.

3. What is your inference? Without going outside, can you be sure that what you have inferred is true?

Applying the Skill

1. The following statements were given to you in report. Some are facts and some are inferences. Circle the letters of the statements that need more data to support them. What questions might you ask the nurse in order to verify the statement?

   a. Mrs. Brady complained about the food.

   b. Geri has not had any visitors this week.

   c. Mr. Jiminez is relieved that the surgery has been postponed.

   d. Ms. McCarthy's incision is infected.

2. State whether the following are facts or inferences:

   a. _____ Patient weighs 250 lb.

   b. _____ Patient is obese.

   c. _____ Temperature is 100° F.

   d. _____ Patient is anxious.

   e. _____ Patient states, "I'm really scared."

3. In the following case, circle the facts (cues).

   _____

   CASE: Maria Gutierrez had a routine surgery and uneventful recovery-room period. She was returned to her room at 4:00 PM, still drowsy, but responding to her name. A Foley catheter was in place, draining clear, pale yellow urine. Her IV was patent; 1,000 mL of D$_5$LR was running at 75 mL/hour. Her skin turgor was good. Her vital signs were: blood pressure 124/76–130/82 mm Hg, pulse 72–86 bpm, and respirations 12–20 throughout the evening. At 8:00 PM, the nurse helped her to sit on the side of the bed for 15 minutes. She moved slowly and complained of incisional pain, which she rated 10 on a scale of 1 to 10 (10 being the worst). She administered her own morphine by use of a patient-controlled analgesia (PCA) pump, and rated her pain as "about 5" when she was lying still. Her abdominal dressing was dry and intact throughout the night. At 9:00 PM she had sips of a carbonated drink. At 9:20 PM she complained of nausea.

4. In the preceding case, the nurse made several inferences. Write the data that led the nurse to make each of the following inferences (use the cues you circled in item 3).

   a. Ms. Gutierrez was drowsy from the anesthetic.

   b. There was no problem with Ms. Gutierrez's urinary functioning.

   c. Ms. Gutierrez was adequately hydrated.

   d. Ms. Gutierrez was experiencing acute incisional pain.

e. The morphine effectively relieved Ms. Gutierrez's incisional pain.

    f. Ms. Gutierrez became nauseated because her gastrointestinal motility had not fully returned after her anesthesia.

5. Do all of these inferences have an equal amount of supporting evidence? Which ones do you think need more evidence?

6. Examine the explanations for each of the following cue clusters. Circle the parts that are inferred and underline the parts that have direct evidence to support them.

    a. *Cues:* Your patient has just had general anesthesia. Bowel sounds are absent to auscultation. Patient drank 100 mL of fluid and immediately vomited. Patient complained of nausea.

Explanation: Patient's nausea and vomiting were caused by decreased gastrointestinal activity secondary to general anesthetic.

b. *Cues*: Your patient has just been admitted to the hospital. He is pale and trembling. His palms are cool and damp. He is speaking rapidly.

Explanation: The patient is anxious owing to being in a strange environment.

c. *Cues*: Your patient is unable to drink anything. He is vomiting and experiencing severe diarrhea. In fact, his fluid output over the past 12 hours has been 500 mL greater than his intake. His skin turgor is poor; his mucous membranes are dry.

Explanation: The patient has a fluid volume deficit caused by being unable to drink and by diarrhea and vomiting.

7. Now, list each inference in Item 6, and write whether you think the evidence is adequate or inadequate. If it is inadequate, what else do you need to know in order to support the inference adequately?

NOTE: Be sure to discuss your answers with your peers or instructors. When using critical thinking, you may find that there is not just *one* correct answer. When someone thinks of a point you hadn't considered, this may cause you to think differently about what is "correct."

Source: Adapted from Wilbraham, et al (1990). "Critical Thinking Worksheets." A Supplement of *Addison-Wesley Chemistry*, Menlo Park, CA: Addison-Wesley.

Case Study: Applying Nursing Process and Critical Thinking

(Discuss with classmates, and look up unfamiliar terms, eg, fractured hip, senile dementia, in a textbook, as needed.) Steven Brown is an 82-year-old man who has been admitted to an extended care facility because he is no longer able to live at home alone. He has a medical diagnosis of senile dementia. On admission, he states his name and knows you are a nurse, but he thinks he is at his daughter's house.

1. What information do you need to gather when planning *safety* measures for Mr. Brown?

2. How is that information different from the information you'd need if everything in the case was the same except that instead of senile dementia, the medical diagnosis is fractured hip, 1 week postoperatively?

3. Refer to Question 1. What data collection method will you use to get each piece of information? What data sources will you use?

4. What special techniques will you use to communicate with Mr. Brown? Write at least 3 questions (or statements) you would use when obtaining information from him.

5. What critical thinking attitudes or skills did you use in this exercise? Refer back to Chapter 2, if necessary, to refresh your memory.

■ SELECTED REFERENCES

Accreditation manual for hospitals (1996). Oakbrook Terrace, IL: Joint Commission on Accreditation of Healthcare Organizations.

Alfaro-LeFevre, R. (1998). *Applying nursing process.* 4th ed. Philadelphia: J. B. Lippincott.

American Nurses Association. (1998). *Standards of clinical nursing practice.* 2nd ed. Washington, DC: ANA.

American Nurses Association. (1991). *Position statement on cultural diversity in nursing practice.* Kansas City, MO: ANA.

American Nurses Association. (1985). *Code for nurses with interpretive statements.* Kansas City, MO: ANA.

Anderson, E. and J. McFarlane (1996). *Community as partner: Theory and practice in nursing,* 2nd ed. Philadelphia: Lippincott-Raven, p. 178.

Andrews, H., and C. Roy (1986). *Essentials of the Roy Adaptation Model.* Norwalk, CT: Appleton-Century-Crofts.

Antai-Otong, D. (1999). Active listening at work. *AJN* 99(2):L24–L25.

Barry, C. (1998). Assessing the older adult in the home. *Home Healthcare Nurse* 16(8): 519–530.

Broughton, V. (1998). Critical thinking: Linking assessment data and knowledge. *Nursing Connections* 11(4):59–65.

Canadian Nurses Association (1987). *CNA: A definition of nursing practice: Standards for nursing practice.* Ottawa, Ontario: CNA.

Cathell, D. (1991). A spiritual assessment without asking spiritual questions. [Lecture] Shawnee Mission Medical Center, Merriam, KS.

Davidhizar, R., and G. A. Bechtel (1998). Assessing the patient from a cultural perspective. *Journal Prac Nursing* 48(3):16–21.

Edelman, C., and C. Mandle (1998). *Health promotion throughout the life span.* 4th ed. St. Louis: Mosby.

Ellis, A., and S. Cavanagh (1992). Aspects of neurosurgical assessment using the Glasgow Coma Scale. *Intensive Crit Care Nurs* 8:94–99.

Eskreis, T. R. (1998). Seven common legal pitfalls in nursing. *AJN* 98(4):34–40.

Feely, M. (1994) Know your patient: The importance of assessment in care delivery. *Prof Nurse* 9(5):318–323.

Giger, J., and R. Davidhizar (1995). *Transcultural nursing: Assessment and intervention.* St. Louis: Mosby.

Gordon, M. (1994). *Nursing diagnosis: Process and application.* 3rd ed. St. Louis: Mosby.

James, L. (1992). Nursing theory made practical. *J Nurs Edu* 31(1):42–44.

Johannsen, J. M. (1992). Self-care assessment: Key to teaching and discharge planning. *Dimen Crit Care Nurs* 11(1):48–56.

Johns, C. (1996). The benefits of a reflective model of nursing. *Nurs Times* 92(27):39–41.

Kacperek, L. (1997). Clinical. Non-verbal communication: The importance of listening. *Brit J Nurs* 6(5):275–279.

Kodadek, M. and M. Boland (1998). Assessing the high-risk pregnant woman at home. *Home Healthcare Nurse* 16(3):157–163.

Koldjeski, D. (1993). A restructured nursing process model. *Nurse Educator* 18(4):33–38.

Kozier, B., G. Erb, A. Berman, et al (2000). *Fundamentals of nursing: Concepts, process, and practice.* 6th ed. Upper Saddle River, NJ: Prentice Hall Health.

Kozier, B., G. Erb, and K. Blais, et al. (1995). *Fundamentals of Nursing.* 5th ed. Redwood City, CA: Addison-Wesley Nursing.

Lindell, D. (1997). Community assessment for the home healthcare nurse. *Home Healthcare Nurse* 15(9):619–628.

Lindsey, E. and G. Hartrick (1996). Health-promoting practice: The demise of the nursing process? *J Advan Nurs* 23:106–112.

Laukhuf, G. and H. Werner (1998). Spirituality: The missing link. *J Neurosci Nurs* 30(1): 60–67.

Mahoney, F. and D. Barthel (1965). Functional evaluation: The Barthel Index. *Maryland Med J* 14(2):61–65.

Maslow, A. H. (1970). *Motivation and personality.* 2nd ed. New York: Harper & Row.

McGourthy, R. J. (1999). A comparative study of outcomes in patients with chronic obstructive pulmonary disease. *Home Care Provider* 4(1):21–25.

McNeal, G. J. (1998). Diversity issues in the homecare setting. *Crit Care Nurs Clin North Am* 10(3):357–368.

Meurier, C. E., C. A. Vincent, and D. G. Parmar (1998). Perception of causes of omissions in the assessment of patients with chest pain. *J Advan Nurs* 28(5):1012–1019.

Moskowitz, E. and C. McCann (1957). Classification of disability in the chronically ill and aging. *J Chronic Dis* 5:342–346.

Murray, R., and J. Zentner (1997). *Health assessment and promotion: Strategies through the life span.* 6th ed. Stamford, CT: Appleton & Lange.

"NANDA. Forging LINKS to the Future." Business meeting of the 14th Biennial Conference on Nursing Diagnosis. April 5–8, 2000. Orlando, FL: North America Nursing Diagnosis Association.

Neal, L. J. (1998). Current functional assessment tools. *Home Healthcare Nurse,* 16(11):766–772.

North American Nursing Diagnosis Association (1986). *Classification of nursing diagnoses. Proceedings of the Sixth Conference.* St. Louis: C. V. Mosby.

Orem, D. E. (1991). *Nursing: Concepts of practice.* 4th ed. St. Louis: Mosby-Year Book.

Pender, N. J. (1996). *Health promotion in nursing practice*. 3rd ed. Stamford, CT: Appleton & Lange.

Pinnell, N., and M. de Meneses (1986). *The nursing process: Theory, application, and related processes*. Norwalk, CT: Appleton & Lange.

Roy, C. (1984). *Introduction to nursing: An adaptation model*. 2nd ed. Englewood Cliffs, NJ: Prentice Hall.

Roy, C. and H. A. Andrews (1991). *The Roy adaptation model: The definitive statement*. Norwalk, CT: Appleton & Lange.

Sarna, L. (1998). Effectiveness of structured nursing assessment of symptom distress in advanced lung cancer. *Oncol Nurs For* 25(6):1041–1048.

Sheehan, J. P. (1998). Assessment delays are a prescription for trouble. *RN* 61(6):56.

Spector, R. (1994). Strategies for multicultural nursing education: Heritage assessment. *Issues in Action Spring* (3):4–5. Redwood City, CA: Addison-Wesley Nursing.

Stewart, C. J. and W. B. Cash, Jr (1991) *Interviewing: Principles and practice*. 6th ed. Dubuque, IA: W. C. Brown.

Stoll, R. (1979). Guidelines for spiritual assessment. *Am J Nurs* 79:1574–77.

Straka, D. A. (1997). Are you listening? Have you heard? *Advan Prac Nurs Quart* 3(2):80–81.

Sumner, C. H. (1998). Recognizing and responding to spiritual distress. *AJN* 98(1):26–30.

Townsend, M. (1996). *Psychiatric mental health nursing*. 2nd ed. Philadelphia: F. A. Davis.

Yancey, R., B. A. Given, N. J. White, et al (1998). Computerized documentation for a rural nursing intervention project . . . the rural partnership linkage for cancer care. *Computers in Nursing* 16(5):275–284.

Ziegler, S. (1993). *Theory-directed nursing practice*. New York: Springer Publishing.

Zimmerman, P. G. (1998). Effective communication with patients with dementia. *J Emerg Nurs* 24(5):412–415.

4

Diagnostic Reasoning

Learning Outcomes

On completion of this chapter you should be able to do the following:

- Explain how diagnosis is related to the other phases of the nursing process.
- Explain what is meant by *present health status*.
- Identify patient strengths, wellness diagnoses, nursing diagnoses, medical diagnoses, and collaborative problems.
- Recognize actual, potential, and possible nursing diagnoses.
- Compare the advantages and disadvantages of computer-aided diagnosis.
- State ways in which nursing diagnoses can be used with critical pathways.
- Describe a process for diagnostic reasoning.
- Use standards of reasoning to evaluate your diagnostic thinking.
- Describe common diagnostic errors and explain how to prevent them with critical thinking.
- Discuss the ethical implications of the diagnostic process.

■ INTRODUCTION

This chapter will: (1) discuss diagnosis as a step of the nursing process; (2) define *patient health status*, (3) help you begin to differentiate between a problem and other phenomena, such as symptoms; and (4) explain the diagnostic reasoning process.

This chapter will help you to identify and describe client health status, including problems, more precisely. The diagnostic process is not just a matter of choosing labels from a list. The labels must accurately reflect the client's health status. This chapter deals with the broad concepts of *problems* and *health status,* not just with nursing diagnoses. Standardized North American Nursing Diagnosis Association (NANDA) terminology will be introduced in Chapter 5.

Both students and practicing nurses tend to see diagnosis as the most difficult aspect of the nursing process. One of the difficulties is that *diagnosis* is both a process and a product, that is:

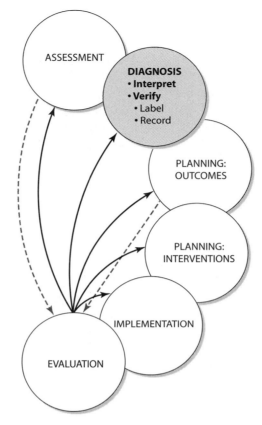

Figure 4–1
The Diagnosis Phase: Interpreting data and verifying the diagnoses

1. *Diagnosis* names a phase of the nursing process.
2. *Diagnosis* (or *diagnostic reasoning*) is a reasoning process that nurses use to interpret patient data.
3. The end product of that reasoning process is a statement of health status that is called a *nursing diagnosis.*
4. In order to write the diagnostic statement, nurses refer to a standardized list of terms that are called *nursing diagnoses* (eg, see the inside front cover of this text).

In the literature, you will see *diagnosis* used in all those ways. To minimize confusion, this text uses the terms as they are shown in Figure 4–2.

■ DIAGNOSIS: SECOND PHASE OF NURSING PROCESS

In the second phase of the nursing process, nurses use diagnostic reasoning to analyze data and draw conclusions about the client's health status. They

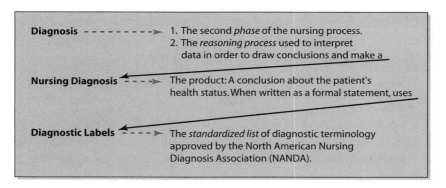

Figure 4–2
Diagnosis Terminology

verify these conclusions with the client, select standardized labels, and record them on the care plan.

Recall from Chapter 1 that the steps of the nursing process are interdependent and overlapping. Diagnosis is a pivotal step. All activities preceding this step are directed toward formulating the nursing diagnoses. All the care-planning activities following this step are based on the nursing diagnoses (see Figure 4–3 below).

Diagnosis depends on the assessment phase because the quality of the data acquired during assessment affects the accuracy of the nursing diagnoses. Also, the two stages overlap. Like most nurses, the nurse in the following example begins to interpret some of the data (diagnosis) at the same time she is collecting it (assessment).

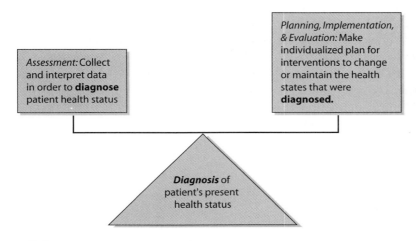

Figure 4–3
Diagnosis: A Pivotal Step in the Nursing Process

EXAMPLE: While interviewing Keisha Mandela, the school nurse notices that the child is speaking hesitantly and softly, giving brief answers and avoiding eye contact. She wonders if Keisha is shy, withdrawn, anxious, or perhaps having difficulty with her self-concept. She continues to gather data to confirm or deny these possibilities. In the diagnosis step, the nurse will critically examine all the data she has gathered, and draw a firmer conclusion about its meaning.

Diagnosis also affects the planning, implementation, and evaluation steps. When specifically and accurately stated, the problems and strengths identified during diagnosis guide the nurse in developing appropriate goals and nursing orders for the care plan (planning). The diagnosis and implementation phases sometimes occur almost simultaneously. For example, in an emergency situation a nurse may take action (implementation) as soon as the urgent problem is recognized—before consciously making a plan or identifying the rest of the problems, or even before completely assessing the patient. Diagnosis also overlaps with the evaluation phase. During evaluation, the nurse determines whether the patient's health status has changed. If not, nursing diagnoses are reexamined to be sure they were diagnosed correctly and completely.

History of Nursing Diagnosis

The term *nursing diagnosis* began to appear in the nursing literature in the 1950s to describe the functions of a professional nurse (McManus 1951). Fry (1953) stated that nursing diagnosis is based on the client's needs for nursing, rather than medical care. Until that time nursing had been seen as a set of tasks, and nursing care was planned around those tasks. Nurses assisted physicians in treating diseases. They gathered data about patients to ensure that doctors could make medical diagnoses, not to plan nursing care.

In the 1960s, diagnosis was becoming an important part of the nursing process, but it was still necessary to establish that diagnosis was a thinking process that nurses could and should use and that they were not encroaching on medical territory.

In 1973, the American Nurses Association (ANA) *Standards of Nursing Practice* included nursing diagnosis as an important nursing activity, making it a legitimate function of professional nurses. During the 1970s and 1980s, the term *nursing diagnosis* was incorporated into nearly all state nurse practice acts, and diagnosis became a nursing obligation as well as a legal right. Diagnosis is now taught in most schools of nursing, commonly used in the literature, and frequently used by nurses to describe their practice. Refer to Box 4–1 for current standards of practice.

Importance of Nursing Diagnosis

Nursing diagnosis can benefit both nurses and healthcare consumers in the following ways:

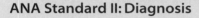 BOX 4–1

Professional Standards of Practice

ANA Standard II: Diagnosis

The nurse analyzes the assessment data in determining diagnoses.

Measurement Criteria

1. Diagnoses are derived from the assessment data.
2. Diagnoses are validated with the patient, family, and other healthcare providers, when possible and appropriate.
3. Diagnoses are documented in a manner that facilitates the determination of expected outcomes and plan of care.

Source: Reprinted with permission from American Nurses Association, *Standards of Clinical Nursing Practice 2nd ed.* (1998). American Nurses Publishing, American Nurses Foundation/American Nurses Association, 600 Maryland Ave. S.W. Washington, DC 20024-2571.

Canadian Nurses Association Standard II

Nursing practice requires the effective use of the nursing process.

Analysis of Data

2. Nurses are required to analyse data collected in accordance with their conception of the goal of nursing, their role, and the source of client difficulty. The nurse in any practice setting:
   2.1 interprets data in accordance with a conceptual model(s) and with knowledge from nursing and related fields.
   2.2 interprets data, taking into account the interdisciplinary plan of care.
   2.3 validates with the client or others, when possible, the interpretation of the data collected.
   2.4 identifies with the client actual or potential problems.
   2.5 sets priorities with the client for resolution of identified problems.
   2.6 communicates with others, when appropriate, about identified problems.

Source: CNA Standards for Nursing Practice (1987). Reprinted with permission of the Canadian Nurses Association: Ottawa, Ontario.

■ **Nursing diagnoses facilitate individualized care.** Driven by cost considerations, today's healthcare organizations emphasize standardized care as a way to promote efficiency and decrease cost. But even though patients with identical medical conditions may need similar nursing interventions, the priorities of care may differ for each (eg, see Box 4–2 on p. 148).

BOX 4–2

Prioritized Nursing Diagnoses for Two Patients with the Same Medical Diagnosis (Myocardial Infarction)

For Mary Chinn

1. Risk for Fluid Volume Deficit related to nausea and vomiting associated with pain and stress
2. Chest Pain related to reduced oxygenation of myocardium

3. Activity Intolerance related to decreased cardiac output

For Donald Schulz

1. Anxiety related to anticipation of financial difficulties because of absence from his business
2. Ineffective Breathing Pattern related to depressant effects of medications
3. Constipation related to decreased mobility, narcotics, and fear that straining will cause another heart attack.

Nursing diagnoses focus attention on a patient's unique needs, which may not be met by standardized plans of care.

- **Nursing diagnoses promote professional accountability and autonomy by defining and describing the independent area of nursing practice.** Nursing diagnosis language makes it clear that nurses do far more than simply carry out orders for medical treatments. It will help you to communicate to legislators, consumers, and insurance providers the unique care you deliver and the specific nature of the health conditions you treat.

- **Nursing diagnoses provide an effective vehicle for communication among nurses and other healthcare professionals.** Because a nursing diagnosis consolidates a great deal of information into a concise statement, it provides a "shorthand" means of communicating client status. For example, imagine you have collected the following data: Patient states his mouth is painful; his tongue is coated and mucous membranes are dry; there are vesicles and ulcerations in his mouth; his mouth has a strong odor. The nursing diagnosis, Altered Oral Mucous Membrane, gives you the same picture of the patient as that entire set of data.

- **Nursing diagnoses help determine assessment parameters.** Using the preceding example, once you have grasped the concept of Altered Oral Mucous Membrane, the term will alert you to other cues related to this diagnosis. For example, when you see that a patient is mouth breathing, you would check to see if his mucous membranes are dry and if he is drinking sufficient fluids.

■ HUMAN RESPONSES

Nurses diagnose **human responses**—reactions to an event or stressor such as disease or injury. Recall from Chapter 1 that *human responses occur in several dimensions.* They can be biological (physical), psychological, interpersonal/social, or spiritual.

> EXAMPLE: Consider the following ways a person might respond to the stressor of a myocardial infarction (heart attack).
>
> | | |
> |---|---|
> | Physical dimension: | Pain |
> | Psychological dimension: | Fear of dying |
> | Interpersonal/social dimension: | Returning to work before full recovery |
> | Spiritual dimension: | Praying |

Human responses occur at different levels: cellular, systemic, organic, or whole person (organismic). A cellular response occurs at the level of individual cells; for example, the ability of a cell to use glucose may change. Systemic responses occur in body systems, such as the circulatory or respiratory system (eg, peripheral vasodilation, increased respiratory rate). Localized skeletal muscle fatigue—in a runner's calves, for instance—is an example of organic response. Nursing occurs at and affects all levels, but nursing diagnosis is usually at the whole person or possibly the systemic level. A single stressor can cause multilevel responses.

> EXAMPLE: A person who is severely burned loses large amounts of body fluids. If the fluids are not replaced, she responds by losing water from the cells into the bloodstream (cellular level). The sympathetic nervous system responds to the trauma by decreasing the activity of the gastrointestinal system (systemic level). The person may respond by perceiving pain (whole-person level) or, later, by social isolation (social level).

KEY POINT
Human responses occur at different levels:

- Cells
- Systems
- Organs
- Whole person

Responses to stressors can be helpful as well as harmful. Human responses may be adaptive, helping to restore health; or they may be maladaptive and damaging to health. In fact, the same response can be helpful at one time and harmful at another.

> EXAMPLE: Mrs. Mason has a "chest cold" and a severe cough. She feels very ill. Her psychological response is *fear* (that she may have pneumonia). The fear motivates her to see her physician for treatment—an adaptive response.

> EXAMPLE: At a later time, Mrs. Mason has an episode of postmenopausal bleeding. Her psychological response is again *fear* (that she may have cancer). This time she is overwhelmed by her fear. She avoids seeing a physician because she is afraid he will tell her she has cancer, thereby making it real. This time the fear was a maladaptive response because it immobilized her instead of motivating her to act.

Refer to Table 4–1 for some examples of stressors and various types and levels of human responses. Notice that a response can become a stressor that produces still another response (eg, Mrs. Mason's fear produced avoidance).

You can recognize a **health problem** (maladaptive/harmful response) by the following characteristics. A health problem:

- is a human response to a life process, event, or stressor.
- is a health-related condition that both the patient and the nurse wish to change.
- requires intervention in order to prevent or resolve illness or to facilitate coping.
- results in ineffective coping, adaptation, or daily living that is unsatisfying to the patient.
- is an undesirable state.

While learning, you may confuse problems with various phenomena that are related but not the same. Table 4–2 provides examples of things that are *not* problems, but which act as stressors to cause a human response that *is* a problem.

■ DIAGNOSING HEALTH STATUS

The purpose of diagnosing is to identify the patient's *present health status*. A comprehensive care plan includes diagnostic statements describing patient health status in terms of (1) strengths, (2) wellness diagnoses, (3) actual,

Table 4–1 Examples of Stressors and Human Responses

Stressor	Human Response	Dimension	Level	Effect
Blocked coronary artery, causing decreased oxygen to heart muscle	Damage to heart muscle (ischemia)	Physical	Cellular and organic	Maladaptive
	Pain	Psychological and physical	Whole-person (organismic)	Adaptive, if causes decreased activity, conserving oxygen; maladaptive, if causes fight-or-flight response, increasing demand for oxygen
	Fear of death	Psychological	Whole-person	Can be adaptive or maladaptive (see above)
Fear of death from heart attack	Increased heart rate	Physical	Systemic	Probably maladaptive
	Praying	Spiritual	Whole-person	Probably adaptive

Table 4–2 Misunderstandings about Problems

A problem is NOT:	Examples (Incorrect)	The Problem (Human Response) is:
A nursing goal or a nursing problem	Urinary drainage device will be kept patent and draining freely.	Bladder distention
	Patient is noisy and disturbs other patients.	Anxiety; confusion, disorientation

Implications for the nurse: View the problem from the patient's perspective. The "problem" is the response (1) that will occur if the nurse's goal is not met, or (2) that is causing the nurse's problem.

A nursing action or routine	Give emotional support.	Anxiety; fear; grief; powerlessness
	Check urinary catheter hourly for patency.	Risk for urinary tract infection

Implications for the nurse: Get the right focus. The incorrect examples focus on *the nurse* (activities to be performed). Problems are statements of client health status—focus is on *the client.*

A diagnostic test, medical treatment, or equipment	Patient is having a barium enema.	Risk for constipation; embarrassment
	New colostomy	Lack of knowledge and skill in caring for the appliance; fear of social contact; impaired skin integrity around the stoma
	Must stay on a salt-free diet	Lack of motivation to change eating habits; lack of knowledge of high-sodium foods
	Patient has cast on leg.	Decreased mobility; itching
	Patient has new dentures.	Change in body image; speech distortion

Implications for the nurse: Patients may respond in many ways to the same treatment. A list of treatments does not provide enough direction for individualizing care. Remember that the problem is the patient's *response* to the test/treatment.

A patient need	Need more sleep	Fatigue; sleep-pattern disturbance; depression
	Needs emotional support	Grief; poor self-concept; anxiety

Implications for the nurse: An unmet need may be the *cause* of a problem; but it is not the same thing as a problem. As a rule, do not use the word "need" in stating problems.

potential, and possible nursing diagnoses, (4) collaborative problems, and (5) medical problems. Although their responsibility is different for each type of problem, nurses analyze data for all types. Nurses cannot legally make definitive medical diagnoses, but they are expected to recognize and refer situations that are beyond their diagnostic and treatment expertise (ie, medical problems). Remember, all problems belong to the *patient.* No one profession "owns" any of the problems. Nursing, collaborative, and medical diagnoses are all addressed, to at least some extent, by all members of the multidisciplinary health team.

Patient Strengths

It is important to integrate patient (family, community) strengths into the plan of care. **Strengths** are those areas of normal, healthy functioning that will help the patient to achieve higher levels of wellness or to prevent, control, or resolve problems. Strengths can be physical (eg, good nutritional status enables a client to heal faster after surgery), psychological (eg, good coping and problem-solving skills), psychosocial (eg, a strong family support system), and spiritual (eg, strong personal values). When identifying spiritual strengths, you might ask questions such as: "What is the most important and powerful thing in your life? Is faith important in your life?" and "What can you do to show love for yourself?" (Burkhardt as cited in Dossey, 1998, p. 45). You can find strengths in the health examination data and the nursing database (eg, information about health practices, home life, education, recreation, exercise, work, friends, and religious beliefs).

KEY POINT
Examples of Strengths

- Sense of humor
- Motivation to change
- Extended family, supportive
- Good knowledge of disease process
- History of successful coping
- Good problem-solving skills
- Good cardiovascular and respiratory reserve
- Balanced diet
- Strong religious faith

Wellness Diagnoses

Wellness diagnoses describe areas in which a healthy client is functioning normally—there is no problem, but the person wishes to achieve a higher level of wellness. For example, a client may be within normal weight limits, but wish to increase the fiber-content of his diet. Or perhaps the client has no apparent problems, but wants to begin an exercise program. In such cases, you would make a wellness diagnosis. A **wellness diagnosis** is a statement reflecting a client's healthy responses in areas where the nurse can intervene to promote growth or maintenance of the healthy response. NANDA defines a wellness diagnosis as describing "human responses to levels of wellness in an individual, family, or community that have a potential for enhancement to a higher state" (1999, p. 149).

KEY POINT
Examples of Wellness Diagnoses

- Effective Breastfeeding related to maternal confidence and experience
- Potential for Enhanced Community Coping related to active civic groups
- Potential for Enhanced Family Coping related to strong social supports

Recognizing Nursing Diagnoses

A **nursing diagnosis** is a statement about the patient's present health status. It describes an actual, potential (risk), or possible problem that nurses can legally diagnose and for which they can prescribe the primary treatment and prevention measures (see Table 4–3 on p. 151). The key term here is *primary*. Nurses may not prescribe *all* the care for a nursing diagnosis (for instance, most patients with a nursing diagnosis of Pain have medical orders for analgesics); but if it is a nursing diagnosis, the nurse can prescribe *most* of the interventions needed to prevent or resolve the problem. Usually the nurse does not need to confer with a physician about treatments for nursing diagnoses.

Table 4–3 Comparison of Nursing Diagnoses, Collaborative Problems, and Medical Diagnoses

Category	Nursing Diagnoses	Collaborative Problems	Medical Diagnoses
Example	Activity Intolerance related to decreased cardiac output	Potential complication of myocardial infarction (heart attack): congestive heart failure	Myocardial infarction
Description	Describe human responses to disease process or stressors; written as one-, two-, or three-part statements.	Describe potential physiologic complications of disease, tests, or treatments; written as two-part statements	Describe disease and pathology; do not consider other human responses; usually written in three words or less
Problem status	Actual, potential, or possible	Always potential	Actual or possible ("rule out")
Duration	Can change frequently; not associated with a particular medical diagnosis	Present when the disease (or medical diagnosis) is present	Remains the same while the pathology exists
Orientation	Oriented to the individual	Oriented to pathophysiology (potential complications)	Oriented to pathology and medical procedures
Responsibility for diagnosing	Nurses are responsible for diagnosing	Nurses are responsible for diagnosing	Physician responsible for diagnosing; diagnosis not within scope of nursing practice
Nursing Focus	Treat and prevent	Prevent and monitor for onset or status of the complication	Implement medical orders for treatment; monitor status of condition
Treatment orders	Nurse can order most interventions to prevent and treat	Requires medical orders for definitive prevention and treatment; nurse may order some preventive measures	Physician orders primary interventions to prevent and treat
Nursing actions	Independent	Some independent actions, but primarily for monitoring	Dependent (primarily)
Classification system	Classification systems (eg, NANDA) are developed and being used, but not universally accepted	No classification system	Well-developed classification universally accepted by the medical profession

Source: Adapted with permission from Kozier et al (2000) *Fundamentals of nursing.* 6th ed. Upper Saddle River, NJ: Prentice Hall Health, p. 295.

Because human responses vary, you cannot predict with certainty which nursing diagnoses will occur with a particular disease or treatment. Any number of nursing diagnoses may—or may not—occur with a particular medical diagnosis (eg, see Box 4–2 on p. 148). You cannot assume, for example, that someone with diabetes will have Fear of Injections or Lack of Knowledge about a diabetic diet.

Actual Nursing Diagnoses

An actual nursing diagnosis is a problem that is actually present at the time you make the assessment. You would recognize it by the presence of associated signs and symptoms (defining characteristics). Nursing care is directed toward relieving, resolving, or coping with actual problems.

EXAMPLE: The Crain family is experiencing many stressors. The parents, Todd and Dana, are caring for their son, Billy, who has leukemia; and Dana has had to quit her job. While making a family visit, the nurse observes that when Todd tries to discipline Billy, Dana interferes to protect him. In a later conversation, Todd tells the nurse, "I mostly just stay out of it. She can take care of Billy better than I can anyway." Dana confirms that Todd has withdrawn from contact with his son. The nurse diagnoses an *actual problem,* Ineffective Family Coping (Compromised) related to family disorganization and role changes.

Potential (Risk) Nursing Diagnoses

A **potential** (or **risk**) **nursing diagnosis** is one that is likely to develop if the nurse does not intervene. You will diagnose them by the presence of risk factors that predispose a patient to developing a problem. Nursing care is directed toward preventing the problem by reducing the risk factors, or toward early detection of the problem to lessen its consequences.

EXAMPLE: Marianne Akiba is a single parent whose child, Janelle, has a new medical diagnosis of leukemia. The nurse knows that Marianne has only one or two people she can turn to for emotional or other support. In an interview, Marianne indicates, "I don't know anything about this disease or how to take care of my child." Although the nurse sees no signs of ineffective coping, she realizes that lack of knowledge and support place this family at risk, so she makes a *potential nursing diagnosis* of Risk for Ineffective Family Coping (Compromised) related to limited support system and lack of knowledge.

A potential (risk) nursing diagnosis should be used only for patients who have a higher than normal risk for developing a problem—those who have more risk factors than the general group to which they belong. NANDA says that a **risk nursing diagnosis:** "describes human responses to health conditions/life processes which may develop in a vulnerable individual, family or community. It is supported by risk factors that contribute to increased vulnerability" (1999, p. 149).

For those who have the same risk as the general population, a collaborative problem (potential complication) can be used (refer to Table 4–3 on p.

153). For example, *all* patients receiving a general anesthetic are at risk for respiratory problems. However, for those who have no risk factors in addition to the surgery, routine postoperative "turn-cough-deep breathe" treatment is adequate; their care planning could be based on the collaborative problem, Potential Complications of Surgery (Respiratory). On the other hand, if a patient is a smoker and is given general anesthesia for a high abdominal incision, his respiratory status merits special attention. He is at higher risk than the general population of surgery patients, so the nurse should write a nursing diagnosis of "Risk for Altered Respiratory Function related to high abdominal incision and smoking."

Possible Nursing Diagnoses

A **possible nursing diagnosis** similar to a physician's "rule-out" diagnosis, is one that you tentatively believe to exist. You have enough data to suspect a problem, but not enough to be sure. A possible problem directs nursing care toward gathering focus data to confirm or eliminate the diagnosis. Using possible problems can help you avoid: (1) omitting an important diagnosis and (2) making an incorrect diagnosis because of insufficient data.

> EXAMPLE: A patient who has had abdominal surgery has no history of smoking and has been adhering to the schedule of turning, coughing, and deep breathing every 2 hours. Still, she is slightly pale and reports that she feels "a little short of breath." The nurse auscultates and finds no abnormal breath sounds. There are no other signs of respiratory distress, but the nurse wants to be sure the situation is carefully evaluated by other shifts, so she diagnoses a *possible problem*: Possible Ineffective Airway Clearance.

Recognizing Collaborative Problems

Carpenito states that **collaborative problems** are "certain physiological complications that nurses monitor to detect their onset or changes in status. Nurses manage collaborative problems by utilizing physician-prescribed and nursing-prescribed interventions to minimize the complications of the events" (1997, p. 27). Independent nursing interventions for collaborative problems focus on monitoring for and minimizing complications. Definitive treatment of the condition requires *both* medical and nursing interventions (see Table 4–3 on page 153).

Because there are a limited number of physiological complications for a given disease, the same collaborative problems—unlike nursing diagnoses—tend to be present any time a particular disease or treatment is present. That is, each disease or treatment has particular complications that are always associated with it. For example, all postpartum patients have similar collaborative problems (potential complications), such as postpartum hemorrhage

KEY POINT
Actual Nursing Diagnosis

- Problem present
- Signs and symptoms present

Potential (Risk) Nursing Diagnosis

- Problem may develop
- Risk factors present

Possible Nursing Diagnosis

- Unsure if problem is present
- Some signs/ symptoms present, but not definitive
- Data incomplete

KEY POINT
Collaborative Problems

- Usually physio-logic complica-tions of a disease or treatment.
- Nurses collabo-rate with other healthcare professionals to treat and prevent.
- Independent nursing actions focus on moni-toring for onset of problem.

and thrombophlebitis. But not all new mothers have the same nursing diagnoses. Some might experience Altered Parent/Infant/Child Attachment (delayed bonding), but most will not. Some might have a Knowledge Deficit problem; others will not.

Collaborative problems (potential complications) are *potential* problems. The patient's medical diagnosis, treatments, and medications are the risk factors (or stressors). The following guidelines will help you to predict and detect potential complications:

1. *Look up the patient's medical diagnosis.* What are the most common complications associated with it? You can find this information in textbooks, journals, and in patient records (eg, diagnostic studies, medical history). Appendix C is a comprehensive list of collaborative problems that are commonly associated with various diseases and pathophysiologies.
2. *Look up all the patient's medications.* Serious side effects, toxicity, drug interactions, and other adverse reactions are potential complications (eg, Potential Complication of Magnesium Sulfate Therapy: Hypermagnesemia).
3. *Look up the most common complications associated with the patient's surgery, treatments, or tests.* Again, you may need to refer to a text or other references. Appendix D lists complications associated with various surgeries. Table 4–4 lists examples of collaborative problems associated with various tests and treatments.
4. *Be sure you know the signs and symptoms of the potential complications, so you will know what assessments are needed.* For example, the early symptoms of Potential Complication of Magnesium Sulfate Therapy: Hypermagnesemia are profound thirst, depressed reflexes, sedation, confusion, and muscle weakness. Thus, in addition to monitoring lab results of plasma magnesium levels, you would regularly assess for those symptoms. Review agency procedures, protocols, and critical paths for your patient's condition (eg, the agency may have a protocol for peritoneal dialysis or oxygen administration).

Recognizing Medical Diagnoses

Although both medical and nursing diagnoses are made by using a diagnostic reasoning process, they are quite different. A **medical diagnosis** identifies a disease process or pathology and is made for the purpose of treating the pathology. It does not necessarily consider the human responses to the pathology.

EXAMPLE: The physician diagnoses hypertension and prescribes antihypertensive medications and a low-salt diet. The nurse will diagnose and treat the patient's and family's responses to the medical diagnosis. Is the patient motivated to change his diet? What changes will the family

Table 4–4   Multidisciplinary (Collaborative) Problems Associated With Tests and Treatments

Test or Treatment	Potential Complications (Collaborative Problems)	
Arteriogram	Allergic reaction Embolism Hemorrhage; hematoma	Paresthesia Renal failure Thrombosis at site
Bone Marrow Studies	Bleeding	Infection
Bronchoscopy	Airway obstruction/bronchoconstriction	Hemorrhage
Cardiac Catheterization	Cardiac arrhythmias Embolism, thrombus Hypervolemia Hypovolemia	Infarction, perforation Paresthesia Site hemorrhage or hematoma
Casts and Traction	Bleeding Edema Impaired circulation	Misalignment of bones Neurological compromise
Chemotherapy (antineoplastic drugs)	Anaphylactic reaction Anemia Central nervous system toxicity Congestive heart failure Electrolyte imbalance Enteritis	Hemorrhagic cystitis Leukopenia Necrosis at IV site Pneumonitis Renal failure Thrombocytopenia
Chest tubes	Bleeding leading to hemothorax Blockage or displacement leading to pneumothorax	Septicemia
Foley catheter	Bladder distention (tube not patent)	Urinary tract infection
Hemodialysis	Air embolism Bleeding Dialysis dementia Electrolyte imbalance Embolism	Transfusion reactions Shunt clotting; fistulas Infection/septicemia Hepatitis B Fluid shifts
Intravenous (IV) therapy	Fluid overload Infiltration	Phlebitis
Medications	Allergic reactions Side effects (specify)	Toxic effects/overdose (specify)
Nasogastric suction	Electrolyte imbalance	
Radiation therapy	Fistulas, tissue necrosis Hemorrhage	Radiation burns Radiation pneumonia
Tracheal suctioning	Bleeding	Hypoxia
Ventilation (assisted)	Acid-base imbalance Airway obstruction (tube plugged or displaced) Ineffective oxygen–carbon dioxide exchange	Pneumothorax Respirator dependence Tracheal necrosis

Source: Wilkinson, J. M. (1999). *Nursing diagnosis handbook—with NIC interventions and NOC outcomes.* 7th ed. Upper Saddle River, NJ: Prentice Hall Health.

need to make to incorporate the diet change into their menu plan? Does the patient understand the importance of taking his medications, even though they may have unpleasant side effects? If the patient is hospitalized, the nurse will give the medications prescribed by the physician.

As long as the disease process is present, the medical diagnosis does not change. Nursing diagnoses, on the other hand, change as the client's responses change. In the preceding example, the nursing diagnosis might initially be "Risk for Noncompliance with medication regimen related to lack of understanding of therapeutic and side effects of the drug." However, as the patient shows knowledge of the drug and takes it as prescribed, this diagnosis would no longer apply. If the patient found the side effects unpleasant and continued to skip doses of the drug, the diagnosis might change to actual "Noncompliance with medication regimen. . . ." Remember that clients who have the same medical diagnosis may have very different nursing diagnoses. Consider the example of Mary Chinn and Donald Schulz, in Box 4–2 on p. 148, who both have a medical diagnosis of myocardial infarction (heart attack), but who have very different nursing diagnoses.

Nurses make observations pertinent to patients' medical diagnoses and perform treatments delegated by the physician. Although nurses do not diagnose or prescribe treatments for medical problems, nursing judgment is required. Nurses must know the pathophysiology of the disease and understand why the medications or treatments are being given.

See Figure 4–4 for a decision tree to help you determine whether a problem is a nursing diagnosis, a collaborative problem, or a medical problem.

??? THINKING POINT

Refer to Figure 4–4 on page 159. Each of the following patients has undergone major abdominal surgery (a medical procedure). Determine whether each set of cues represents a nursing diagnosis, a medical diagnosis, or a collaborative problem.

Patient A. Four days after surgery, incision is red, oozing pus, and not healing—symptoms of an infection.

Patient B. Two days after surgery, the patient's vital signs are normal, but he is breathing shallowly and not moving very much. These cues represent risk factors for postoperative pneumonia.

Patient C. The patient has just returned from surgery. The surgical dressing is dry, but must be monitored to assure that surgical hemostasis was obtained and that no excessive bleeding will occur.

Computer-Assisted Diagnosis

In some agencies, nurses use computers to classify and interpret assessment data. Such application programs, called **expert** (or **knowledge based**) **systems,**

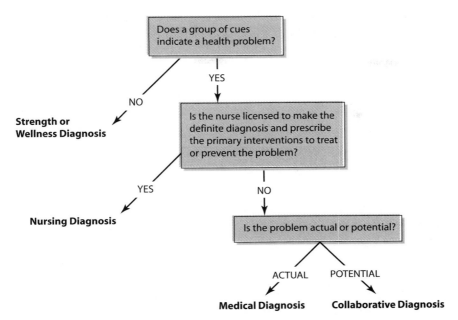

Figure 4–4

Decision Tree for Nursing Diagnoses and Collaborative Problems

are a kind of artificial intelligence that uses reasoning to infer conclusions from stored facts. After the nurse enters the data, the software compares the cues to those that are associated with each nursing diagnosis in its database. It then generates a list of abnormal cues or a list of possible diagnoses (see Figure 4–5), and the nurse chooses which diagnoses to accept or reject or add to the list. When the nurse chooses a diagnostic label, the next screen shows that label with all its associated signs and symptoms so that the nurse can compare them to the actual patient data (see Figure 4–6). If the nurse accepts the diagnostic label, she completes the problem statement by choosing the appropriate etiologies (causes) of the problem from the next screen (see Figure 4–7).

The advantages of computer-assisted diagnosis are that computers are consistent, systematic, and organized. They do not experience fatigue, distraction, or other human weaknesses; therefore, they are able to identify patterns the nurse might overlook. You must use professional judgment in evaluating the computer-generated diagnoses, however. The computer will assume that all the patient data is true, correct, and current. You must be sure this is so. Furthermore, patients respond to health problems in infinite ways, so it is impossible to predict all combinations of cues and all possible diagnoses. And finally, some NANDA nursing diagnoses have very small databases, making accurate diagnosis difficult.

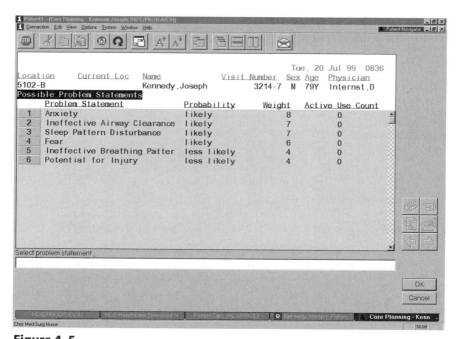

Figure 4–5

List of Suggested Nursing Diagnoses (NANDA), Computer Generated From Assessment Data (Courtesy of Per-Se Technologies, Atlanta, GA)

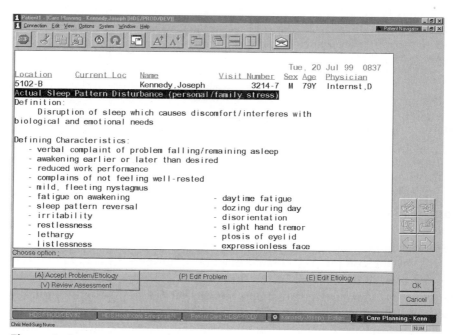

Figure 4–6

Definition and Defining Characteristics of a Selected NANDA Diagnostic Label (Courtesy of Per-Se Technologies, Atlanta, GA)

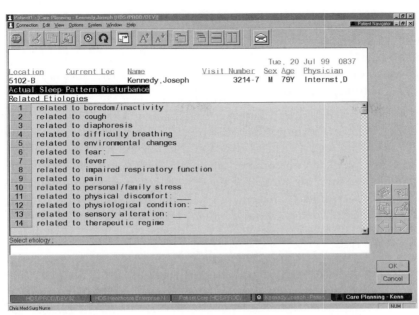

Figure 4–7

The Nurse Chooses the "Related Factors" for the Selected Nursing Diagnosis From the List Prompted by the System (Courtesy of Per-Se Technologies, Atlanta, GA)

Using Nursing Diagnoses with Critical Pathways

Many organizations use a system called *managed care* to standardize care for the medical diagnoses they treat most often. Each common medical diagnosis has a preprinted, standardized care plan called a **critical pathway** that indicates the patient and family outcomes that should occur within a specified time frame. The critical pathway is a multidisciplinary plan that outlines the crucial care to be given for all patients of a certain type (eg, all patients undergoing cardiac catheterization). Critical pathways are not designed to meet the unique needs of individual patients. Nevertheless, nursing diagnoses can be used successfully with critical pathways.

Nursing Diagnosis Incorporated Into Critical Pathway

The critical pathway replaces the traditional (nursing diagnosis) care plan for many clients. It is a standardized plan for outcomes and care for "all" clients. Nursing diagnoses are unique to the individual and cannot really be predicted to occur in the presence of particular diseases and treatments. However, some agencies do include in the critical pathway the nursing diagnoses most often seen with the medical diagnosis (eg, a critical pathway for total knee replacement might include nursing diagnoses of Pain and Impaired Mobility).

Nursing Diagnosis Used to Name Variance

Some agencies use nursing diagnoses to name variances from the predicted outcomes and time frames and to develop an individualized plan for achieving revised outcomes. A **variance** occurs when the patient does not achieve a goal in the time predicted by the critical pathway.

> EXAMPLE: The critical pathway for a patient with newly diagnosed type 1 diabetes would not include a nursing diagnosis, but rather would list "teaching needs" for each day. On day 5, if the patient is unable to meet the predicted outcome of self-injection, the nurse would identify and analyze this "variance." The nurse would then write a nursing diagnosis of "Ineffective Management of Therapeutic Regimen . . ." to individualize the nursing care and hasten outcome achievement.

Nursing Diagnosis Used for Problems Not on the Critical Pathway

You should use nursing diagnoses to individualize care to meet unique patient needs that are not addressed by the standardized critical pathway. If *only* the standardized care is given, that care can probably be given by someone other than a nurse.

> EXAMPLE: Al Collins has had a myocardial infarction. He is also blind. The critical pathway outlines care only for his heart condition. The nurse writes a separate nursing diagnosis to provide information about the amount of help Mr. Collins needs with eating, ambulating, and other activities of daily living.

Critical pathways can improve care by indicating the most important care for a specific condition (eg, for a patient with pneumonia). However, they can impede care if task-oriented nurses use them in place of thinking. Busy caregivers who know the "routine" care on the pathway may rush through assessments and outcomes evaluation. Do not let the critical pathway, or any standardized approach, make a robot of you. Be alert for patient care needs that are *not* addressed by the critical pathway.

■ DIAGNOSTIC REASONING

Diagnosing is an intellectual activity in which nurses use critical thinking skills to identify patterns and draw conclusions about data. It is the same reasoning process that experts of any discipline use to draw conclusions about their phenomena of concern (that is, what they "work on"). Speech therapists diagnose speaking problems, teachers diagnose learning problems, and automobile mechanics diagnose engine problems. Diagnostic reasoning can be divided into three broad stages: (1) interpreting the data, (2) verifying the diagnosis, and (3) labeling (and recording) the diagnosis. Refer to Box 4–3 on page 164 for an overview of these processes.

Use of Nursing Models

How you define and recognize patient problems depends somewhat on the nursing model you use. For example, in the Roy model (1984) you would recognize a problem as a failure to adapt. In the Gordon (1994) model, you would recognize it as a dysfunctional health pattern; that is, a group of related cues that do not meet expected norms. The theory you use also helps determine problem etiologies—the "causes" of the problem.

Using a physiology theory, the cause of infant colic is swallowed air and intestinal gas. Using a psychology theory, the cause of colic might be excessive parental anxiety and tension. The concepts of a framework help you to recognize relationships between isolated pieces of data. Concepts cause clusters to stand out for your attention. For example, the concept of *fluid volume deficit* would help Luisa Sanchez's nurse (Chapter 3, Figure 3–2, on pp. 86–87) to notice that Luisa's decreased urine output, poor skin turgor, and elevated temperature were somehow related. This chapter will use Gordon's Functional Health Patterns as a framework for data analysis, continuing the example of Luisa Sanchez from Chapter 3.

Interpreting Data

After you organize and record the assessment data, you must analyze and interpret it in order to determine what it means. This section presents data interpretation as a series of steps in order to help you understand the process. In reality, it is a complex process, not a rigid set of linear steps to be accomplished one at a time. You must, of course, take some steps before others; but you should use these steps as guidelines, realizing you will do some of them simultaneously, move back and forth among them, and perhaps even intuit portions of them, especially as you gain clinical experience.

Data interpretation occurs at four levels (see Box 4–3 on page 164). In the first level, you identify significant cues; in the second level, you cluster cues and identify data gaps; in the third level, you identify the client's health status; and in the final level, you determine the probable causes of the problems.

Level I: Identify Significant Cues

In your initial analysis (level one), you will organize data and compare them to established norms to identify significant cues (Steps 1 and 2).

Step I. Organize the data. If you have made an initial, comprehensive assessment, the data will already be grouped by your data collection form.

a. *Rewrite all the database information according to your preferred framework* (see Box 4–4 on pages 165–166). While you are learning, this will make

BOX 4-3

Overview of Diagnostic Reasoning

Interpret the Data

Level I—Identify significant cues

1. *Organize data* in concise format, using a nursing framework.
2. *Compare individual data to standards and norms* to identify significant cues.

Level II—Cluster cues and identify data gaps

3. *Cluster significant cues;* look for patterns and relationships.
4. *Categorize clusters* according to your framework.
5. *Identify data gaps and inconsistencies.*

Level III—Draw conclusions about present health status.

6. *Think of as many explanations as possible for each cue cluster. Then decide which hypothesis best explains it.* (Note: You can sometimes identify both problem and etiology in this step.)
7. *Identify wellness diagnoses; actual, potential, and possible nursing diagnoses; collaborative problems; and medical problems.*
8. *Identify patient and family strengths.*

Level IV—Determine Etiologies and Categorize Problems

9. *Determine the etiologies of the problems.*
10. *Categorize problems according to your framework.*

Verify the Diagnoses

11. *Verify diagnoses and strengths* with patient, family, other professionals and references.

Label the Diagnoses

12. *Choose standardized problem label.* Write the formal health status statements: nursing and wellness diagnoses, collaborative problems, and strengths.
13. *Prioritize the problems.*

Record the Data

14. *Record the problem statements* on the appropriate documents: patient care plan, chart, etc.

BOX 4–4

Data for Luisa Sanchez, Organized According to Gordon's Functional Health Patterns

Luisa Sanchez, 28 years old, was admitted to the hospital with a productive cough and rapid, labored respirations. She stated that she has had a "chest cold" for 2 weeks and has been short of breath on exertion. Yesterday she began to experience a fever and "pain in my lungs." (See Figure 3–2 on pp. 86–87).

Health Perception/Health Management

Knows her medical diagnosis
Gives thorough medical history
Complying with Synthroid regimen
Relates progression of illness in detail
Realistic expectations (to have antibiotics and "go home in a day or two")
States usually eats "3 meals a day"

Nutritional/Metabolic

5 ft. 2 in. (158 cm) tall; weight 125 lb (56 kg)
"No appetite" since having "cold"
Reports nausea
Oral temp 103°F (39.4°C)
Decreased skin turgor
Mucous membranes dry and pale
Skin hot and pale, cheeks flushed
Synthroid 0.1 mg per day
History of appendectomy and partial thyroidectomy
Old surgical scars: anterior neck, RLQ abdomen
Has not eaten today; last fluids at noon today

Elimination

Last bowel movement yesterday: formed, "normal"
Urinary frequency and amount decreased × 2 days
Abdomen soft, not distended
Diaphoretic

Activity/Exercise

No musculoskeletal impairment
States, "I feel weak"
Short of breath on exertion
Exercises daily
Respirations shallow; chest expansion <3 cm
Blood pressure 122/80 sitting
Radial pulse weak, regular, rate = 92
Cough productive of pale, pink sputum
Inspiratory crackles auscultated throughout right upper and lower chest
Diminished breath sounds on right side

Sleep/Rest

Difficulty sleeping because of cough
"Can't breathe lying down"

Cognitive-Perceptual

No sensory deficits
Pupils 3 mm, equal, brisk reaction
Oriented to time, place, and person
Responsive, but fatigued
Responds appropriately to verbal and physical stimuli
Recent and remote memory intact
"I can think OK. Just weak."
States "short of breath" on exertion
"Pain in lungs," especially when coughing
Experiencing chills
Reports nausea

BOX 4–4

Data for Luisa Sanchez, Organized According to Gordon's Functional Health Patterns *(continued)*

Roles/Relationships

Lives with husband and 3-year-old daughter

Sexual relationship "satisfactory"

<u>Husband out of town;</u> will be back tomorrow

<u>Child with neighbor</u> until husband returns

States "good" relationships with friends and coworkers

Working mother, attorney

Husband helps "some" at home

Self-Perception/Self-Concept

<u>Expresses "concern" and "worry" about leaving daughter with neighbors until tomorrow</u>

Well-groomed; says, <u>"Too tired to mess with hair and makeup"</u>

Coping-Stress Tolerance

<u>Anxious: "I can't breathe"</u>

<u>Facial muscles tense; trembling</u>

"I can think OK. <u>Just weak.</u>"

<u>Expresses concerns about work: "I'll never get caught up"</u>

Value/Belief

Catholic. No special practices desired except last rites

Middle-class, professional orientation

No wish to see chaplain or priest at present

---

data gaps and inconsistencies more obvious and help you to see relationships among the cues.

b. *You do not have to use the same framework as the data collection form.* Luisa Sanchez's admission assessment (Figure 3–2 in Chapter 3) was organized according to body systems and specific nursing concerns (eg, screening for falls). In Box 4–4, those data are organized according to Gordon's Functional Health Patterns. As a rule, nurses use the assessment form categories to organize data. However, different models are used here to show differences in organizing frameworks and to demonstrate that you are not limited to the framework of the data collection form.

Step 2. Compare individual data to standards and norms (see Table 4–5 for examples). In this step you will use your knowledge of anatomy, physiology, psychology, developmental theory, and so on to *find significant cues.* Compare all data to such standards as norms for height and weight, lab values, nutritional requirements, social functioning, and coping skills. It may help you to *highlight, circle, or underline significant (abnormal) data,* as in Box 4–4.

Table 4–5 Comparing Cues to Standards and Norms (Examples)

Type of Cue	Client Cues (Examples)	Standard/Norm
Deviation from population norms	Height is 158 cm (5 ft 2 in). Woman with small frame. Weighs 109 kg (240 lbs).	Height and weight tables indicate the "ideal" weight for a woman 158 cm tall with a small frame is 49–53 kg (108–121 lbs).
Developmental delay	Child is 18 months old. Parents state child has not yet attempted to speak. Child laughs aloud and makes cooing sounds.	Children usually speak their first word by 10 to 12 months of age.
Changes in client's usual health status	States, "I'm just not hungry these days." Ate only 15% of food on breakfast tray. Has lost 13 kg (30 lbs) in past 3 months.	Client usually eats three balanced meals per day. Adults typically maintain stable weight.
Dysfunctional behavior	Amy's mother reports that Amy has not left her room for 2 days. Amy is 16 years old. Amy has stopped attending school and has withdrawn from social contact.	Adolescents usually like to be with their peers; social group very important. Functional behavior includes school attendance.
Changes in usual behavior	Mrs. Stuart reports that lately her husband angers easily. "Yesterday he even yelled at the dog." "He just seems too tense now."	Mr. Stuart is usually relaxed and easygoing. He is friendly and kind to animals.

Source: Adapted with permission from Kozier et al (2000). *Fundamentals of nursing* (6th ed). Upper Saddle River, NJ: Prentice Hall Health, p. 296.

Level II: Cluster Cues and Identify Data Gaps

The second level of analysis involves grouping the significant cues and identifying missing and inconsistent data (Steps 3–5).

Step 3. Cluster significant cues, looking for patterns and relationships among them.

a. *To begin clustering, look for cues that are repeated in more than one category (or pattern).* For example, Mrs. Sanchez reports being "too tired to mess with hair and makeup" in the Self-Perception/Self-Concept pattern. She reports "weakness" in both the Cognitive/Perceptual and Activity/Exercise patterns as well. Therefore, weakness is probably an important diagnostic cue.

b. *Next, group together (cluster) the cues that seem related.* Think about the relationships between facts.
  - Does Mrs. Sanchez's report of decreased urinary frequency (Elimination pattern) have anything to do with her decreased skin turgor and elevated temperature (Nutritional/Metabolic pattern)?

■ Why is she feeling weak? Is it related to her nausea (Nutritional/Metabolic), her cough (Activity/Exercise), or both? Or neither?

As you compare data across the categories of your framework, some seemingly normal data may take on new significance. In Box 4–4, in the Roles/Relationships pattern, the fact that Mrs. Sanchez's husband is out of town is, by itself, not a concern. However, taken with her expression of worry (Self-Perception/Self-Concept) and her anxiety (Coping/Stress), the information about her husband seems more significant. That is why it is underlined in Box 4–4, even though it seems normal when considered by itself.

c. *While you are learning, you should make another written list, using only the significant (abnormal) clustered data.* The way you form cue clusters will depend on whether you reason deductively or inductively (refer to "Reasoning" in Chapter 2, on pages 56–57).

If you use *deductive reasoning,* you would list all the significant cues, underlined in Box 4–4, under the appropriate categories of your framework. For example, the abnormal cues from two categories in Box 4–4 would be listed as follows:

Self-Perception/Self-Concept
Expresses "concern" and "worry" about leaving daughter with neighbors until tomorrow
"Too tired to mess with hair and makeup"

Roles/Relationships
Husband out of town (back tomorrow)
Child with neighbor

Using *inductive reasoning,* as shown in Table 4–6, you would make your new list of cue clusters by grouping all significant cues (underlined in Box 4–4) that are related, regardless of the pattern in which individual cues are found. For each significant cue, look for all other data that seem related to it. You may find the same cue appearing in more than one cluster (eg, in Table 4–6, "Can't breathe lying down" appears in Cluster 4 and Cluster 6). The remainder of this chapter illustrates an inductive approach to data interpretation.

???

THINKING POINT

Think about each of the following cue clusters. Do the cues fit together? Explain your reasoning.

Cluster 1—Osteoarthritis, difficulty getting out of bed, stiff joints, walks with walker

Cluster 2—Longstanding diabetes, legally blind, states feels lonely, wears glasses

Cluster 3—Incontinent of urine, wears incontinence pants, drinks adequate fluids, reddened area over coccyx

Cluster 4—Has bowel movement only every 3–4 days, sedentary lifestyle, history of urinary tract infections

Table 4–6 Luisa Sanchez Data—Related Cues Suggesting Problem Responses (Clustered Inductively)

Related Cues (Clusters)	Functional Health Pattern	Tentative Problem Statement (Inference)
Cluster 1 No significant cues	Health Perception/ Health Management	*Strength:* Healthy lifestyle; understanding and compliance with treatment regimens
Cluster 2 "No appetite" since having "cold" Reports nausea × 2 days Has not eaten today; last fluids at noon today	Nutritional/Metabolic Requirements	*(Nursing diagnosis)* Altered Nutrition: Less than Body
Cluster 3 "No appetite" since having "cold" Reports nausea × 2 days Last fluids at noon today Oral temp 103°F (39.4°C) Skin hot and pale, cheeks flushed Mucous membranes dry Poor skin turgor Decreased urinary frequency and amount × 2 days Diaphoresis	Nutritional/Metabolic (includes hydration) or ~~Elimination~~	*(Nursing diagnosis)* Fluid Volume Deficit. Cues include elimination *data,* but are not an elimination *problem.* Decreased urine is a symptom of a fluid volume problem.
Cluster 4 Difficulty sleeping because of cough "Can't breathe lying down" States, "I feel weak" Short of breath on exertion	Sleep/Rest or ~~Activity-Exercise~~	*(Nursing diagnosis)* Sleep Pattern Disturbance
Cluster 5 Taking Synthroid 0.1 mg/day Old surgical scar on anterior neck	Nutritional/Metabolic	*(Medical treatment)* Not a problem as long as patient follows regimen.
Cluster 6 Difficulty sleeping because of cough "Can't breathe lying down" Short of breath on exertion States, "I feel weak" Responsive but fatigued "I can think OK, just weak" Radial pulse rate 92, weak	~~Sleep/Rest~~ or Activity/Exercise or ~~Cognitive/Perceptual~~	*(Nursing diagnosis)* Activity Intolerance or Self-Care Deficit (needs help with hygiene, etc. because of weakness). Cues from other patterns are contributing to the problem in the Activity/Exercise pattern.
Cluster 7 Reports chills Oral temp 103°F (39.4°C) Diaphoretic	Cognitive/Perceptual or ~~Nutritional/Metabolic~~	*(Nursing diagnosis)* Problem is altered comfort (chills); elevated temp is contributing to problem

Table 4-6 *(continued)*

Related Cues (Clusters)	Functional Health Pattern	Tentative Problem Statement (Inference)
Cluster 8 Husband out of town; will be back tomorrow Child with neighbor until husband returns	Roles/Relationships or ~~Coping/Stress~~	*(Nursing diagnosis)* Altered Family Processes because parents temporarily unavailable to care for child
Cluster 9 Husband out of town; will be back tomorrow Child with neighbor until husband returns Expresses "concern" and "worry" over leaving child with neighbors until husband returns Anxious: "I can't breathe" Facial muscles tense; trembling Concerns about work: "I'll never get caught up"	~~Roles/Relationships~~ or Self-Perception/ Self-Concept or ~~Coping/Stress~~	*(Nursing diagnosis)* Anxiety is a problem; the Roles/Relationships and Coping/Stress cues are contributing to (causing) the anxiety
Cluster 10 "Pain in lungs," especially when coughing Cough productive of pale, pink sputum	Cognitive/Perceptual	*(Nursing diagnosis)* Chest pain
Cluster 11 Skin hot and pale Respirations shallow; chest expansion < 3 cm (1¼ in.) Cough productive of pale, pink sputum Inspiratory crackles auscultated throughout right upper and lower chest Diminished breath sounds on right side Mucous membranes pale	Activity/Exercise (pattern includes respiratory and cardiovascular status)	*(Medical problem)* Pneumonia *(Collaborative problems:* respiratory insufficiency, septic shock) *(Nursing diagnosis)* Ineffective Airway Clearance caused by disease process

Step 4. Next, decide which framework category (pattern) is represented by each new cue cluster. Identifying the category in which the problem occurs helps to narrow your search for the specific problem. Clustering is "messy" because there are many ways to group cues and they do not fall neatly into a single category.

■ *You may have more than one cue cluster in a pattern* (eg, in Table 4–6, on page 169, Clusters 2 and 3 represent the Nutritional/Metabolic pattern)

- *A cue cluster may suggest more than one pattern.* If so, list them all—it may be that the cue cluster represents more than one problem. Cluster 3, for example, yields two problems: a fluid volume problem and a potential oral mucous membrane problem.
- *A cue cluster may fit only one pattern, but you may not be sure at first which one.* If this occurs, list all the patterns that seem to fit (as in Table 4–6). After you think more about the relationships among the cues and recognize specific problems, you may be better able to identify the pattern. For example, some Cluster 3 cues fit in both the Nutritional/Metabolic and the Elimination patterns. Only as you begin to determine cause and effect does it become clear that the problem response occurs in the Nutritional/Metabolic pattern, and that the Elimination cues are merely symptoms of the problem.

Look for overlap in the clusters. If there is overlap, see if you can find a way to combine the clusters or the cues differently. The goal is to find a set of clusters that is thorough and efficient—that addresses all the patient's strengths and problems, but does not include problems the nurse can do nothing about. Be sure to consider various ways to group the cues.

Step 5. Identify data gaps and inconsistencies. Ideally, data will have been completed and validated during the assessment phase. However, the need for certain data may not be apparent until you cluster and begin to look for meaning in the data.

- *Look for inconsistencies.* Does the information in one cue cluster contradict that in another? Do your objective findings conflict with what the patient has said? Has the client given you the same information about concerns and strengths as other team members?
- *See if you have enough data to support or rule out your hunches about the meaning of the clusters.* For example, if in Clusters 8 and 9 you did not know that Mrs. Sanchez's husband was "out of town and coming back tomorrow," you would probably look at the clusters and think, "I wonder where her husband has gone and when he'll return. How long will the child need to stay with the neighbors? Why is she worried about leaving the child with them?"

Your patient complains of abdominal cramping. He states that even though he takes a laxative every day, he must strain to have a bowel movement. What is your first hunch about the meaning of these data? Is there a problem? What is it? What data do you still need to feel more confident about your diagnosis? (Hint: Look up "Constipation" and "Perceived Constipation" in a nursing diagnosis handbook.)

???
THINKING POINT

Level III. Draw Conclusions About Present Health Status

In Steps 6–8 you determine the meaning of the cue clusters. Begin by making initial judgments about the meaning of each cue cluster. Does the cluster represent a problem? Or the cause of a problem in another cluster? The following discussion continues to use an inductive process. It would vary slightly if you were using a deductive approach.

Step 6. Think of as many explanations as possible for each cue cluster. This helps keep you from drawing premature conclusions about the meaning of the data. Continue looking for data gaps. You may rule out some hypotheses because of insufficient data and confirm others based on your knowledge and experience. For Cluster 3 in Table 4–6, two possible explanations are:

1. Mrs. Sanchez's decreased urine output could represent a urinary tract problem. She also has chills and a fever, which are symptoms of a kidney infection. However, she has already been seen by a physician and has a medical diagnosis of pneumonia; and she shows no other signs of a urinary tract problem. So this explanation is unlikely.
2. Mrs. Sanchez's decreased urine output could be a result of a Nutrition/Metabolic problem. Inadequate fluid intake, combined with fluid loss from fever and diaphoresis, may mean there is scant fluid for her kidneys to eliminate. In this explanation, her fever is the cause, rather than a symptom, of a problem.

Step 7. Identify problems and wellness diagnoses. In this step, you choose the best explanation for each cue cluster, making a judgment about whether each cluster represents:

- *No problem* and no need for nursing intervention.
- *A wellness diagnosis.* (Patient wishes to achieve a higher level of wellness.)
- *A medical problem* (and possible need for referral).
- *A collaborative problem.* (Patient's medical diagnosis indicates the need to monitor for development of predictable complications.)
- *An actual nursing diagnosis.* (Client data indicate a need for nursing assistance.)
- *A potential (risk) nursing diagnosis.* (There are no signs or symptoms of an actual problem, but risk factors exist; a problem may occur if you do not intervene.)
- *A possible nursing diagnosis.* (You have reason to suspect a problem, but not enough data to confirm it.)

Table 4–6 includes the inferences made about all eight cue clusters. For the explanations for Cluster 3 (proposed in Step 6, preceding), you would probably conclude:

1. There is no Elimination problem.
2. There is an actual nursing diagnosis: Fluid Volume Deficit, in the Nutritional/Metabolic category.

All but three of Luisa Sanchez's problems are nursing diagnoses. The nurse can order the definitive actions to prevent or treat all except these three problems. Cluster 5 is a medical problem: hypothyroidism as a result of having had a thyroidectomy. This problem is being controlled by the Synthroid, prescribed by a physician. Cluster 11 reflects the medical diagnosis of pneumonia, which had already been made by a physician. It will be managed medically and need not be written on a nursing care plan (there may even be a critical pathway for pneumonia). Cluster 11 also contains some collaborative problems (Potential Complications of Pneumonia: Respiratory Insufficiency and Septic Shock) that are not apparent from the cue clusters in Table 4–6. They are identified from the fact that Mrs. Sanchez has pneumonia, and would be included in the care plan or critical pathway for *any* patient with pneumonia.

KEY POINT
Wellness Diagnoses:

Used to develop care plans to support a healthy patient's change to a higher level of wellness (eg, Potential for Enhanced Breastfeeding)

Strengths:

Characteristics that help patients overcome problems or reach wellness goals. No care plan made to change patient status (eg, motivation, knowledge)

Step 8. Identify patient and family strengths. You should integrate strengths into the plan of care. Examine your *original* list of cues (see Box 4–4 on pp. 165–166); you cannot use the clustered cues because they consist of abnormal data. Ask the client and family how they have coped successfully in the past and what they see as their strengths. The following are some of Mrs. Sanchez's strengths:

Pattern	Strength
Health Perception/Health Management	Shows healthy lifestyle, understanding of and compliance with treatment regimen
Nutritional/Metabolic	Normal weight for height
Roles/Relationships	Husband supportive; neighbors available and willing to help

> What other strengths can you identify for Mrs. Sanchez?

???
THINKING POINT

Level IV. Determine Etiologies and Categorize Problems

This is the final level of the diagnostic reasoning process. Refer to Box 4–3 on page 164.

Step 9. Determine the etiologies of nursing diagnoses. In this step, you determine the most likely causes of the nursing diagnoses you identified in Step 8. These are the problem **etiologies**—the physiological, psychological, sociological, spiritual, or environmental factors believed to be causing or contributing to

KEY POINT
Sources of Etiologies:

Environmental

Socioeconomic

Personal loss

Religious, ethical

Physiological

Psychological

Legal

Congenital malformations

Hereditary/genetic

Role changes

Political

Cultural

Communication difficulties

Lack of education/information

the problem. The etiologies must be correctly identified in order for your nursing actions to be effective. Ask yourself the following questions:

- What is causing this problem?
- Which is the problem and which is the etiology?
- How likely is it that this etiology is contributing to the problem?
- What data, knowledge, or past clinical experience support the link between the etiology and this problem? Or do not support it?

You must make inferences in this step, because you cannot actually *observe* the link between problem and cause. For example, in Cluster 3, you can observe that Mrs. Sanchez has dry mucous membranes, decreased urine output, hot skin, and poor skin turgor, and conclude that she has a problem: Fluid Volume Deficit. However, you cannot observe that the elevated temperature, diaphoresis, and limited fluid intake are the *causes* of this problem. You must infer this link between the problem and cause based on your knowledge of the metabolic effects of a fever and the physiology of fluid balance in the body, as well as your experience with similar patients.

You will not always find the etiology within the same pattern as the problem. In the following example from Table 4–6, a problem in the Activity/Exercise pattern is caused by stressors in the Nutritional/Metabolic, Activity/Exercise, and Cognitive/Perceptual patterns.

Problem:	**Functional Health Pattern**
Ineffective airway clearance	Activity/Exercise
Etiology:	
(1) Viscous secretions because of fluid volume deficit	Nutritional/Metabolic
(2) Shallow chest expansion because of pain, weakness, and fatigue	Cognitive/Perceptual Activity/Exercise

Although patients may have the same problem, the etiologies may be different.

EXAMPLE   All three patients have "Noncompliance with prescribed medication regimen" as their problem.

Patient A, etiology: Denial of illness
Patient B, etiology: Forgetfulness
Patient C, etiology: *Both* forgetfulness and denial of illness

When writing a nursing diagnosis, you should focus on those etiologies that can be influenced by independent nursing interventions.

Step 10: For each problem, make the final decision about which framework pattern it represents.   Relating problems to framework patterns (see Table 4–6, center column) can help you to choose a label when you begin to write your diagnostic statements. It may help you to look back at the discussion of nursing frameworks in Chapter 3.

Cluster 3 at first appears to involve both the Nutritional/Metabolic and Elimination patterns. However, the most reasonable explanation of the cues is that Mrs. Sanchez's fluid volume deficit (Nutritional/Metabolic) is causing her decreased urine output (Elimination). Her fluid volume deficit is the problem—the human response that needs to be changed. In this step, you are categorizing the problem, not the etiology; so Cluster 3 fits best in the Nutritional/Metabolic pattern. When you write your formal diagnoses (in a later step) you will look first at the diagnostic labels in the Nutritional/Metabolic pattern. Follow this same process for each group of cues until you have listed and identified the appropriate pattern for all the patient's problems (see "Tentative Problem" column of Table 4–6).

Verifying Diagnoses

After identifying the client's health status, you should verify your conclusions with the patient. A diagnosis is your interpretation of the data; and interpretation is not the same as fact. You can never be *certain* that an interpretation is correct, even after verifying it. Try not to think of diagnoses as right or wrong, but as being on a continuum of more or less accurate. Make your diagnoses as accurate as possible, but remain open to changing them as you obtain new data or insights. If the client is unable to participate in the decision making, you may be able to verify your diagnoses with significant others.

> EXAMPLE   You might say to Mrs. Sanchez, "It seems to me that you are worried about getting behind in your work, but that your main worry is about leaving your daughter with your neighbors. Does this seem accurate to you?"

If the patient confirms your hypothesis, you will include the problem on her care plan. If the patient does not agree with the problems you have identified you will clarify and restate them until they accurately reflect her health status. You may occasionally include a problem in a care plan even though the patient does not verify it. It may be a problem the patient is not aware of (as in the case of an unconscious patient) or one she is denying.

> EXAMPLE   A client may not perceive that she has Low Self-Esteem. Yet, because your data strongly suggest it, you may wish to continue to assess for this problem and use nursing interventions to promote self-esteem. If you want to assure that other nurses will also do this, you must include the problem in the care plan as a possible problem.

You should further validate each diagnosis by comparing it with the criteria in Box 4–5. If the client verifies it and it meets the criteria, your diagnosis should be high on the accuracy continuum.

BOX 4–5

Criteria for Validating Diagnoses

- The database is complete and accurate.
- The data analysis is based on a nursing framework.
- The cue clusters demonstrate the existence of a pattern.
- The cues are truly characteristic of the problems hypothesized.
- There are enough cues present to demonstrate the existence of the problem.
- The tentative cause-and-effect relationship is based on scientific nursing knowledge and clinical experience.

Labeling and Recording Diagnoses

After identifying and verifying the client's problems and strengths, the final step is to state them formally. To choose the labels for the nursing diagnoses, you simply compare the cue clusters with the definitions and defining characteristics of the NANDA **diagnostic labels** in a nursing diagnosis handbook. The process of selecting labels and writing diagnostic statements for nursing diagnoses and collaborative problems is covered in detail in Chapter 5.

Health Promotion: Diagnosing Wellness

Nurses engaged in health promotion may use a slightly different diagnostic process. Because clients are basically well, a health-promotion process considers them to be their own experts. Therefore, much of the power and responsibility for defining health needs belongs to those experiencing them. The nurse merely facilitates the process. The nurse engages in a "participatory dialogue" with the client, reflecting on the client's experiences and raising critical questions. Together the client and nurse begin to see behavioral patterns that facilitate or hinder the client's potential for healing. Health promotion focuses not on client problems, but on client potential, positioning the client in a better position to manage his own health and healing (Lindsey and Hartrick 1996). Statements of client potential may take the form of wellness diagnoses.

■ CRITICAL THINKING AND DIAGNOSIS

When diagnosing, you will use critical thinking to analyze and synthesize data, apply knowledge, recognize patterns, and draw conclusions. To check the quality of your thinking in the diagnosis phase of the nursing process, ask yourself the questions in Table 4–7 (review "Standards of Reasoning" in Table 2–3, on page 65, as needed).

Table 4–7 Diagnosis: Think About Your Thinking

Standard of Reasoning	Questions to Ask Yourself
Clarity—A statement must be clear in order to know whether it is accurate, relevant, etc.	■ Have I clustered the cues without too much overlap? ■ How have I clustered these cues in the past? ■ When I verified my diagnoses, did the patient understand my descriptions of his problems and strengths? ■ Have I expressed the problems and strengths clearly? ■ Do they give a clear picture of the patient's health status?
Accuracy—A statement can be clear, but not accurate.	■ Is this the best explanation for the cue cluster? ■ Do I have enough data to support my diagnoses? Did I identify all the data gaps? ■ Did the patient verify my diagnoses?
Precision—A statement can be both clear and accurate, but not precise.	■ Did I use the most specific description of the patient's health status (eg, "severe headache" is more specific than "pain")?
Relevance—A statement can be clear, accurate, and precise, but not relevant to the issue.	■ Have I focused on the significant cues? What data are outside normal ranges? Is it normal for this patient? ■ Have I omitted any relevant cues from the clusters? ■ Are the problems within the domain of nursing practice?
Significance—Related to relevance. What is *most* important?	■ Considering the whole situation, what are the most important problems right now? ■ What problems can I realistically deal with? ■ Do I need to refer or report any problems immediately?
Depth—A statement can be clear, accurate, precise, and relevant, but superficial.	■ What are the different possibilities for clustering the cues? ■ Am I qualified to determine what the problem is, or do I need help? ■ Is my diagnosis within the domain of nursing practice? ■ Did I consider social, cultural, and spiritual factors? ■ For problems and etiologies, did I look beyond the medical diagnosis to consider human responses?
Breadth—A line of reasoning can meet all of the other standards, but be one-sided.	■ What other problems do the cue clusters suggest? ■ Did I verify the diagnoses with the client and family? ■ Do I have biases, stereotypes, or preconceived notions about the patient's health status? ■ Did I identify wellness diagnoses, strengths, and collaborative problems, as well as nursing diagnoses?
Logic—Reasoning brings various thoughts together in some kind of order. If the thoughts make sense in combination, then thinking is logical.	■ *How* are the cues related within each cluster? ■ *How* is the etiology related to the problem? Would it really produce that human response? ■ Did I jump to conclusions about the patient's health status? Or did I take the time to think carefully about the data analysis/synthesis?

Source: Based on R. Paul (1996). *Critical thinking workshop handbook.* Dillon Beach, CA: Foundation for Critical Thinking. See www.critical thinking.org.

Reflective Practice

Critical thinking includes "a commitment to look for the best way" (Alfaro-LeFevre 1998, p. 14). In the diagnosis phase, you will look for the "best way" to describe the patient's health status. The core questions for reflection are:

- ■ *What is the most useful and accurate way to describe the patient's present health state?*
- ■ *What is the central issue (theme) for this patient?*

Finding the central issue will help you to prioritize your care and decide which problems should be the main focus for care. First reflect on the cue clusters to find a balance between omitting clusters and having too many overlapping clusters; then reflect on the diagnoses. Look for a theme. For example, Luisa Sanchez's problems (see Table 4–6 on pp. 169–170) include Ineffective Airway Clearance, Anxiety, and Sleep Pattern Disturbance. Ineffective Airway Clearance is a part of the etiology of both Anxiety and Sleep Pattern Disturbance. As you reflect, you will notice Ineffective Airway Clearance (or its effects) in other diagnoses. It emerges as a theme—as the central issue. If Mrs. Sanchez's airway clearance improves, she will be less anxious and able to sleep better. As you can see, intervening effectively for a central problem also relieves some peripheral problems. Think about the total picture for the patient at the same time you examine each diagnosis. Truly, you need to think about everything at once during this part of the process—that is why reflection is needed.

Avoiding Diagnostic Errors

Although you can never be absolutely certain a diagnosis is correct, it is important for diagnoses to be accurate. The following suggestions may help you to avoid diagnostic errors. Keep in mind that most sources of diagnostic error are also legitimate sources of hypotheses about the meaning of patient data. They cause errors only when you rely too heavily on them. See Box 4–6 for common diagnostic errors.

1. *Don't jump to conclusions based on just a few cues.* *Look for patterns in the data, and look at behavior over time rather than at isolated incidents.* For example, in Table 4–6 on pp. 169–170, you would not diagnose Altered Family Processes on the basis of the two cues in Cluster 8. There are no data to show that the family was ever before disrupted or that it will ever be again. You would need to see if the situation persists or if other data were found to support such a hypothesis.

Suspend judgment when data is incomplete. In the following example, the nurse should have gathered more data before interpreting the cues to mean Pain.

EXAMPLE: On entering the room for a scheduled postoperative observation, the nurse sees that Ms. Foley is crying. The nurse quickly

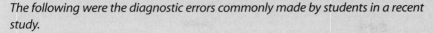

Common Diagnostic Errors

The following were the diagnostic errors commonly made by students in a recent study.

Accepting label definition alone without comparing patient data to defining characteristics for the diagnosis

Missing etiological or related factors

Inferring beyond the data

Misinterpreting a realistic worry (eg, calling it anxiety or impaired judgment)

Reading data or diagnostic criteria inaccurately

Missing cues because of lack of knowledge and experience

Reference: J. A. O'Neil (1997). The consequences of meeting "Mrs. Wisdom": Teaching the nursing diagnostic process with case studies. In M. J. Rantz and P. LeMone (Eds.). *Classification of Nursing Diagnoses: Proceedings of the Twelfth Conference North American Nursing Diagnosis Association.* Philadelphia: NANDA, pp. 131–138.

leaves the room, saying, "I'll be right back with your pain medication." On checking the medication record, the nurse discovers that the patient has already received an analgesic. The patient actually was crying because she had just received bad news from the surgeon about the results of her operation.

2. ***Build a good knowledge base and acquire clinical experience.*** Principles from other disciplines (eg, physiology) help you to understand patient data in different ways, thereby improving the accuracy of your diagnoses.

A good knowledge base helps you recognize significant cues and patterns. You need to know what is normal for most people, for such things as vital signs, lab tests, speech development, breath sounds, and so on. In addition, you must determine what is normal for a particular person, taking into account age, physical makeup, lifestyle, culture, and the person's own perception of normal. Compare findings to the patient's baseline data when possible. For example, normal blood pressure for adults ranges from 110/60 to 140/80 mm Hg. However, a blood pressure of 90/50 mm Hg may be perfectly normal for a particular individual. For a person with long-standing hypertension, 150/90 mm Hg may be not be a significant cue.

A good knowledge base helps you to have faith in your own reasoning and keeps you from relying too much on authority figures. You should certainly consult experienced nurses for input about the meaning of patient data. But realize that even experienced nurses can make errors. Patient problems you identify with the help of an authority must be verified in the same manner as any other problem.

3. *Examine your beliefs and values.* Beliefs are not usually acquired rationally, and they can be misleading. We tend to believe what those around us believe, what we are rewarded for believing, what serves our own interests, and what makes us comfortable. Reflect on your beliefs, keeping the ones that are supported by good reasons and evidence, to help you avoid the errors of bias and stereotyping.

Bias is the tendency to slant one's judgment in a particular way. We all have ideas about what people are like and what causes them to behave in certain ways, and even why they become ill. Some people believe they will catch a cold if they get their feet wet; others believe that illness is punishment for wrongdoing. Such ideas are based on life experience, not evidence, and may or may not be accurate.

> EXAMPLE   A nurse feels strongly that people are responsible for their own health. This nurse makes biased judgments about a patient with lung cancer who has a 40-year smoking history, and about a patient with emphysema who asks to have his ventilator shut off. The nurse's personal theory likewise affects his data interpretation for patients with AIDS and other sexually transmitted diseases.

Stereotypes are expectations about a person based on beliefs about his group (eg, physicians, elderly people, nurses, drug users). Two examples of stereotypes are (a) fat people are jolly and (b) women are emotional. A negative stereotype is a **prejudice**. Stereotypes are based more on hearsay than on fact or experience. If you rely on stereotypes instead of patient data, you will miss the uniqueness of each person. A common example of this is referring to patients as "the hysterectomy patient," or "the teenager in room 220."

4. *Keep your mind open to all possible explanations of the data clusters.* Remember that diagnoses are only tentative conclusions. Be ready to change your diagnoses as you reflect on and acquire more data. This will help you to avoid the following thinking errors:

a. *Forming premature conclusions based on context.* Nurses sometimes make judgments before even meeting the client, based on the client's medical diagnosis, the setting they are in, the chart, or what others say about the client (eg, "she's a complainer"). Such information can help you to think of possible meanings in the data, but be careful not to let it bias your thinking. For example, Nurse Thomas has read that grief is a response to loss of a body part. She also knows the theory that childbearing is an important aspect of a woman's identity. She therefore expects that patients having a hysterectomy will grieve over the loss of childbearing ability. This nurse fails to see each patient as an individual and is quick to develop a diagnosis of grieving at the first sign of crying, sadness, or other emotional upset—based on what she "knows." Patients become upset for many reasons, and Nurse Thomas's inference of grief is highly inaccurate for some of them.

b. *Relying too much on past experience.* This is different from stereotyping, because stereotypes are formed on the basis of little or no experience. Basing conclusions on past experience with similar situations is a common and legitimate practice. Generalizing from experience can help you to formulate tentative diagnoses, but it can also lead to error unless you validate your assumptions.

EXAMPLE: In the past 6 months, Nurse Thomas has cared for several women who have undergone hysterectomy. All of her patients have experienced at least some level of grief after surgery. Unconsciously, she has used the specific cases in her experience to generalize a rule about *all* cases. She now expects to see a grief reaction after hysterectomy and frequently identifies cue clusters in that manner.

5. *Validate all diagnoses with data; don't rely on intuition alone.* Be able to back your diagnosis up with patient data (signs and symptoms), and verify your conclusions with the patient and family. You may have "a feeling," but no evidence, that a problem exists. This should be a signal for you to watch the patient more closely than usual for signs and symptoms that the problem is developing. You may want to share your feeling with another nurse, the patient, or the physician—"I can't put my finger on it, but I just have a feeling that something is going on."

6. *Develop cultural sensitivity.* A situation may be considered a problem in one culture but not another. For example, in the mainstream United States culture, it is acceptable to bottle-feed a baby. However, some cultures (eg, Navajo) believe that breastfeeding promotes respect and obedience, while bottle feeding does not. From that cultural perspective, bottle-feeding might be considered a problem or a symptom of a problem. The key is to understand that personal and cultural meanings are attached cue clusters. The following guidelines will improve the accuracy of your diagnoses:

- Learn about the cultural or ethnic groups in your area.
- Do not assume the meaning of a behavior (cue) without considering the patient's culture and ethnicity.
- Be aware of your own beliefs and attitudes about health; examine their logic and origins.

■ ETHICAL CONSIDERATIONS

The nursing process deals with persons rather than things/objects. Therefore, every act of nursing, including diagnosis, has a moral or value dimension. Your values, especially about nursing roles and responsibilities, determine your choices about what data are even worthy of collection, especially when you are pressed for time. For example, when a nurse values decreased length of stay, assessments for the medical diagnosis, which are required by the critical pathway, may be a higher priority than a more holistic nursing assessment (Gordon et al 1994).

When analyzing assessment data, you may interpret some of that data to represent moral/ethical problems—for the patient and family, other healthcare professionals, or yourself. For example, if a cue cluster suggests Impaired Reasoning as a nursing diagnosis, then ethical questions arise about the patient's ability to give informed consent for treatments. Identification of an actual or potential ethical problem signals the need to gather information about all involved parties, what they want to happen, and the moral basis for their claims. You would then formulate a problem statement, the same as for other aspects of health status.

Defining or describing ethical problems requires sensitivity to the needs of others and awareness of your own moral duties or obligations to others in a situation. You also need some general knowledge about ethical principles and problems. That, of course, is beyond the scope of this text. Refer to a fundamentals of nursing or an ethics text for that information.

■ SUMMARY

The diagnostic process is summarized in Box 4–3 on page 164.

Diagnosis

- is a pivotal step in the nursing process.
- is the process of *interpreting data, verifying* hypotheses about the data (with the client or other professionals), *labeling* the problems, and *recording* the diagnoses.
- may identify nursing diagnoses, collaborative problems, other health problems, or wellness diagnoses.
- may identify actual risk, or possible problems, as well as patient strengths.
- requires knowledge, critical thinking, *not* making premature judgments, and keeping an open mind.
- may identify ethical problems.

Nursing diagnoses

- involve human responses to disease and other stressors in the area of health.
- are problems that nurses can independently treat or prevent.
- are culturally influenced.
- can be used to individualize standardized care plans such as critical pathways.

❏ Is the problem correctly identified?
❏ Does it describe the patient's health status?
❏ Is there anything I can do to help with it?

Nursing Process Practice

1. Place a check mark (✓) beside the words or phrases that are patient problems. Underline those that are probably nursing diagnoses.

   a. _____ Appendicitis

   b. _____ Catheter obstruction

   c. _____ Decreased peripheral circulation

   d. _____ Asthma

   e. _____ Delayed parent-infant bonding

   f. _____ Undergoing bowel resection surgery

   g. _____ NPO (nothing by mouth)

   h. _____ Constipation

   i. _____ Activity intolerance

   j. _____ Needs skin care

   k. _____ Low white blood cell count

   l. _____ Uncooperative

   m. _____ Needs constant attention

2. You are head nurse on a hospital unit, and your job is to encourage the staff nurses to begin using nursing diagnoses on their care plans and in their charting. One nurse says, "I didn't learn that when I went to school, and I've done just fine without it all these years. I can't see any reason to do all that extra work." What would you say to persuade her that nursing diagnosis is important to her practice?

3. In the following situation, circle the stressors and underline the responses.

> A blood clot developed in Ms. Sato's right thigh. Her thigh was swollen and warm to the touch. It was also slightly red. An intravenous catheter was inserted in her right forearm, and she was started on a heparin drip. She was placed on complete bedrest. That evening, she rang for the nurse several times, asking to have her leg checked and requesting pain medication. She was observed reading her Bible each time the nurse entered the room. Twenty-four hours later, when her clotting time returned to normal, the heparin was discontinued.

4. Now list Ms. Sato's *responses* (from Question 3) below. Write whether each occurred at the cellular, systemic, organic, or whole-person *level*. Also indicate whether it was in the physical, psychological, interpersonal, or spiritual *dimension*. The first one is done for you.

Response	Level	Dimension
Thigh swollen	Organic	Physical

5. Complete the following nursing diagnoses by adding etiologies to the problems given. Remember that a problem can be caused by several different etiologies. Use your knowledge of the medical condition to suggest appropriate etiologies.

For a client with a medical diagnosis of:	Problem	Etiology
Fractured femur	**a.** Acute Pain related to	
	b. Risk for Impaired Skin Integrity: pressure sores or excoriation related to	
Pneumonia	**a.** Ineffective Breathing Patterns related to	
	b. Activity intolerance related to	

6. Match the terms to the correct statements.

   N—Nursing diagnosis   **C**—Collaborative problem

   a. _____ Deals mainly with physiological complications.

   b. _____ A two-part or three-part statement about a client response to a situation or health problem.

   c. _____ A physiological complication resulting from pathophysiology or disease process.

   d. _____ Independent nursing interventions are mainly to monitor for symptoms and prevent condition.

   e. _____ Nurse can order definitive treatment.

   f. _____ Requires medical intervention.

   g. _____ Can be expected to be present any time the disease or treatment is present.

   h. _____ Can be a physiological, psychosocial, spiritual, or interpersonal problem.

   i. _____ The patient is receiving heparin. The nurse is monitoring lab values and other signs that abnormal bleeding may be developing.

   j. _____ The patient's knee is red and swollen. Because of the pain, he cannot bear weight on that leg and must have help to walk to the bathroom.

   k. _____ The patient record shows that Mr. Jonas has fallen several times in the nursing home. He has just been admitted to the hospital and is mildly confused. The nurse believes he will need special attention to assure his safety.

   l. _____ The patient has several severely fractured bones. The nurses are monitoring for the development of fatty emboli, which sometimes occur after a fracture and are a life-threatening emergency.

7. Fill in the blanks with the status of each of the following problems.

   A—Actual problem   **Pot**—Potential (risk) problem   **Pos**—Possible problem

   a. _____ A client states he is experiencing stomach pain.

   b. _____ A blind client is at risk for falls in an unfamiliar environment.

   c. _____ The problem is likely to occur if certain preventive nursing actions are not begun.

   d. _____ Risk factors are the etiology for the problem.

   e. _____ Data are not sufficient to confirm or rule out the diagnosis; more data are needed.

f. _____ Client has a group of related signs and symptoms.

g. _____ Similar to a physicians differential ("rule-out") diagnosis.

h. _____ Nurse prescribes interventions to prevent by reducing risk factors or monitoring status and onset of the problem.

i. _____ Nurse prescribes interventions to treat the problem as well as monitor status.

j. _____ Problem is identified mainly to assure additional data collection.

k. _____ The patient has arthritis. Her knee is red and swollen. She states that it is very painful. She has a/an _____ problem of Pain.

l. _____ The patient has arthritis. Her knee is red and swollen. The status of her Pain diagnosis is _____.

m. _____ The patient has arthritis. Her knee is red and swollen. You see she is limping. The status of her Pain diagnosis is _____.

8. Place an *N* beside the problem statements that are nursing diagnoses. Some have etiologies and some do not. Circle the part(s) of the statements that the nurse can independently treat or prevent.

   a. _____ potential arrhythmia related to myocardial infarction

   b. _____ low self-esteem related to perceived sexual inadequacy

   c. _____ risk for skin breakdown

   d. _____ perineal rash and excoriation related to urinary incontinence

   e. _____ confusion and disorientation related to inadequate cerebral oxygenation 2° cerebrovascular accident (CVA).

9. Using the NANDA framework (see Table 3–13 on page 108), group the following cues *inductively* and classify each cluster in the correct pattern of the framework. The patterns are Health Promotion, Nutrition, Elimination, Activity/Rest, Perception/Cognition, Self-perception, Role Relationships, Sexuality, Coping/Stress Tolerance, Life Principles, Safety/Protection, Comfort, Growth/Development. Decide the NANDA pattern in which the *problem* occurs. (You will probably have two or three cue clusters.)

   Cues: Ms. Petersen's blood pressure is 190/100 mm Hg. She says she hasn't been taking her "blood-pressure pills" because "they don't make me feel any better." She says she also has trouble remembering to take them. She is 50 lb overweight. She says she works long hours and doesn't have time to cook—tends to eat fast food and snacks a lot. Her job is sedentary, and she does not engage in any physical exercise. For fun, she likes to "eat at a nice restaurant."

Cue Clusters	Pattern in Which Problem Occurs

10. Now look at the problems and etiologies you have identified for the cue clusters in Exercise 9. Write nursing diagnoses for the cue clusters (Problem r/t etiology). Use NANDA terminology if you wish, or simply state the problem and its etiology in your own words. You should have two nursing diagnoses.

11. Match the diagnostic error with the case that illustrates it.

   a. _____ Mike Skarda actually hears very well; but because he is elderly, his new nurse speaks loudly when talking to him.

   b. _____ Sharon Weiss feels it is cruel to prolong life by using heroic technology. When Mr. Ivanov's family will not agree to a "Do not resuscitate" order, Sharon fails to identify their guilt feelings and need for support.

   c. _____ All the cesarean birth moms Susan Stone has cared for have been ambulatory 24 hours postoperatively. Her nursing text indicates that this is the norm. When Susan asks her patient to walk to the chair so she can make her bed, the patient says, "You will need to help me." Assuming the patient is being overly anxious, Susan says, "You can do it. Just go slow." However, this particular mom cannot walk without her cane and leg braces.

   d. _____ When a young woman with long, blond hair is brought to the emergency department in critical condition, the nurse (herself a young woman) becomes immobilized, thinking "Poor thing. That could be me!"

   1. Premature data interpretation
   2. Personal bias
   3. Stereotyping
   4. Generalizing from past experience
   5. Relying on authority
   6. Empathy

12. In your own words, write the most likely explanation for each of the following cue clusters.

   a. An elderly client with left-side paralysis has a red, broken area of skin over his sacrum.

   b. Larry VanHuff has had severe diarrhea for 2 days. Today he has been vomiting each time he takes fluids by mouth. He does not yet have such symptoms as poor skin turgor or dry, sticky, mucous membranes in his mouth.

Critical Thinking Practice: Analysis and Synthesis

In diagnostic reasoning, you will use both the skills of analysis and synthesis.

Learning the Skill of Analysis

Analysis is the cognitive process of breaking material down into component parts and identifying the relationships among them. Every day you hear or read many statements. Some seem correct at first, yet as you think about them, you find you disagree. It is important to analyze why you agree or disagree. The following is a process you can use to help you.

Step 1: Study the statement to make sure you understand what is being said (eg, Has the author or speaker used key words in the same way you use them?).

Step 2: Determine whether or not you agree with the statement (eg, Has the author made an assumption that you do not agree with? Has the author made a mistake, such as faulty logic or incorrect mathematics?).

Step 3: State clearly whether or not you agree, and give reasons for your judgment.

Analyze the following statement. State clearly whether you agree or not and give your reasons. Try to go through the three steps mentally before writing.

Nursing diagnoses provide an effective form of communication among nurses and other healthcare professionals.

Step 1. Study the statement to make sure you understand what is being said (eg, Has the person used key words in the same way you use them?).

1. Underline the key words in the statement.

2. What do you think the author means by those words? Do you agree with the author's meanings?

Step 2. Determine whether or not you agree with the statement.

3. What assumptions has the author made?

4. Do you agree with the assumptions? Why or why not?

5. Has the author left anything out of the argument?

Step 3. State clearly whether you agree or not and give reasons for your judgment.

6.

Applying the Skill of Analysis

7. Analyze the following statement. In your response, clearly state whether you agree or not and state your reasons. Try to go through the three steps mentally before writing.

Nurses should examine and be aware of their values so they will be able to keep them from influencing their decisions and judgments.

Learning the Skill of Synthesis

Synthesis means putting things together to form something new. Chemists combine various substances to synthesize new compounds for use as medicines. We can also link concepts, data, and ideas from one source with those from other sources to develop new ideas. This is an important skill because it allows us to come up with new ideas to deal with the constantly changing situations we find in everyday life—and in nursing. Nurses use synthesis to take ideas from nursing and related fields (eg, nutrition) and combine them to bring patient data together into meaningful relationships—as is done in the diagnostic process.

Step 1. Cluster cues by using your knowledge to discover how cues are related.
Step 2. Use knowledge of physiological and psychological processes and other concepts to explain the clustered data.
Step 3. Form the explanations and information into a meaningful whole: the nursing diagnosis.

Read the following case. Seven facts/principles are listed for you to consider along with the data in the case:

CASE: Max Dupree is 75 years old. He has a medical diagnosis of peripheral arterial disease, characterized by decreased circulation in both lower legs. Mr. Dupree has atherosclerosis and artriosclerosis, which have caused his arteries to become stiff, resistant, and smaller in diameter. He is a heavy smoker.

Even if you are not familiar with the nursing care of a patient with peripheral arterial disease, you should be able to synthesize a potential (risk) nursing diagnosis (problem + etiology) for Mr. Dupree, based on the following facts:

All body cells need oxygen and nutrients and are sensitive to any reduction in their supply.

Oxygen and nutrients are carried to the tissues in the arterial blood.

Vessel resistance (including vessel size) is one of the most important factors in determining arterial blood flow.

The physiological effects of decreased peripheral circulation depend on the degree to which *reduced blood flow exceeds tissue demands* for oxygen and nutrients. If tissue needs are high, then even a small reduction in flow can create symptoms.

Metabolic rate is a measure of the rate at which energy is being expended. An increased metabolic rate causes an increase in oxygen use.

Physical exercise greatly increases the metabolic rate.

Metabolic activity in poorly oxygenated muscles results in hypoxia and a buildup of metabolites, producing muscle spasms.

(NOTE: Do not write a nursing diagnosis of Altered Peripheral Tissue Perfusion, because independent nursing interventions for that diagnosis are limited in this case. Additionally, if you use this diagnosis, the etiology will either consist of pathophysiology or a medical diagnosis, neither of which can be addressed by nursing orders.)

As you work your way through the following questions, you will practice the skill of synthesizing a new idea by combining the seven original ideas you were given.

A. First, use synthesis to determine a potential (risk) problem for Mr. Dupree.

1. What is the connection between the diameter of the arteries/arterioles and the amount of blood flow to the tissues?

2. What is the connection between decreased blood flow and the amount of oxygen that reaches the tissues?

3. Knowing Mr. Dupree's diagnosis, and using the facts in (1) and (2), what can you say about the probable state of oxygenation of the muscle tissues in Mr. Dupree's lower legs?

4. What is the connection between hypoxia, muscle spasms, and pain?

5. How does the balance (imbalance) between reduced blood flow and tissue demands affect the severity of symptoms or the likelihood that the patient will have symptoms?

6. Taking (4) and (5) into account, you could say that Mr. Dupree will probably have Pain **if**

7. Therefore, you could diagnose the problem as _____.

B. Now use synthesis to determine an etiology for Mr. Dupree's potential problem of Pain.

1. What determines the likelihood that a symptom will be produced by a reduction in peripheral blood flow?

2. What is the connection between metabolic rate and oxygen use?

3. What is the connection between exercise and metabolic rate?

4. Combine the ideas in (1) and (2). What is the connection between exercise and the demands of the skeletal muscle tissues for oxygen (especially in Mr. Dupree's legs)?

5. Combine the ideas in (1) and (4). Under what circumstances is Mr. Dupree most likely to experience the problem (symptom) of pain?

6. Therefore, for Mr. Dupree, the etiology of risk for pain in lower legs is _____.

Reviewing What You Have Learned

In your own words, explain what synthesizing an idea means.

Compare your nursing diagnosis with those of your peers. If they are different, compare your answers to Questions A1–7 and B1–6. Were all of your facts correct? Or did you draw different conclusions about the facts? Can you support your reasoning, or do you wish to change your diagnosis?

Source: Adapted from *Critical Thinking Worksheets,* a Supplement of *Addison-Wesley Chemistry,* by Wilbraham et al. (Menlo Park, CA: Addison-Wesley, 1990).

Case Study: Applying Nursing Process and Critical Thinking

Discuss the following case with classmates. Look up unfamiliar terms (eg, emphysema) as needed.

Imagine that you are providing home care for a client who has chronic obstructive pulmonary disease (COPD). He has often been admitted to the hospital for acute respiratory distress, and at times even requires mechanical ventilation. His activities are always limited because of his inadequate oxygenation; he requires assistance from home health aides for cooking and bathing. His home smells of stale cigarette smoke and you see ashtrays full of ashes and cigarette stubs. The client begins smoking a cigarette during your visit.

1. What feeling would you have? (Just identify your feelings at this time.)

2. What thoughts, perhaps about past experiences, might be contributing to your feelings?

3. What values do you have that might influence the way you see this situation? (Examples of values are, "Mothers should take good care of their children," "It is important to be honest.")

4. With items 1–3 in mind, what, if anything, would you say to this client when he lights the cigarette?

When you begin to discuss smoking with the client (in item #4), he becomes very angry. He bangs his fist on the table and shouts, "I wish you would mind your own business!"

5. What do you think the client is feeling?

6. What thoughts or past experiences may have contributed to his anger?

7. Would you make a nursing diagnosis of Noncompliance for this patient? If so, what is the etiology? If not, why not?

8. Would you make a nursing diagnosis of Knowledge Deficit (effects of smoking on COPD) for this patient? Why or why not?

9. Are there any other nursing diagnoses you would want to make, based on the available data?

■ SELECTED REFERENCES

Alfaro-Lefevre, R. (1998). Continuing education: improving your ability to think critically. *Nursing Spectrum (Illinois ed.)*, 11(4):14–16.

American Nurses Association (1998). *Standards of clinical nursing practice.* 2nd ed. Washington, DC: ANA.

American Nurses Association (1973). *Standards of nursing practice.* Kansas City, MO: ANA.

Anderson, L. (1998). Exploring the diagnostic reasoning process to improve advanced physical assessments. *Perspectives.* 22(1):17–22.

Caputo, L. A. and S. A. Mior (1998). The role of clinical experience and knowledge in clinical decision making. *Topics Clin Chiro* 5(2):10–18, 69–72.

Carpenito, L. (1997). *Nursing diagnosis.* 7th ed. Philadelphia: J. B. Lippincott.

Dossey, B. M. (1998). Holistic modalities and healing moments. *Amer J Nurs* 98(6):44–47.

Fry, V. (1953). The creative approach to nursing. *Amer J Nurs* 53(3):301–302.

Goehner, E. D. (1997). Integrating nursing diagnosis into clinical pathways. In M. A. Rantz & P. LeMone (Eds). In *Classification of Nursing Diagnoses: Proceedings of the Twelfth Conference North American Nursing Diagnosis Association.* Philadelphia: NANDA, pp. 285–292.

Gordon, M. (1994). *Nursing diagnosis: Process and application.* 3rd ed. St. Louis: Mosby.

Gordon, M., C. Murphy, D. Candee, et al (1994). Clinical judgment: An integrated model. *Advan Nurs Sci* 16(4):55–70.

Harding, W. T., R. T. Redmond, M. C. Corley, et al (1996). Techniques in evaluating nursing expert systems: A case study. *Nurs Forum* 31(4):13–20.

Hirsch, M., B. Chang, and K. Jensen (1993). Concurrent validity of a rule-based system. *Computers Nurs* 11(3):134–139.

Lavin, M. A., G. Meyer, and J. H. Carlson (1999). A review of the use of nursing diagnosis in U.S. nurse practice acts. *Nurs Diag.* 10(2):57–64.

Lindsey, E., and G. Hartrick (1996). Health-promoting nursing practice: The demise of the nursing process? *J Advanc Nurs* 23:106–112.

Lobley, L. S. (1997). Using nursing diagnoses to achieve desired outcomes for hemodialysis clients. *Advanc Renal Replace Ther* 4(2):112–124.

London, S. (1998). DXplain: A web-based diagnostic decision support system for medical students. *Medical Reference Services Quarterly.* 17(2):17–28.

McManus, L. (1951). Assumption of functions of nursing. In: *Regional Planning for Nursing and Nursing Education.* New York: Teachers College Press.

North American Nursing Diagnosis Association (1990). *Taxonomy I—Revised 1990.* St. Louis: NANDA.

North American Nursing Diagnosis Association (1999). *NANDA Nursing Diagnoses: Definitions & Classification, 1999–2000.* Philadelphia: NANDA.

O'Neill, J. A. (1997). The consequences of meeting "Mrs. Wisdom": Teaching the nursing diagnostic process with case studies. In M. A. Rantz & P. LeMone (Eds.). In *Classification of Nursing Diagnoses: Proceedings of the Twelfth Conference North American Nursing Diagnosis Association.* Philadelphia: NANDA, pp. 131–138.

O'Neill, E. S., and Dluhy, N. M. (1997). A longitudinal framework for fostering critical thinking and diagnostic reasoning. *J Advan Nurs* 26:825–832.

Roy, Sr. C. (1984). *Introduction to nursing: An adaptation model.* Englewood Cliffs, NJ: Prentice Hall.

Szaflarski, N. L. (1997). Diagnostic reasoning in acute and critical care. *AACN Clin Issues.* 8(3):291–302.

Taylor, C. (1997). Problem solving in clinical nursing practice. *J Advan Nurs* 26:329–336.

Wilkinson, J. M. (1999) *Nursing diagnosis handbook: With NIC interventions and NOC outcomes.* Upper Saddle River, NJ: Prentice Hall Health.

Wilbraham, A. et al. (1990) *Critical thinking worksheets,* a supplement of *Addison-Wesley Chemistry.* Menlo Park, CA: Addison-Wesley.

Zeigler, S. (1993). *Theory-directed nursing practice.* New York: Springer.

5

Diagnostic Language

Learning Outcomes

On completing this chapter, you should be able to do the following:

- Briefly describe the history of the nursing diagnosis movement in North America.
- Discuss the importance of using standardized nursing language for writing diagnostic statements.
- Name and describe four nursing diagnosis language systems (taxonomies) currently in use.
- Use North American Nursing Diagnosis Association (NANDA) diagnostic labels to write precise, concise, and accurate nursing diagnoses for individuals, families, and communities.
- Write collaborative problem statements in correct format.
- Describe the ethical issues involved in writing diagnostic statements.
- Write diagnostic statements describing wellness states.
- Recognize the cultural implications inherent in many nursing diagnoses.
- Write nursing diagnoses to describe human responses in the spiritual dimension.
- Prioritize client problems using a basic needs or a preservation of life framework.
- Use "standards of reasoning" to think critically about diagnostic statements.

■ INTRODUCTION

In Chapter 4 you learned to identify and verify nursing diagnoses, collaborative problems, and patient strengths. This chapter explains how to use the North American Nursing Diagnosis Association (NANDA) standardized terminology to write nursing diagnoses, describes formats for collaborative problems, and presents frameworks for prioritizing patient problems. Figure 5–1 highlights the aspects of the diagnosis phase that are emphasized in this chapter.

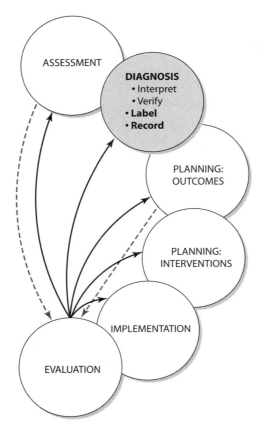

Figure 5–1
The Diagnosis Phase: Writing the diagnostic statement.

■ STANDARDIZED NURSING LANGUAGES

Standardized languages are essential for structuring and communicating knowledge and practice, as well as for evaluating the cost and quality of nursing care. Some examples of standardized languages include the musical scale, Arabic numerals, and symbols of chemical elements. As nursing knowledge has developed, nurse theorists and scientists have begun to develop vocabularies to describe and explain what nurses know and do, and systems to organize that knowledge for practice, education, and research.

Classification Systems

A **classification system** (also called a **taxonomy**) identifies and classifies ideas or objects on the basis of their similarities. For example, in anatomy, parts of the body are named and then classified according to body systems—the radius and ulna are bones in the skeletal system. Classification systems are created and used for various purposes. The following are examples of some non-nursing classification systems used in healthcare.

- The *International Classification of Disease (ICD)* names and classifies medical conditions, including mental disorders (World Health Organization 1992).
- The *Current Procedural Terminology (CPT)* names and defines all services and procedures performed by physicians. It is used for reimbursement of physician services (American Medical Association 1993).
- The *Diagnostic and Statistical Manual (DSM)* of the American Psychiatric Association is used by mental health professionals to name and describe psychiatric disorders.

The Need for Uniform Nursing Language

Well-developed classifications of standardized nursing languages are needed for the following reasons:

1. **Expanding Nursing Knowledge**. Taxonomies structure memory, thinking, and decision making. Their systematic organization structures a body of knowledge, making it possible to identify gaps and relationships in the knowledge. Existing nursing taxonomies have already collected and organized the major concepts needed to construct practice-level theories for nursing (Blegen and Tripp-Reimer 1997).
2. **Supporting Computerized Records**. Computer information systems and computerized patient records require standardized languages that can be converted to numerical codes. A common nursing language is required in order for nursing data and documentation to be included in patient records and research databases.
3. **Defining and Communicating Unique Nursing Knowledge**. Nurses are the largest group of healthcare professionals in the United States. Nevertheless, there is confusion, even among nurses, about what nurses do. A common language could be used by all nurses to communicate with each other and with those outside of nursing, enabling nurses to describe what they do for patients and to show the difference it makes in patient outcomes.

    In an effort to reduce costs, most healthcare institutions are reorganizing and questioning traditional roles, especially those of nurses. If nursing is to survive as a discipline, we need to answer two questions: (1) What do nurses do? and (2) Do nurses' actions make a difference in patient outcomes? This requires research-based findings, which depend on standardized nursing languages to reflect nursing contributions.
4. **Improving Nursing Care Quality**. Each discipline should delineate the data elements needed to define and evaluate a clinical encounter. For nursing, the data elements are diagnoses, interventions, and outcomes.

When standardized nursing vocabularies are included in clinical documentation systems, data can be generated to evaluate the effectiveness of nursing interventions.

5. **Influencing Health Policy Decisions**. Standardized terms would "generate data that more accurately represent nursing practice than outcomes-related measures currently used to support important policy decisions" (Keenan and Aquilino 1998, p. 81). Such data would make it possible to compare the effectiveness and cost of nursing treatments, not just in an institution, but across locations. Results from such studies could be used to influence health policy decisions locally, regionally, and nationally.

Existing Nursing Taxonomies

Table 5–1 contains a list of standardized nursing languages presently recognized by the American Nurses Association (ANA) and used in the United States. Each system will be discussed in more detail throughout this and subsequent chapters. NANDA, Nursing Interventions Classification (NIC), and Nursing Outcomes Classification (NOC) each focus on only one element of nursing. The Home Health Care and Omaha classifications contain all three elements: diagnoses, outcomes, and interventions. Because this chapter focuses on nursing diagnoses, NANDA and the NANDA taxonomy are discussed in more detail than the other classification systems.

In addition to the US taxonomies, the International Council of Nurses (ICN) is developing an International Classification for Nursing Practice (ICNP) that classifies nursing phenomena (diagnoses), nursing outcomes, and nursing actions (ICNP Update, Sept. 13, 1999, p. 2). This classification intends to provide a common language for nurses throughout the world.

■ THE NORTH AMERICAN NURSING DIAGNOSIS ASSOCIATION (NANDA)

In the 1950s and 1960s, nursing leaders recognized the need to describe nursing work and nursing knowledge. Several studies were done to identify patient problems requiring nursing intervention. These evolved into lists of *nursing problems* (Abdellah 1957) and *client needs* that might require basic nursing care (Henderson 1964). While neither of these was actually a list of patient problems as we now define them, they did demonstrate that nursing care focuses on something other than disease processes. In 1973, the American Nurses Association identified nursing diagnosis as an important function of the professional nurse.

Before 1973, there was no language to describe the conclusions that nurses reached through assessment. Although NANDA is a volunteer organization and mostly unfunded, it pioneered the work in nursing language and classification with its classification of nursing diagnoses. It began in

Table 5-1 Nursing Taxonomies Recognized by the American Nurses Association

Taxonomy	Elements Classified	Comments
NANDA (North American Nursing Diagnosis Association)	Diagnoses	The first nursing language taxonomy in the United States. Development of standardized language systems for nursing-sensitive outcomes and nursing interventions followed. Comprehensive across specialty and practice areas. See "North American Nursing Diagnosis Association," pages 200–202.
NIC (Nursing Interventions Classification)	Interventions	The first comprehensive standardized classification of nursing interventions. Developed by a research team at the University of Iowa, it describes both direct and indirect care activities performed by nurses (McCloskey and Bulechek 1992). Comprehensive across specialty and practice areas.
NOC (Nursing Outcomes Classification)	Outcomes	The first standardized classification of nursing-sensitive patient outcomes. Developed by a research team at the University of Iowa, it describes outcomes that can be influenced by independent nursing actions (Johnson and Maas 1997). Comprehensive across specialty and practice areas.
Home Health Care Classification	Diagnoses, Outcomes (expected and actual), Interventions	Designed for home health or ambulatory care. Specifically designed for computer-based documentation systems. Developed from research conducted at Georgetown University School of Nursing (Saba 1995, 1997).
Omaha System	Diagnoses, Interventions, Outcomes	A system for classifying and coding problems, outcomes, and nursing interventions for patients receiving care in the community. Developed by the Visiting Nurses Association of Omaha, Nebraska (Martin and Scheet 1992).

Source: Nursing Information and Data Set Evaluation Center, 11/4/99.

1973, when nursing faculty at St. Louis University, led by Kristine Gebbie and Mary Ann Lavin, called the first conference on classification. A national task force was formed and 100 nurses attended the First Conference on Nursing Diagnosis (Gebbie 1976). This group continued to meet every two years and, at the Fifth Conference in 1982 (Kim et al 1984), formally became the North American Nursing Diagnosis Association. NANDA membership consists of nurses from education, practice, research, and administration, as well as from all nursing specialty areas (eg, intensive care, maternal-child, home health). This diversity assures input from a variety of perspectives.

The major functions of the early groups were to generate, name, and implement diagnostic categories. Emphasis then shifted to clarifying existing labels and developing etiologies and defining characteristics. These priorities still exist, along with others, such as revising the taxonomy, promoting research to validate the diagnostic labels, and encouraging nurses to use standardized language in their practice.

In 1994, **The Nursing Diagnosis Extension Classification** (NDEC) research team at the University of Iowa reached a collaborative agreement with NANDA to extend and refine the NANDA work by addressing some of the issues about comprehensiveness, specificity, clinical usefulness, and clinical testing of the NANDA taxonomy. Many of the diagnoses on the official NANDA list have been tested only minimally.

The NANDA Taxonomy

Any number of ordering principles can be used to classify things (eg, size, weight, color). The first NANDA taxonomy was alphabetical and nonhierarchical (as in the list inside the front cover of this text). A new framework (shown in Table 3–13 on page 109) was accepted at the 2000 conference and will be used to organize the more than 150 NANDA diagnostic labels.

NANDA has been working with the ANA and other organizations to include the NANDA labels in other classification systems, for example the World Health Organization International Classification of Diseases (ICD). NANDA diagnosis-related articles are presently indexed in the Cumulative Index of Nursing and Allied Health (CINAHL) and in the National Library of Medicine Medical Metathesaurus for a Unified Medical Language.

NANDA Review Process

Review and refinement of diagnostic labels is ongoing. New and modified labels are discussed at each biannual conference. All individual nurses can submit diagnoses to NANDA. Diagnoses are also submitted by NDEC and nursing specialty organizations (eg, the Association of Operating Room Nurses). The elected Diagnostic Review Committee "stages" each diagnosis according to how well it is developed and supported (eg, by concept analysis or research). Diagnoses on the official NANDA list are not finished products, but are approved for clinical use and further study. NANDA reports ongoing work in its official journal, *Nursing Diagnosis: The International Journal of Nursing Language and Classification.*

■ CHOOSING A PROBLEM LABEL

The NANDA diagnostic labels provide a common language for all nurses to use in describing health problems for any type of client and in all healthcare settings. You must understand the meaning of the NANDA labels if your written statements are to accurately reflect your clinical judgments.

Components of a NANDA Diagnosis

Each NANDA diagnosis has four components: label, definition, defining characteristics, and either related factors or risk factors.

Label

Also referred to as the *title* or *name*, the **label** is a concise word or phrase describing the client's health. Labels can be used as either the problem or the etiology in a diagnostic statement. Many labels include qualifying terms such as *Actual, Risk, Ineffective, Impaired,* or *Increased*. NANDA has provided a list of definitions for these qualifiers (see Table 5–2).

After *Taxonomy II* becomes more widely used these qualifiers may not be needed. *Taxonomy II* includes 6 "axes" that will be used to describe a diagnosis:

Axis 1—The diagnostic concept (eg, *parenting*)

Axis 2—Time: Acute to chronic (long term, short term)

Table 5–2   Qualifiers for Diagnoses

Qualifier	Definition
(Suggested but not limited to the following)	
Acute	Severe but short of duration
Altered	A change from baseline
Chronic	Lasting a long time; recurring; habitual; constant
Decreased	Lessened; lesser in size, amount, or degree
Deficient	Inadequate in amount, quality, or degree; defective; not sufficient; incomplete
Depleted	Emptied wholly or in part; exhausted of
Disturbed	Agitated; interrupted, interfered with
Dysfunctional	Abnormal; incomplete functioning
Excessive	Characterized by an amount or quantity that is greater than is necessary, desirable, or useful
Increased	Greater in size, amount, or degree
Impaired	Made worse, weakened; damaged, reduced; deteriorated
Ineffective	Not producing the desired effect
Intermittent	Stopping or starting again at intervals; periodic; cyclic
Potential for Enhanced	Made greater, to increase in quality, or more desired (for use with wellness diagnoses)

Source: North American Nursing Diagnosis Association (1999). *NANDA Nursing Diagnoses: Definitions and Classification 1999–2000.* Philadelphia: NANDA, pp. 152–153.

Axis 3—Unit of care: Individual, family, community, target group (eg, *parents*)

Axis 4—Age: Fetus to elder (eg, *adolescent*)

Axis 5—Potentiality: Actual, risk for, opportunity or potential for growth/enhancement (eg, *risk for*)

Axis 6—Descriptor: Altered, decreased, increased, excess, deficit, depleted, excessive, defective, disturbed, impaired, ineffective, effective, ability, inability, intermittent, continuous, dysfunctional, functional, loss, gain, management, imbalance, deprivation, delayed (more descriptors can be added as needed) (eg, *altered*)

Using the preceding examples (in italics), you would write a diagnosis of *Risk for Altered Parenting by an individual adolescent.*

??? THINKING POINT

> Use the *Taxonomy II* axes to write a problem statement for the following data: An elderly client with left-sided paralysis has a red area of abraded ("broken") skin over his sacrum. (The concept, Axis 1, is Skin Integrity.)

Notice that many of the labels are very general; you cannot know what a diagnostic concept includes by looking at the label alone. For example, do you think "Activity Intolerance" means that the patient tires easily when playing football, or that he has chest pain when he walks up the stairs? What is the difference between the labels "Activity Intolerance" and "Fatigue"? The other components of a NANDA diagnosis help to clarify these questions.

Definition

The **definition** expresses clearly and precisely the essential nature of the diagnostic label; it differentiates the label from all others. For example, Activity Intolerance and Fatigue both involve decreased energy and abilities; however, the Activity Intolerance definition focuses on the inability to "complete . . . daily activities," whereas the Fatigue definition requires the presence of "an overwhelming sustained sense of exhaustion."

Defining Characteristics

Defining characteristics are the *cues* (subjective and objective data) that indicate the presence of the diagnostic label. For actual diagnoses, the defining characteristics are the patient's *signs and symptoms*; for risk diagnoses, they are *risk factors*. It is not necessary for all of the defining characteristics to be present in order to use a label; usually the presence of two or three confirms a diagnosis.

EXAMPLE: You could diagnose Constipation if only one or two of the following major defining characteristics were present:

a. Decreased frequency
b. Hard, dry formed stool
c. Straining with defecation
d. Pain with defecation
e. Abdominal distention
f. Palpable abdominal mass

It is easy to see that a client with a diagnosis of Constipation might experience one or more of these symptoms in various combinations. A palpable mass is present in most clients who have Constipation, but some clients may not have a palpable mass. Furthermore, you would probably diagnose Constipation for a client who had only symptoms *b* and *c*, but you would not make that diagnosis for a client who had only symptoms *a* and *e*.

Related or Risk Factors

Related or **risk factors** are the conditions or situations that are associated with the problem in some way. They are conditions that precede, influence, cause, or contribute to the problem. They can be biological, psychological, social, developmental, treatment-related, situational, and so on. Each diagnosis lists the related factors seen most often; however, do not interpret this as a complete list of factors that *could* be associated with the label. Imagine, for example, the variety of situations or factors that could contribute in some way to Anxiety; it would be impossible to list them all.

Related factors are often, but not always, used as the etiologies of a diagnostic statement. A related factor may be a part of the etiology for several problems, or a single problem may have several related factors as its etiology ("cause").

EXAMPLES:

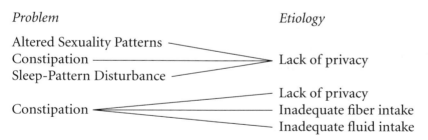

Problem — *Etiology*

Altered Sexuality Patterns
Constipation ——————→ Lack of privacy
Sleep-Pattern Disturbance

Constipation ←—— Lack of privacy
Inadequate fiber intake
Inadequate fluid intake

For potential nursing diagnoses, such as Risk for Fluid Volume Deficit, risk factors are similar to defining characteristics: they are the cues that must be present in order to make the diagnosis. Risk factors are nearly always at least a part of the etiology of the risk diagnostic statement.

EXAMPLE: Using the factors below, you might write the following diagnosis for a patient: "Risk for Fluid Volume Deficit related to increased urinary output secondary to diuretic medications."

Risk factors for the label Risk for Fluid Volume Deficit are: excessive fluid losses through both normal and abnormal routes, medications (eg, diuretics); factors influencing fluid needs (eg, hypermetabolic state), deviations affecting access to or intake or absorption of fluids (eg, physical immobility), extremes of weight, and knowledge deficiency related to fluid volume.

The related factors listed in handbooks are written in general terms and are used only as suggestions. Related factors are unique to each person, so you will usually need to individualize them. For example, one of the related factors for Impaired Physical Mobility is "prescribed movement restrictions." For a given patient, it is important to know exactly what the restrictions are, so you would need to write the diagnostic statement as, "Impaired Physical Mobility related to prescribed bed rest," or ". . . related to medical order for no weight-bearing on right leg," for example.

How to Choose a Label

To choose the correct label, you simply match patient symptoms (cues) with the definitions and defining characteristics of one of the NANDA labels. Remember, though, that there are over 150 different labels, so random searching is not practical. By the time you are ready to choose a label, you should already have narrowed the possibilities. Recall that during data interpretation you identified the most likely explanation (problem and etiology) for each cluster of cues and decided which of your framework patterns fit it best. Finding labels on the list that appear to have the same meaning as your hypothesized explanation should then be a simple matter. Refer again to Table 4–6 on pp. 169–170 in Chapter 4, the clustered abnormal cues for Luisa Sanchez. Cluster 11 is shown as follows:

Cluster 11 from Table 4–6
1. Cough productive of pale, pink sputum
2. Respirations shallow
3. Chest expansion < 3 cm
4. Inspiratory crackles through right chest
5. Mucous membranes pale
6. Diminished breath sounds on right side
7. Skin hot and pale

Functional Health Pattern
Activity/Exercise (pattern includes respiratory status)

The nurse hypothesized the following explanation for Cluster 11:

Cues 1 through 4 are defining characteristics for Ineffective Airway Clearance. This problem may be causing inadequate oxygenation, resulting in Cue 5. Cues 1, 6, and 7 are indicators of pneumonia, the medical problem that is creating the Ineffective Airway Clearance. Other problems are contributing as well: Fluid Volume Deficit is probably causing the patient's mucus to be thick and hard to bring up (Cues 4 and 6); Pain and weakness are contributing to Cues 2 and 3.

The nurse concluded that this explanation represented an actual problem, and that the problem is a nursing diagnosis not a collaborative or medical problem. Her informal problem statement was "ineffective airway clearance."

To find the appropriate NANDA label for this problem, you could simply look at an alphabetized list (such as the one inside the front cover of this text) for labels that seem related in some way to the explanation. You would, in this case, look for labels with words like *airway, breathing,* or *respiration,* and then find the labels in a nursing diagnosis handbook and compare them to your cluster of cues.

It is more efficient, however, to organize your list of diagnostic labels according to a theoretical framework (the same one you used to organize your data), so that related diagnoses are listed together. Since Luisa Sanchez's data analysis used the Gordon Functional Health Patterns, you would look for your labels under the Activity/Exercise pattern in that table (see inside back cover). There are quite a few titles under this pattern, but certainly fewer than the 150 listed in the alphabetical table on the inside front cover. Of the labels under Activity/Exercise, the only ones with possible connections (and some are remote, indeed) to Cluster 11 are the following:

Ineffective Airway Clearance   Impaired Gas Exchange

Ineffective Breathing Pattern

Next, look up the most likely sounding label. Does the definition for Ineffective Airway Clearance match the nurse's explanation of the cues (Cluster 11)? Do the cues match the defining characteristics of that label? How about Ineffective Breathing Pattern? Does that fit better?

For Mrs. Sanchez, Ineffective Airway Clearance is the best-fitting label. She does not have enough of the defining characteristics for Impaired Gas Exchange or Ineffective Breathing Pattern. Notice, too, that one of Mrs. Sanchez's cues is found in the related factors listed for Ineffective Airway Clearance: infection. The complete nursing diagnosis for Mrs. Sanchez would be: Ineffective Airway Clearance related to thick secretions and shallow chest expansion secondary to pain, fluid volume deficit, and fatigue.

The diagnostic statements for Mrs. Sanchez's other cue clusters are given below. Compare the cue clusters in Table 4–6, on pp. 169–170, to the definitions and defining characteristics in your handbook. Notice that NANDA labels can be used for both problems and etiologies. Review information on human responses in Chapters 1 and 4 as needed. Recall that responses occur on many levels, and that a response can function as a stimulus that produces another response.

Cluster 1   No problem. Strengths are healthy lifestyle and understanding of and compliance with treatment regimens.

Cluster 2   Altered Nutrition: Less than Body Requirements related to decreased appetite and nausea, and increased metabolism secondary to disease process. (Note that this is a short-term problem that will be corrected primarily by medical treatment of her pneumonia. Meanwhile, though, she will need nutritional assessment and support.)

Cluster 3   Fluid Volume Deficit related to intake insufficient to replace fluid loss secondary to fever, diaphoresis, and nausea.

Cluster 4   Sleep Pattern Disturbance related to cough, pain, orthopnea, fever, and diaphoresis.

Cluster 5   No problem as long as medical regimen is followed.

Cluster 6   Self-Care Deficit (Level 2) related to Activity Intolerance secondary to Ineffective Airway Clearance and Sleep Pattern Disturbance.

Cluster 7   Altered Comfort: Chills related to fever and diaphoresis.

Cluster 8   Risk for Altered Family Processes related to mother's illness and temporary unavailability of father to provide child care. (Note that the defining characteristics for this diagnosis are not present in Cluster 8; however, there are risk factors.)

Cluster 9   Anxiety related to difficulty breathing and concerns over work and parenting roles.

Cluster 10   Chest Pain related to cough secondary to pneumonia.

Cluster 11   (See discussion on pages 206 to 207.)

The following collaborative problems (potential complications) complete the list of problems for Mrs. Sanchez:

Potential Complications of pneumonia: (1) Respiratory insufficiency, (2) Septic shock

Potential Complications of intravenous therapy: (1) Inflammation, (2) Phlebitis, (3) Infiltration

Potential Complications of antibiotic therapy: (1) Allergic reactions, (2) Gastrointestinal upset, (3) Other side effects, depending on specific medication

Mrs. Sanchez's potential complications do not require collaboration unless they develop into actual problems. The nurse independently monitors for all three, and can take independent action to prevent the potential complications of intravenous therapy. Because Mrs. Sanchez is not at higher risk than the normal population of pneumonia patients, individualized nursing diagnoses (such as Risk for Infection) are not written for these problems. They are prevented by agency routines and standards of care and will require no special interventions. This will be explained further in Chapter 10, "Creating a Care Plan."

Learning to Recognize the NANDA Labels

As you become familiar with the NANDA problem labels, it will be easier to recognize cue clusters in your patients—it is always easier to see something if you know what you are looking for. The best way to learn the labels is by using them; however, like most clinical skills, you need a certain degree of familiarity in order to use them. "Nursing Process Practice," at the end of this chapter, will help you learn what the labels mean. Refer to a nursing diagnosis handbook frequently for definitions, defining characteristics, and related/risk factors.

■ FORMAT FOR WRITING DIAGNOSTIC STATEMENTS

As shown in Box 5–1, ANA Standards of Care specifically address format and content of diagnostic statements. As you have already learned, a diagnostic statement describes the patient's problem and the related or risk factors. This basic *Problem + Etiology* format varies slightly depending on whether you are writing a nursing diagnosis, wellness diagnosis, or a collaborative problem, and depending on nursing diagnosis status (actual, risk, or possible). Briefly, the *basic* components of a diagnostic statement are:

1. **Problem**. The problem describes the client's health status clearly and concisely. Remember that it identifies what should be changed about the client's health status, so it should suggest client goals/outcomes. Use a NANDA label for this part of your statement when possible.
2. **Etiology**. The etiology describes factors causing or contributing to actual problems. For potential problems, it describes the risk factors that are present. The etiology may include a NANDA label; some of the defining characteristics; a NANDA risk factor or related factor; or something entirely outside the NANDA standardized language. The etiology enables you to individualize nursing care for a client. For example, even though the problem is the same, Impaired Verbal Communication related to *inability to speak English* would suggest different interventions than Impaired Verbal Communication secondary to *tracheostomy.*
3. **Related to (r/t)**. This phrase connects the two parts of the statement. The phrase *due to* is not used because it implies a direct cause-and-effect relationship, which is hard to prove in a nursing diagnosis. Human beings

Table 5–3 NANDA Components in Diagnostic Statements

Diagnostic Statement	NANDA Components	
	Actual Diagnoses	Potential Diagnoses
Problem:	Label	Label
Etiology:	Related factors, other diagnostic labels	Risk Factors
"A.M.B.":	Defining characteristics	None

and human responses are complex. Usually there are multiple factors that interact to "cause" a problem, and it is possible that even if those factors were eliminated, the problem response might still exist. At best, you can say that it is highly likely that the factors are influencing, creating, or contributing to the problem.

Actual Nursing Diagnoses

When a client's signs and symptoms match the defining characteristics of a label, an actual diagnosis is present. Note that the word *actual* is assumed and not written in the diagnostic statement. This section presents the basic format, and several variations, for actual diagnoses.

Basic Format: Two-Part Statement

The basic format for an actual nursing diagnosis consists of two parts: the problem and the etiology.

Problem	r/t	Etiology
↓		↓
(NANDA label)	r/t	(Related factors)
↓		↓
Self-Esteem Disturbance	r/t	Being rejected by husband

Some NANDA labels contain the word *Specify*. For these you need to add words to indicate more specifically what the problem is.

EXAMPLE: Noncompliance *(specify)*
Noncompliance *(diabetic diet)* r/t unresolved anger about having diabetes

The NANDA labels in most listings are arranged with the qualifiers after the main word (Infection, Risk for) for ease of alphabetizing. Do not write your diagnoses in that manner; write them as you would say them in normal conversation.

EXAMPLE: *Incorrect*: Airway Clearance, Ineffective r/t weak cough reflex

Correct: Ineffective Airway Clearance r/t weak cough reflex

P.E.S. Format

Besides *Problem + Etiology*, you may wish to include the defining characteristics as a part of your diagnostic statement. This is called the *P.E.S. format*, for "problem, etiology, and symptom." The P.E.S. format is especially recommended when you are first learning to write nursing diagnoses. If you use this method, simply add *as manifested by (A.M.B.)*, followed by the patient's signs and symptoms that led you to make the diagnosis. Use the following format:

Problem	(r/t)	Etiology	(A.M.B.)	Symptoms
↓	↓	↓	↓	↓
(NANDA label)		(Related factors)		(Defining characteristics)
↓	↓	↓	↓	↓
Self-Esteem Disturbance	r/t	Being rejected by husband	A.M.B.	Hypersensitive to criticism; states, "I don't know if I can manage by myself." Rejects positive feedback.

Another example of the P.E.S. format follows. Notice that this method creates a very long statement.

EXAMPLE: Noncompliance (diabetic diet) r/t unresolved anger about diagnosis A.M.B. elevated blood pressure, 10-lb weight gain, and statements: "forget to take my pills," and "can't live without salt on my food."

Patient symptoms are helpful in planning interventions, so it is important that they be easily accessible. If they result in a statement that is too long, you can record them in the nursing progress notes when you first make the diagnosis. Another possibility, recommended for students, is to record the signs and symptoms *below* the nursing diagnosis, grouping the subjective and objective data.

EXAMPLE: Noncompliance (diabetic diet) r/t unresolved anger about diagnosis.
S—"I forget to take my pills."
"I can't live without salt on my food."
O—Weight 215 (gain of 10 lb)
B/P 190/100

A common error among beginning diagnosticians who use the P.E.S. format is to write a vague, nonspecific problem and etiology, hoping that the client's health status will be explained by listing the signs and symptoms. Guard against this tendency by making the Problem + Etiology as specific and descriptive as possible before adding the signs and symptoms. Your diagnostic statement should present a clear picture of your client's health status even without the listing of symptoms.

"Secondary to"

Sometimes the diagnostic statement is clearer if the etiology is divided into two parts with the words *secondary to* (2°). The part following secondary to is often a pathophysiology or a disease process, as in "Risk for impaired skin integrity r/t decreased peripheral circulation 2° diabetes." Use "2°" only if it is the only way to make your statement precise.

"Unknown Etiology"

You can make a diagnosis when the defining characteristics are present, even if you do not know the cause or contributing factors. For instance, you might write, "Noncompliance (medication regimen) r/t unknown etiology." If you think you know an etiology, but still need more data to confirm it, use the phrase *possibly related to*. When you have confirming data you can rewrite the diagnosis more positively. You might say, for example, "Noncompliance (medication regimen) *possibly r/t* unresolved anger about diagnosis."

"Complex Etiology"

Occasionally there are too many etiological factors or they are too complex to be stated in a brief phrase. The actual causes of Decisional Conflict or Chronic Low Self-Esteem, for instance, may be long-term and complex. In such unusual cases, you can omit the etiology and replace it with the phrase *complex factors* (eg, Chronic Low Self-Esteem *r/t complex factors*).

Three-Part and Four-Part Statements

Some diagnostic labels consist of two parts: the first indicates a general response, and the second makes it more specific. Adding an etiology to these labels creates a three-part diagnosis; adding *secondary to* makes it four parts.

EXAMPLES:

Labels:	Ineffective Family Coping: Disabling
	Altered Nutrition: Less than Body Requirements
	Feeding Self-Care Deficit (Level 3)
Nursing Diagnosis:	Altered Nutrition: Less than Body Requirements
	r/t nausea 2° chemotherapy

You may need to add a third part to other NANDA labels as well. Diagnostic statements must precisely describe the client's health concern because general concepts and categorizations are ineffective for planning nursing care. Not all NANDA labels provide this level of precision. You can sometimes make them more descriptive by using the P.E.S. format or by using a two-part etiology with *secondary to*, as in the preceding example. Sometimes, however, you may need to add a colon and third part, using your own words. Notice that the following example does not indicate the *degree* of mobility, even though the etiology is very descriptive. Can the patient turn herself in bed? Can she transfer to the chair unassisted? Or can she not move her legs at all? In some cases, the label definition makes the problem more specific, but in this instance it does not offer much help.

KEY POINT
Actual Nursing Diagnoses

1-Part Statement
Problem

2-Part Statement
Problem r/t etiology

P.E.S. Format
Problem r/t etiology A.M.B. symptoms

3-Part Statement
General problem: Specific description r/t etiology

4-Part Statement
General problem: Specific description r/t etiology 2° pathophysiology

EXAMPLE: Impaired Physical Mobility r/t knee-joint stiffness and pain secondary to muscle atrophy.

Label Definition: A limitation in independent purposeful physical movement of the body or of one or more extremities.

To make the nursing diagnosis more specific, you should add a third part (descriptor):

Problem	*Descriptor* +	*Etiology*
↓	↓	↓
(NANDA label)	(Specific problem description)	r/t (related factors)
↓	↓	↓
Impaired Physical Mobility	*Inability to walk*	r/t knee-joint stiffness and pain 2° muscle atrophy

In the Impaired Physical Mobility example, using the P.E.S. format does not help, because the signs and symptoms are the same as the etiology: inability to walk. The statement can be improved by adding *secondary to* the etiology: *2° muscle atrophy*. However, inability to walk is really a *type* of mobility problem rather than the *cause* of a mobility problem; therefore, it should not be used on the right side of the diagnostic statement in the etiology phrase. The most logical way to write the diagnosis is to add a colon and a more specific description to the general problem of Impaired Physical Mobility.

EXAMPLE:	Impaired Physical Mobility r/t inability to walk
P.E.S.:	Impaired Physical Mobility r/t inability to walk A.M.B. inability to walk
Better:	Impaired Physical Mobility r/t inability to walk 2° muscle atrophy
Best:	Impaired Physical Mobility: Inability to walk 2° muscle atrophy
Format:	*General Problem: (Specific Descriptor) r/t Etiology*

Pain is another label that often needs an added third-part descriptor. Even when considered with its etiology and definition, it does not always fully specify the client's problem. In the following example, you cannot tell how severe the pain is or where it is located. In the *Better* example, words are added to make the diagnosis thoroughly descriptive and specific to the client. Notice that in the *Better* example, the NANDA label describes the general area of the problem, and the descriptor describes the specific type of problem in that area.

EXAMPLE:	Pain related to fear of addiction to narcotics
Better:	Pain: Severe headache r/t fear of addiction to narcotics

You may see this diagnosis written as "Pain r/t severe headache." However, headache is a *type* of pain, not the *cause* of pain; the second part of the statement is supposed to consist of etiological factors, not problems. Furthermore, while this statement clarifies the location and severity of the pain, it does not indicate the cause.

"Risk for Infection" and "Altered Family Processes" are other labels that may need a third part added to make them more specific. Risk for Infection can often be made more specific by adding *secondary to*. However, in the following example, the first statement does not indicate whether the client is at risk for systemic infection or a localized infection of a wound or incision.

EXAMPLE:	Risk for Infection r/t susceptibility to pathogens 2° compromised immune system
Better:	Risk for Infection: Systemic r/t susceptibility to pathogens 2° compromised immune system, or
	Risk for Infection: Abdominal Incision r/t susceptibility to pathogens 2° compromised immune system

Remember that the diagnostic statement must thoroughly and specifically describe the problem and its causes (or risk factors). This is what dictates your format. In order to be fully descriptive, you will use *secondary to*, the P.E.S. format, qualifying words, a third-part descriptor, or a combination of these as needed.

One-Part Statements

A few NANDA labels are so specific that you do not need an etiology in the diagnostic statement. Most nurses write *wellness diagnoses* (eg, Effective Breastfeeding, Potential for Enhanced Spiritual Well-Being) without etiologies. The following NANDA *syndrome diagnoses* are also written without an etiology (a **syndrome diagnosis** is actually a collection of several nursing diagnoses grouped under one label):

Disuse Syndrome
Environmental Interpretation
   Syndrome
Post-Trauma Syndrome

Rape-Trauma Syndrome
Relocation Stress Syndrome

In addition, for the following labels it is difficult to think of an etiology other than a medical diagnosis, or if an etiology is written it is somewhat redundant:

Death Anxiety
Decreased Cardiac Output
Defensive Coping

Latex Allergy Response
Unilateral Neglect

Death Anxiety, for instance is fully described by its definition, which states that it is fear related to dying. In a statement such as "Death Anxiety r/t fear of dying," the etiology adds nothing to the understanding of the problem.

Potential (Risk) Nursing Diagnoses

A potential (risk) nursing diagnosis is one that is likely to develop if you do not intervene to prevent it. It is diagnosed by the presence of risk factors rather than defining characteristics. Risk nursing diagnoses have the same Problem + Etiology format as actual diagnoses—the client's risk factors form the etiology.

> EXAMPLE: Risk for Impaired Skin Integrity (pressure sores) r/t *immobility 2° casts and traction*

Risk diagnoses may have most of the previously mentioned variations in format (eg, one-part statement, three-part statement, multiple etiology). Of course, the P.E.S. format cannot be used because the patient does not have any defining characteristics of the diagnosis—if signs and symptoms are present, the diagnosis is actual, not risk.

Possible Nursing Diagnoses

When you do not have enough data to confirm a diagnosis that you suspect is present, or when you can confirm the problem but not the etiology, write a *possible* nursing diagnosis. The word *possible* can be used in either the problem or the etiology. As in other kinds of diagnoses, the etiology may be multiple, complex, or unknown.

EXAMPLES: *Possible Situational Low Self-Esteem* related to loss of job and rejection by family

Altered Thought Processes *possibly related to unfamiliar surroundings*

Possible Low Self-Esteem related to unknown etiology

Use *r/t unknown etiology* if you do not know the etiology; use *possibly r/t* if you suspect but cannot confirm the etiology. Remember, though, that etiologies are inferred, so you can never be *absolutely* certain an etiology is correct.

Wellness Diagnoses (Format)

New NANDA wellness labels are preceded by the phrase *Potential for Enhanced*, and will be one-part statements (eg, Potential for Enhanced Parenting). However, there are still some wellness labels that have different one-part formats (eg, *Enhanced* Breastfeeding, *Potential for Growth* in Family Coping, and *Health-seeking Behaviors*).

Collaborative Problems

Collaborative problems are complications of a disease, test, or treatment that nurses cannot treat independently. Nurses focus mainly on monitoring and preventing such problems. The etiologies of collaborative problems are likely to be diseases, treatments, or pathologies. Notice in the following example that if you use the usual *Problem + Etiology* format, the etiology suggests the need for medical interventions.

EXAMPLE: (Incorrect) Potential for Increased Intracranial Pressure r/t head injury

The problem statement should include both the possible complication for which you are monitoring and the disease, treatment, or other factors that produce it. In the following example, you would monitor for signs and symptoms of increased intracranial pressure that might result from the patient's head injury.

EXAMPLE: Potential Complication of Head Injury: Increased Intracranial Pressure

Sometimes you will be monitoring for a *group* of complications associated with a disease or pathology. In that case, state the disease and follow it with a list of the complications.

EXAMPLE: Potential Complications of Pregnancy-Induced Hypertension:

Seizures	Premature labor
Fetal distress	Central nervous system (CNS)
Pulmonary edema	hemorrhage
Hepatic or renal failure	

You cannot use the P.E.S. format for collaborative diagnoses because they are usually potential problems. The patient does not have the signs and symptoms—you are monitoring to see if they occur. However, for some collaborative problems an etiology can be helpful in planning interventions; for example, the complication may be caused by something more specific than a disease process. While you are a student, you should write the etiology, as in the following examples, (1) when it clarifies your statement, (2) when it can be concisely stated, or (3) when it helps to suggest nursing actions.

EXAMPLE:

Disease/Situation	*Complication*	*r/t Etiology*
↓	↓	↓
Potential complication of *childbirth*:	Hemorrhage	r/t 1. uterine atony 2. retained placental fragments 3. bladder distention
↓	↓	↓
Potential complication of *diuretic therapy*:	Arrhythmias	r/t low serum potassium

■ RELATIONSHIP OF NURSING DIAGNOSES TO OUTCOMES AND NURSING ORDERS

The first part of the diagnostic statement (the problem) states what needs to change; thus, it determines the patient outcomes needed to measure this change. In the example below, the goal would be to relieve the anxiety. This suggests a need to observe for symptoms such as rapid speech and shakiness.

EXAMPLE: Anxiety r/t lack of knowledge of scheduled venogram
↓
Goals (Outcomes)

The second part of the diagnostic statement (the etiology) identifies factors contributing to the actual problem, or the risk factors for a risk problem. In many cases, the etiology directs the choice of nursing interventions. In the preceding example, the etiology suggests a nursing order for patient teaching. In addition to teaching the patient about the venogram, however, the nurse would probably intervene more directly to relieve the anxiety—for instance, by helping the patient to recognize and express his anxiety. As you can see, nursing interventions can be suggested by either part of the diagnostic statement.

EXAMPLE: Anxiety   r/t   lack of knowledge of scheduled venogram
↓   ↓

Nursing   **Nursing**
Orders   **Orders**

A few other problem labels also call for particular nursing interventions regardless of the cause of the problem, for example: Decisional Conflict, Fear, Hopelessness, Ineffective Denial, and Risk for Violence.

As the NANDA labels become more specific, you will probably discover more instances in which the etiology cannot be treated by independent nursing actions, and both the goals and nursing orders will be determined by the problem. In the following example, the nurse cannot treat a spinal cord lesion. Both the outcome and nursing orders are suggested by "Reflex Incontinence."

EXAMPLE: Reflex Incontinence   r/t   spinal cord lesion
↙ ↘

Outcomes and Nursing Orders

When possible, though, you should rewrite the etiology so that it will provide direction for nursing intervention. Usually this means replacing a disease or medical condition with a principle or pathophysiology. This is not necessary for experienced nurses.

EXAMPLE: Risk for Infection r/t *surgical incision*

Rewritten: Risk for Infection r/t *portal of entry for pathogens 2°*
                   surgical incision

In every case, the nurse should be able to prescribe definitive prevention and treatment for at least one side of the nursing diagnosis.

■ THINKING CRITICALLY ABOUT THE CONTENT OF DIAGNOSTIC STATEMENTS

In addition to using the correct format for your diagnostic statements, you must consider the quality of their content—reflect on their meaning. After writing your diagnoses, judge them against the following criteria, which are based on the "Standards of Reasoning" set forth in preceding chapters. If you need to review these standards, refer to Chapter 2 and Table 4–7 on page 177.

1. **(Standard: Clarity) The statement is stated clearly and gives a clear picture of the patient's situation.** It uses terminology generally understood by other professionals and limits jargon and abbreviations.

   EXAMPLE:

   Incorrect: Toileting *SCD* r/t inability to get *OOB w/o help*
   Correct: Toileting *Self-Care Deficit* r/t inability to get *out of bed without* help.

2. **(Standard: Clarity) The statement is concise.** Wordy statements are often unclear. Using NANDA labels helps to keep the problem statement brief.
   a. If etiological factors are long and complicated, use "r/t complex etiology."
   b. If P.E.S. format produces a long statement, list the signs and symptoms under the diagnostic statement.

   EXAMPLE: Self-Esteem Disturbance related to longstanding feelings of failure aggravated by recently being rejected by her husband as manifested by being hypersensitive to criticism, stating, "I don't know if I can manage by myself," rejecting positive feedback, and not making eye contact.

   Better: Self-Esteem Disturbance r/t complex factors, A.M.B.
          S—"I don't know if I can manage by myself."
          O—Hypersensitive to criticism, rejects positive feedback, no eye contact

3. **(Standard: Accuracy) The statement is accurate and valid.** Diagnostic statements should meet the following criteria:
   - Patient signs and symptoms match NANDA defining characteristics.
   - For potential problems, patient risk factors match NANDA risk factors.
   - The cue cluster fits the NANDA label definition.
   - The patient has validated the diagnosis.

4. **(Standard: Precision) The statement is descriptive and specific.** The statement should fully describe the client's problem. Meet this criterion even if it makes the statement longer than you would like. The NANDA labels are always made more specific by:
   a. Knowledge of the label definition (If you know the definition, you may realize the label is more precise than you thought.)
   b. Adding the etiology to make the complete problem statement.
   c. Adding the patient's defining characteristics (P.E.S. format)

   If the statement still is not descriptive enough, make it more specific by:
   d. Adding qualifying words (eg, *mild, moderate, intermittent*).
   e. Adding "secondary to" in the etiology.
   f. Adding a third part (a colon and more specific problem)

EXAMPLE: Pain r/t fear of addiction to narcotics

Better: Pain: *Severe Headache* r/t fear of addiction to narcotics

5. **(Standard: Depth) The statement uses legally advisable language**. Ask yourself, "What are some of the complexities of this diagnosis?" (eg, legal implications). The statement should not affix blame or refer negatively to aspects of patient care.

EXAMPLE:

Incorrect	*Correct*
Impaired Skin Integrity:	Impaired Skin Integrity:
Pressure Sores	Pressure Sores
r/t *not being turned*	r/t *inability to turn self*
frequently enough	

6. **(Standards: Depth, Breadth) The complete list of nursing diagnoses and collaborative problems reflects the client's overall health status**. Although collaborative problems are not always written on the care plan, the master problem list for the patient should include all the patient's collaborative problems, as well as the actual, risk, and possible nursing diagnoses and client strengths. A complete list will enable you to plan all the nursing care the patient requires.

7. **(Standard: Breadth) The statement uses nonjudgmental language**. Remember to ask, "Do I have preconceived notions or values that affect how I see the problem?"

EXAMPLE:

Incorrect: Risk for Injury: Falls *r/t poor housekeeping*
Better: Risk for Injury: Falls r/t *cluttered floors*

8. **(Standard: Logic) Cause and effect are correctly stated**. That is, the etiology "causes" the problem, or puts the client at risk for the problem.

EXAMPLE:

Correct: Altered Oral Mucous Membrane r/t fluid volume deficit
         A.M.B. xerostomia and oral lesions
Incorrect: Fluid Volume Deficit r/t altered oral mucous membrane
         A.M.B. xerostomia and oral lesions

To check this logic, insert the parts of your statement in this sentence format (you are reading your diagnosis backwards, actually):

"(Etiology) causes (Problem)"

EXAMPLE: Dysfunctional Grieving r/t inability to accept death of spouse.

Read backwards:

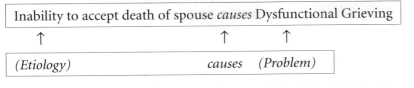

Inability to accept death of spouse *causes* Dysfunctional Grieving

↑ ↑ ↑

| *(Etiology)* | *causes* | *(Problem)* |

EXAMPLE: Risk for infection r/t interruption of body's first line of defense 2° abdominal incision

Read backwards:

Abd. incision *causes* break in 1st line of defense, *which causes* Risk for Infection

↑ ↑ ↑ ↑ ↑

| *(Secondary) causes* | *(Etiology)* | *which then causes* | *(Problem)* |

9. **(Standard: Logic) The problem side of the statement contains only one diagnostic label.**

EXAMPLE:

Incorrect
Risk for Fluid Volume Deficit and Constipation r/t inadequate fluid intake

Correct
Constipation r/t inadequate fluid intake

10. **(Standard: Logic) The etiology is not merely a rewording of the problem.**

EXAMPLE:

Incorrect
Chronic Pain r/t headache

Correct
Chronic Pain (Headache) r/t unknown etiology

11. **(Standard: Logic) At least one side of the statement provides direction for nursing actions.** If you cannot prescribe the interventions to change either the problem or the etiology, then you should reevaluate the statement. Perhaps what you have identified as the problem is actually the stimulus for other problem responses. In the following example, the nurse cannot change what was first identified as a "hearing problem." However, the hearing problem produced a social interaction problem, which the nurse *can* address.

EXAMPLE:

Incorrect: Sensory/Perceptual Alteration (Auditory) r/t progressive hearing loss 2° nerve degeneration

Correct: Impaired Social Interaction r/t embarrassment at being unable to follow conversations because of progressive hearing loss 2° nerve degeneration

a. Nursing diagnoses suggest independent nursing actions to treat or prevent.

b. Collaborative problems suggest independent nursing actions to detect and prevent.

12. **The statement does not include any of the errors described in Table 4–2 on page 151** (ie, stating a patient need; a nursing goal or action; or medical test, equipment, or treatment, rather than a problematic human response).

■ WELLNESS DIAGNOSES

Wellness diagnoses are especially useful for healthy clients, such as school children or new parents, who require teaching for health promotion, disease prevention, and personal growth. Following is the NANDA definition of wellness diagnosis.

> **Wellness diagnoses** "describe human responses to levels of wellness in an individual, family, or community that have a potential for enhancement to a higher state" (1999, p. 149).

All new wellness diagnoses are preceded by the phrase *Potential for Enhanced*, and will be one-part statements. The following wellness labels are included in the NANDA taxonomy, but most NANDA labels could be used to express wellness states by adding "Potential for enhanced" (eg, Potential for enhanced parenting):

Anticipatory Grieving

Effective Breastfeeding

Effective Management of Therapeutic Regimen: Individual

Family Coping: Potential for growth

Health-Seeking Behaviors

Potential for Enhanced Community Coping

Potential for Enhanced Organized Infant Behavior

Potential for Enhanced Spiritual Well-Being

The Omaha classification system for community health nursing (see Table 5–1 on p. 201) deals with wellness diagnoses by using modifiers. For each diagnosis used, the nurse must describe the status as "health promotion, potential, or actual." When no signs, symptoms, or risk factors are present, the nurse identifies a health promotion status (eg, Emotional stability: Health promotion).

Wellness diagnoses provide a clear focus for planning interventions without indicating that a problem exists. For some nurses, health promotion is their primary role. However, even patients with many health problems may have health promotion needs or areas of wellness. For example, you might use a wellness diagnosis for the following:

- Chronically ill clients in long-term care settings, for whom you wish to improve functioning and quality of life by providing physical exercise to improve strength and flexibility
- Acute-care patients in ambulatory care settings, such as clinics and emergency departments, for whom your secondary role would be to prevent further problems and enhance well-being, perhaps by referring patients to preventive or health promotion services.

Examples of processes where you might use a wellness diagnosis include patients who are gaining new information, learning new skills, improving physical functional status, weaning from ventilators, acquiring new roles, achieving maturational or developmental tasks, or experiencing wound healing (Stolte 1997, pp. 16B, 16H).

Describing healthy states for acutely ill hospitalized patients presents some difficulties. Hospitalized patients often have many nursing diagnoses and collaborative problems. From a practical standpoint, you can address only a limited number of problems during a workday, so you will usually address the high-priority diagnoses first. Because wellness diagnoses are usually lower in priority, the acute care nurse may never find the time to carry out the health-promotion interventions that a wellness diagnosis suggests. For hospitalized patients, it may be better to describe healthy responses by identifying strengths to use in planning interventions for the problems you identify. Concluding that a set of cues represents "no problem" does not necessarily mean you need to write a wellness diagnosis for that set. It is quite acceptable to identify health responses as strengths, rather than writing them as wellness diagnoses, especially in short-term situations. Some examples of strengths include: communicates adequately in dominant language, stable family situation, and adequate financial support. For a discussion of patient strengths, see Chapter 4, page 173, "Step 8: Identify Patient and Family Strengths."

■ SPIRITUAL DIAGNOSES

Spirituality both affects and is affected by a person's health status. Thus, from a holistic perspective, nurses need to be able to describe problems of spirituality. Two NANDA labels that relate to spiritual problems are Spiritual Distress and Risk for Spiritual Distress. Potential for Enhanced Spiritual Well-Being is a NANDA wellness diagnosis. The following NANDA diagnoses may also be helpful in describing a client's spiritual status:

Anticipatory Grieving
Death Anxiety
Decisional Conflict
Dysfunctional Grieving
Fear
Hopelessness

Ineffective Denial
Ineffective Individual or Family Coping
Powerlessness
Self-Esteem Disturbance
Sleep-Pattern Disturbance

If the patient does not have the defining characteristics for these diagnoses, you may be able to use one of the following O'Brien or Sumner terms to describe the patient's spiritual status. O'Brien (1982, p. 81) further categorizes spiritual distress as follows:

- *Spiritual pain*: Difficulty accepting the loss of a loved one or intense physical or emotional suffering
- *Spiritual alienation*: Separation from religious or faith community
- *Spiritual anxiety*: Challenge to beliefs and value systems (eg, by moral implications of therapy, such as abortion or blood transfusion)
- *Spiritual guilt*: Failure to abide by religious rules
- *Spiritual anger*: Difficulty accepting illness, loss, or suffering
- *Spiritual loss*: Difficulty finding comfort in religion
- *Spiritual despair*: Feeling that no one cares

Others describe spiritual problems on a continuum from mild to severe:

- *Spiritual concerns*—In which the patient shows mild anxiety and discouragement and expresses concerns about relationships with God.
- *Spiritual distress*—In which anxiety is more severe; the patient cries, expresses guilt; feels anger toward staff, family, or higher power; and experiences loss of meaning/purpose in life.
- *Spiritual despair*—In which patient loses hope and spiritual belief, is severely depressed, refuses to participate in treatment, does not communicate with family, and wishes to die. (Sumner 1998).

Spiritual Distress may be the etiology of the preceding problems, and others as well. For example:

- Self-Esteem Disturbance r/t Spiritual Distress 2° failure to live according to the principles of one's religion
- Sleep-Pattern Disturbance r/t Spiritual Distress

■ FAMILY AND HOME HEALTH DIAGNOSES

Efforts are being made to incorporate family diagnoses into the NANDA classification system. The labels in Box 5–2 could be used to describe family health status, and others could be adapted by adding "family" (eg, Family Decisional Conflict, Family Social Isolation). Home health nurses use both individual and family diagnoses. Box 5–3 shows the labels used most often by home healthcare nurses in a recent study. Because Medicare and other insurers consider client education to be a reimbursable skill, it is especially important to include a Knowledge Deficit diagnosis in a home health plan of care.

The Home Health Care Classification (HHCC) System (see Table 5–1, p. 201) includes 145 nursing diagnoses appropriate for individuals, families, or communities. The HHCC uses the NANDA definition of "nursing

---

BOX 5–2

NANDA Family Diagnoses

Effective Breastfeeding
Interrupted Breastfeeding
Ineffective Breastfeeding
Ineffective Management of
Therapeutic Regimen (Families)
Parental Role Conflict

Altered Family Processes
Ineffective Family Coping
(Compromised, Disabling, or
Potential for Growth)
Altered Family Processes,
Alcoholism
Parent/Infant/Child attach-
ment (Altered/Risk for)

---

diagnosis," and most of its diagnoses were adapted from NANDA labels (Saba 1995, 1997).

■ COMMUNITY HEALTH DIAGNOSES

Community health nurses need labels to describe the health status of individuals, families, groups (eg, all pregnant adolescents in the community), and entire communities. For example, a community may have high levels of

---

BOX 5–3

Frequently Used Home Health Diagnoses

A recent survey of 96 home healthcare nurses found the following diagnoses were rated as high frequency–high treatment priority. They represent four diagnostic areas: health management, activity, nutrition, and cognitive-perceptual patterns. The highest ranked label was Knowledge Deficit.

Knowledge Deficit
Self-Care Deficit: Bathing/Hygiene
Self-Care Deficit: Dressing/Grooming
Risk for Infection
Risk for Impaired Skin Integrity
Impaired Skin Integrity

Pain
Nutritional Deficit (Specify)
Risk for Injury
Impaired Mobility
Activity Intolerance
Decreased Cardiac Output

Source: From Gordon, M. and B. Butler-Schmidt (1997). High frequency–high treatment priority nursing diagnoses in home health care nursing. In: Rantz, M. J. and P. LeMone (eds.). *Classification of Nursing Diagnoses. Proceedings of the Twelfth Conference. North American Nursing Diagnosis Association.* Glendale, CA: Cinahl Information Systems.

KEY POINT
"Top Ten" nursing diagnoses reported by 36 public health nurses (Lesh 1997)

Inadequate Income

Knowledge Deficit

Health Management Deficit

Altered Parenting

Altered Health Maintenance

Potential for Altered Parenting

Potential Noncompliance

Impaired Home Maintenance Management

Support System Deficit

Compliance with Immunization Regulations

air pollution, or widespread unemployment, both of which have implications for the health of its citizens. Efforts are being made to incorporate community diagnoses into the NANDA classification system. Presently the following are the only NANDA labels to describe the health status of communities:

Ineffective Community Coping

Potential for Enhanced Community Coping

Ineffective Management of Therapeutic Regimen: Community

The Omaha System was developed by community health nurses (see Table 5–1 on page 201) for use in settings such as home care, public health, school health, and prisons (Martin and Norris 1996). It consists of 40 diagnostic labels organized into four categories (see Table 5–4 below). There are two sets of modifiers that the nurse must use with each diagnosis:

- Health promotion, Potential deficit, Deficit
- Family, Individual

So, for example, a family diagnosis might read "*Deficit* in *Family* Income." Even with this system, there are no terms to describe the health status of communities or groups. It has been suggested that the term "Group" should be added to the modifiers (Martin and Scheet 1992, p. 67). A possible diagnosis, then might be "*Deficit* in *Group* (shelter for the homeless) Income."

Table 5–4 The Omaha System Domains and Problems

Domains	Problem Labels
Environmental	Income, sanitation, residence, neighborhood/workplace safety, other
Psychosocial	Communication with community resources, social contact, role change, interpersonal relationship, spiritual distress, grief, emotional stability, human sexuality, caretaking/parenting, neglected child/adult, abused child/adult, growth and development, other
Physiological	Hearing, vision, speech and language, dentition, cognition, pain, consciousness, integument, neuro-musculo-skeletal function, respiration, circulation, digestion/hydration, bowel function, genitourinary function, antepartum/postpartum, other
Health-Related Behaviors	Nutrition, sleep/rest patterns, physical activity, personal hygiene, substance abuse, family planning, healthcare supervision, prescribed medication regimen, technical procedure, other

Source: Martin, K. S. and N. J. Scheet (1992). *The Omaha system: Applications for community health nursing.* Philadelphia: W. B. Saunders, pp. 67–74. Used with permission.

■ ISSUES ASSOCIATED WITH THE NANDA CLASSIFICATION

There are various criticisms of the NANDA taxonomy and of individual labels: they are unclear, too abstract (eg, Altered Parenting), too medical (eg, Decreased Cardiac Output), not understood by others, and so on. These problems probably will be corrected as the system evolves and diagnoses are refined. Meanwhile, if you disagree with a diagnostic label, you do not have to use it; or you can add words to make it more specific and clear. You should not reject the idea of standardized diagnostic language just because of a few awkward diagnoses. The system is evolving, as do all classification systems. In the medical diagnosis taxonomy, only in recent years was *toxemia of pregnancy* changed to *preeclampsia/eclampsia*; and only recently has *AIDS* become a medical diagnosis. Both NANDA and NDEC continue working to test, refine, and clarify the diagnoses and the classification structure.

Unrealistic Expectations

The more serious issues involve the whole system, rather than individual diagnoses. We may be expecting too much from nursing diagnosis in terms of what it can do for the profession and for patients. Does it truly define nursing? If so, will that make any difference in the long run? Nursing is changing rapidly and being shaped by events outside the profession (eg, technology, the economy). We must remember that nursing diagnosis is simply an important part of nursing. Do not expect it to singlehandedly remedy such problems as lack of autonomy and third-party payment; other (political) measures will be necessary.

Effect on Holistic Perspective

Some believe that using a list of ready-made labels causes nurses to miss creative inferences they would otherwise make. Others believe that a step-by-step, scientific approach inhibits intuitive problem solving and prevents a holistic perspective. Certainly we have all seen examples of the dehumanizing effects of science and technology. However, we can use our science in a humanistic manner. According to Kritek, "Naming our phenomena of concern does not narrow our perception of clients, but broadens it . . . . When a child weeps, you work hard to discover why. You try to solve the problem. But of course, you always comfort the entire child, not just the problem. Nursing will retain its fidelity to holism if it chooses to do so" (1985, p. 396). Using a common language and logical thinking should actually help nurses to identify and communicate unique aspects of patients that they might otherwise miss.

Ethical Considerations

Neither the diagnostic process nor diagnostic statements are value-free. A nurse's values may lead him to emphasize or ignore certain data during assessment, resulting in inaccurate or missed diagnoses. Because nursing diagnoses direct the way others view and relate to the patient, as well as the nursing care that is given, inaccurate diagnoses mean that the most effective interventions may not be selected.

EXAMPLE: A nurse's highest patient-care value is safety. Autonomy has never been a big issue in his life. When he cares for an elderly client, he diagnoses Risk for Injury r/t Altered Thought Processes 2° aging A.M.B. confusion and disorientation. He did not take into account that confusion is a side effect of one of the client's medications. Seeing this diagnosis, other nurses begin to perceive the client as needing more supervision than he actually does. Gradually, the client loses his autonomy and becomes more dependent.

Even if it were possible for the diagnostic *process* to be value-neutral, the *phrasing* of a diagnostic statement can have ethical implications. A diagnosis stated in value-laden terms may influence how other caregivers treat the patient. The etiology is the part of the diagnosis most likely to harbor negative or judgmental terms, because it is often complex and not stated in standardized language.

EXAMPLES: Ineffective Family Coping r/t *sexual promiscuity of the mother*

Anxiety r/t *unrealistic expectations of others*

The problem side of the statement can also create difficulty because the NANDA diagnostic labels are not entirely value-free. For example, *Noncompliance* may imply that the patient is not cooperating as he "should"; this can negatively affect nurses' attitudes toward the patient (Keeling et al 1993). You may be able to remove some of the stigma from such problem labels by writing the etiology carefully, as in the following: "Noncompliance with clinic appointments r/t inability to find reliable transportation for long trip." Geissler (1991) suggests *Nonadherence* as a less negative term than *Noncompliance*.

Some NANDA labels are not negative in and of themselves, but can be perceived as negative by nurses because of their own values. *Anxiety* carries a negative connotation for those who value strength and self-control; they may see an "anxious" patient as weak or unworthy of attention. *Knowledge Deficit* may imply lack of ability or lack of motivation to learn, either of which could evoke a negative reaction from caregivers who place a high value on learning.

Remember that it is the nurse, not the diagnostic statement, who determines the quality and the morality of a patient's care. Some nurses were surely making value judgments about their patients long before nursing diagnoses existed. As a part of their role, nurses interpret patient experiences, regardless of whether these interpretations are named as nursing diagnoses; and, like all interpretations, nursing judgments are influenced by values. Many judgments go unstated as assumptions, and are never examined. By writing a diagnostic statement, the nurse's judgment at least becomes open and explicit, and is available for examination by the nurse and by others.

Even though it is impossible to be value-neutral, diagnosing does not need to be unethical. To diagnose in an ethical manner, you must be aware of your values and their influence on the diagnostic process. You must realize the effect of your nursing diagnoses on other caregivers and try to phrase them in neutral, nonjudgmental language. And finally, you should validate your nursing diagnoses with the patient, to be sure that, in the *patient's* judgment, the cue cluster represents a *problem* (dysfunction, impairment) and not just a difference in perspectives and values. The ill person is vulnerable and in a position of inequality with healthcare providers, so you need to promote a relationship in which the patient feels free to voice disagreement.

Cultural Considerations

Many nurses (for example, Geissler 1992, Leininger 1990) believe that NANDA nursing diagnoses are not culturally sensitive. This characteristic can lead to misdiagnosis of problems and etiologies. Remember that diagnoses represent responses that clients and families find problematic from *their* perspective, cultural or otherwise. Undoubtedly, all problems and etiologies are influenced by cultural factors. However, it is especially easy to see how the following labels would be interpreted differently from different cultural perspectives:

Altered Health Maintenance
Altered Role Performance
Decisional Conflict
Impaired Social Interaction
Ineffective Denial
Ineffective Individual Coping

Altered Nutrition
Anxiety
Effective/Ineffective Breastfeeding
Impaired Verbal Communication
Ineffective Family Coping
Pain

???

THINKING POINT

In Culture A, pain is considered a punishment for sins, so the person is expected to tolerate pain without complaint in order to make atonement. In Culture B, expressions of pain elicit attention and sympathy. Suppose you are caring for a client with a fractured arm. He is holding his arm, pacing the floor, cursing, and complaining loudly of unbearable pain.

- If you are from Culture A, what would be your most likely interpretation of these cues?
- If you are from Culture B, what would be your most likely interpretation?
- If you and the client are both from culture A, would your interpretation be accurate?
- If you are from Culture A and the client is from Culture B, would your interpretation be accurate?

■ RECORDING NURSING DIAGNOSES

After validating and labeling the nursing diagnoses, you will write them in priority order in the appropriate documents (or computer): either the client's chart or the care plan. Some documentation systems include a multidisciplinary problem list at the front of the client record (chart). In many agencies the care plan becomes a part of the client's permanent record on dismissal, so diagnoses should be written in ink. When a diagnosis is resolved or changed, you can draw a single line through it or mark over it with a highlighter pen. Some care plans include a space beside the diagnosis to write the date the diagnosis is resolved or discontinued. Refer to Box 5–1, p. 209, for ANA standards for documenting nursing diagnoses.

Prioritizing Diagnoses

Prioritizing is sometimes considered a part of the planning phase of the nursing process, but if the diagnoses are to be recorded in priority order, then prioritizing must occur in the diagnosis phase. Priorities are assigned on the basis of the nurse's judgment and the client's preferences. You can rank the diagnoses from highest to lowest priority (1, 2, 3, etc.), or you can assign each problem a high, medium, or low priority. Prioritizing problems helps to assure that care is given first for the more important problems. This does not necessarily mean that one problem must be resolved before you address another.

> EXAMPLE: Bathing Self-Care Deficit might be a long-term problem for a patient. This does not mean you should wait until the patient can bathe himself before addressing the next highest priority, Risk for Constipation.

You should also consider risk problems when setting priorities. It is often as important to prevent a problem as it is to treat an actual one.

> EXAMPLE: For a poorly nourished, immobile patient, Risk for Impaired Skin Integrity is of higher priority than actual Diversional Activity Deficit.

Preservation of Life

If you use preservation of life as a criterion, you would rate the client's diagnoses based on the amount of threat they pose to the client's life. Life-threatening problems would take priority over those that cause pain or discomfort. A **high-priority problem** is one that is life-threatening, such as severe fluid and electrolyte loss or respiratory obstruction. A **medium-priority problem** does not directly threaten life, but it may produce destructive physical or emotional changes (eg, Rape-Trauma Syndrome). A **low-priority problem** is one that arises from normal developmental needs, or requires only minimal supportive nursing intervention (eg, Altered Sexuality Patterns related to knowledge deficit). After assigning high, medium, and low priorities, you can rank the diagnoses from most to least important.

EXAMPLE:

Rank	Diagnosis	Priority
1	Fluid Volume Deficit related to vomiting	Medium
2	Sleep Pattern disturbance . . .	Low
3	Diversional Activity Deficit . . .	Low

Maslow's Hierarchy

Maslow's Hierarchy of Human Needs also provides a good framework for prioritizing nursing diagnoses. Recall from Chapter 3 that in Maslow's model there are five levels of human needs. Starting with the most basic (highest priority) need, they are: physiologic, safety and security, social, esteem, and self-actualization. As a rule, the more basic needs must be met before the client can deal with the higher needs.

Kalish (1983) has made Maslow's system even more useful by dividing the physiological needs into survival and stimulation needs. Survival needs are the most basic; only when they are satisfied can the client be concerned about higher level needs. When survival needs are met, the client tries to meet stimulation needs before moving up the hierarchy to safety, social, and other higher needs. Kalish's division of physiological needs includes the following:

Survival needs: Food, air, water, temperature, elimination, rest, pain avoidance

Stimulation Needs: Sex, activity, exploration, manipulation, novelty

In this framework, diagnoses involving survival needs have priority over those involving stimulation needs.

EXAMPLE: The following diagnoses are ranked from highest to lowest priority:

Need	Nursing Diagnosis
Survival	Altered Nutrition: Less Than Body Requirements related to fatigue
Stimulation	Diversional Activity Deficit related to infectious disease isolation
Esteem	Chronic Low Self-Esteem related to inability to perform role functions

Patient Preference

Consider patient preference as much as possible when setting priorities. Give high priority to the problems the patient feels are important, as long as this

KEY POINT
Maslow Priorities:

Physiologic
Safety & Security
Social
Esteem
Self-Actualization

KEY POINT
Kalish Priorities:

Survival
Stimulation
Safety & Security
Social
Esteem
Self-Actualization

KEY POINT
"Patient Preference" Priorities:

Balance patient preferences with therapeutic and safety needs

KEY POINT
Canadian Nurses Association Nursing Process Standard 2.5

The nurse in any practice setting sets priorities with the client for resolution of identified problems.
Source: CNA (1987). Used with permission

does not interfere with survival needs or medical treatments. Because she is exhausted after delivery, a new mother's first priority may be to sleep. However, you must observe her closely for signs of postpartum hemorrhage, so you cannot safely follow her priorities in this situation. If you explain your priorities, you may be able to persuade the patient to agree with them.

Attending to problems that are high priorities for the patient increases the likelihood that they will be successfully resolved: patients will cooperate most enthusiastically to solve problems they consider important. As in the following example, patients may not be motivated to address other problems until their main concerns are dealt with.

EXAMPLE: Pat Sams is an 18-year-old who has just had her first baby. The nurse knows she must teach Ms. Sams how to bathe her infant before she is dismissed—within 24 hours after delivery. The nurse has given highest priority to Ms. Sams' Knowledge Deficit diagnosis. However, Ms. Sams finds it difficult to concentrate on the bath demonstration because she has a different priority. She is hoping the baby's father will come to visit, and has been washing her hair and putting on makeup. She has not heard from him since coming to the hospital, and she is worried he will not want to see her and the baby.

■ SUMMARY

- Standardized nursing languages are essential for developing and communicating nursing knowledge and practice, and for evaluating the cost and quality of nursing care.
- Five standardized nursing languages are recognized by the American Nurses Association: North American Nursing Diagnosis Association (NANDA), Nursing Interventions Classification (NIC), Nursing Outcomes Classification (NOC), the Home Health Care System, and the Omaha System.

Nursing diagnosis statements

- use NANDA labels.
- use the format of Problem related to (r/t) Etiology (or the P.E.S. variation).
- are varied by one-part statements, use of *secondary to*, unknown and complex etiologies, and three- and four-part statements.
- should be descriptive, accurate, and specific using nonjudgmental, legally advisable language.
- can be used to describe the health responses of individuals, families, or communities.
- are not value-free and require nurses to be aware of their own values and the perceptions of others.

- have ethical, cultural, and spiritual dimensions.
- may describe wellness states as well as health problems.
- should be recorded on the care plan in priority order.

Collaborative problems

- use the format of Potential Complication of (<u>disease</u>, <u>test</u>, or <u>treatment</u>): (<u>complication</u>)

Nursing Process Practice

Refer to a nursing diagnosis handbook as often as necessary when working the following exercises. Many of the exercises are designed to help you become familiar with the NANDA labels.

1. Identify the underlined parts of the nursing diagnoses by writing the correct terms beneath them. Use these terms:

    Label   Related factors   Qualifying term
    Defining characteristics   Risk factors

    a. Risk for <u>Body Image Disturbance</u> r/t amputation of right leg
        _____

    b. Risk for Body Image Disturbance r/t <u>amputation of right leg</u>
        _____

    c. Severe <u>Chronic Pain</u> r/t knowledge deficit (effects of exercise and rest)
        _____

    d. <u>Severe</u> Chronic Pain r/t knowledge deficit (effects of exercise and rest)
        _____

    e. Severe Chronic Pain r/t <u>knowledge deficit (effects of exercise and rest)</u>
        _____

2. Choose the most likely etiology for each of the following problems from the numbered list.

    a. Risk for Infection r/t _____

    b. Activity Intolerance r/t _____

    c. Altered Parenting r/t _____

    d. Fluid Volume Deficit r/t _____

    e. Possible Sexual Dysfunction r/t _____

    1. insufficient oxygenation for activities of daily living

    2. compromised immune system

    3. increased fluid loss secondary to vomiting

    4. delayed parent-infant contact 2° illness of infant

    5. body image disturbance 2° mastectomy

3. Place a *C* beside the correctly written nursing diagnoses.

   a. _____ Risk for Infection Transmission r/t lack of knowledge about communicable nature of the disease

   b. _____ Altered Oral Mucous Membrane r/t dry mouth

   c. _____ Elevated Temperature r/t infectious process

   d. _____ Constipation r/t inadequate fiber intake and prolonged bedrest

   e. _____ Risk for Impaired Skin Integrity r/t prescribed bedrest

   f. _____ Impaired Skin Integrity r/t prescribed bedrest

   g. _____ Rape-Trauma Syndrome

   h. _____ Acute Back Pain r/t unknown etiology

   i. _____ Impaired Skin Integrity r/t not being repositioned often enough

   j. _____ Crying r/t anxiety

4. Circle the risk factors. Underline the related factors.

   a. Fear r/t progressive loss of vision

   b. Risk for Anxiety r/t possibility of going blind

   c. Possible Fluid Volume Deficit r/t post-op NPO

   d. Pain r/t effects of surgery

   e. Grieving r/t recent loss of job

5. Write a diagnostic statement for each of the following cases. Refer to a nursing diagnosis handbook.

   a. A hypertensive client states that she hasn't been taking her medication because it doesn't make her feel any better. Also, she says she intends to take it, but has difficulty remembering.

   b. An elderly patient with left-side paralysis has a red, broken area on the skin over his coccyx. The patient cannot turn himself in bed.

c. The client is 45 pounds overweight. He states that he is in a high-stress job and doesn't have time to cook regular meals—he tends to eat fast food and snacks a lot. His job is sedentary and he does not engage in any type of physical exercise or sport. For fun, he likes to "eat at a nice restaurant."

d. A client is 2 hours postoperative vaginal hysterectomy. Her blood pressure has dropped from 130/80 to 100/60 mm Hg, and her pulse is 90 bpm. She is slightly pale, but not cyanotic. She has a 4 cm^2 spot of blood on her vaginal pad. Her abdomen is firm and tender to the touch, but not distended.

e. A client with pelvic inflammatory disease has just tested positive for gonorrhea. She states that she has unprotected intercourse.

6. Circle the labels that are NANDA-approved terminology.

Altered Nutrition: More Than
    Body Requirements
Altered Body Temperature
Diarrhea

Risk for Infection
Altered Bowel Elimination
Risk for Aspiration
Social Isolation

Anorexia
Constipation
Altered Protection
Activity Intolerance

7. Circle the labels that require additional words to make the problem more specific (eg, Feeding Self-Care Deficit, *Level 3*).

a. Activity Intolerance

b. Stress Incontinence

c. Sensory/Perceptual Alteration

d. Chronic Pain

e. Impaired Physical Mobility

f. Fatigue

g. Ineffective Breastfeeding

h. Constipation

8. For each of the labels you circled in item 7, write an example of words you might add to make the problem more specific.

9. Supply the label that fits the following definitions. Refer to a nursing diagnosis handbook as needed.

a. _____ Change in normal bowel habits characterized by involuntary passage of stool

b. _____ Passage of loose, unformed stools

c. _____ An overwhelming sustained sense of exhaustion and decreased capacity for physical and mental work at usual level

d. _____ The state in which an individual is at risk for entry of gastrointestinal secretions, oropharyngeal secretions, or solids or fluids into tracheobronchial passages

e. _____ Inability to clear secretions or obstructions from the respiratory tract to maintain a clear airway

10. Match the diagnostic label with the defining characteristics.

a. Ineffective Airway Clearance

b. Ineffective Breathing Patterns

c. Sensory/Perceptual Alterations (specify)

d. Social Isolation

e. Impaired Social Interactions

f. Impaired Swallowing

_____ 1. Diminished breath sounds, orthopnea, ineffective or absent cough, sputum, cyanosis, dyspnea, changes in respiratory rate and rhythm

_____ 2. Restlessness, poor concentration, visual distortions, irritability, change in usual response to stimuli

_____ 3. Expressed feelings of aloneness imposed by others, absence of supportive significant others, feels rejected; says time passes slowly

_____ 4. Orthopnea, use of accessory muscles to breathe, dyspnea, shortness of breath, pursed lip breathing, nasal flaring

_____ 5. Reports inability to receive or communicate a satisfying sense of belonging, caring, interest, or shared history

_____ 6. Coughing, choking, or gagging; food falls from mouth; drooling

11. Write the label that fits the following cue clusters. Compare the cue clusters to the defining characteristics in a nursing diagnosis handbook. You do not need to write etiologies.

a. _____

Mr. Maier has been hospitalized with a heart attack. He has been told he needs to rest and avoid stress. He says his advertising agency cannot run without him, and he phones the office several times a day to check on things and give instructions. He tells them he will be back to work "in a few days." He says he doesn't believe this is really a heart problem; "it feels like indigestion to me." He says he does not intend to change to a low-fat diet: "I'm too old to change my ways now." He does not seem anxious: He laughs and jokes a lot.

b. _____

Althea Harper has severe, chronic arthritis in her hands. When the nurse makes a home visit, Ms. Harper meets her at the door in a robe and slippers. Her hair is uncombed. She apologizes to the nurse for her appearance, saying, "I'm sorry I'm such a mess. It's just too hard to get dressed; I can't seem to work the buttons and zippers, or even tie my shoes. It hurts even to hold a hairbrush."

c. _____

Ms. Turner has been blind in her right eye for several years. Lately, her nurse has noticed that Ms. Turner does not seem to hear him when he speaks to her while standing to her right. The aide has reported several times that Ms. Turner ate only about half the food on her tray. The nurse observes that the food remaining is on the right side of the tray. To validate his findings, he pats Ms. Turner's right shoulder; Ms. Turner does not respond.

d. _____

The client reports that she must wear a vaginal pad because she leaks urine when she laughs or lifts heavy objects.

e. _____

The client reports that he must void every 30 minutes, but only small amounts. When he feels the need to void, he must hurry to the bathroom because he cannot wait. He also reports that he gets up three or four times during the night to void.

f. _____

A 70-year-old client has a medical diagnosis of arteriosclerosis. His left foot is blue and cold to the touch. The nurse finds a weak pedal pulse. She validates the findings by elevating his leg. It becomes pale, and the color does not return when she lowers it to a dependent position. She notes that the skin is shiny on both of his lower legs.

g. _____

Lorraine Richards' 3-week-old son has a temperature of 104°F. She says he has been having diarrhea and is not nursing well. His fontanels are still firm, and his skin turgor is good.

h. _____

Mr. and Ms. Welytok have a baby with myelomeningocele. They have been attempting to care for the baby at home for the past 2 weeks. Ms. Welytok confides to the visiting nurse that she doesn't feel she can care for the baby adequately. "I feel guilty, but I'm afraid to touch her, much less turn her. My husband just comes home from work and goes straight to bed, so he's no help at all. I can't give the other kids the attention they need now because I have to spend all my time with Jill. I don't feel like a very good mom right now."

i. _____

Tresa Liu is 12 weeks pregnant. She is 17 years old. She says, "I want to keep the baby, but my parents won't let me. They think I need to finish school. They want me to have an abortion. I think maybe they're right, but then I've heard sometimes you can't ever get pregnant after that. But I hate to quit school and miss all the basketball games and stuff. So I want to do it and then I don't. I should have made up my mind before this, I know."

j. _____

The client has been on prolonged bedrest. While ambulating, he complains of fatigue and dyspnea; he leans on the nurse for support. When she checks his vital signs, his heart rate is 120 bpm and irregular.

12. Circle the related factors identified by NANDA for the label Hopelessness.

Long-term stress	Loss of belief in God
Multiple caretakers	Prolonged activity restriction creating isolation
Pain	Decrease in circulation to the brain

13. Circle the correct client in each situation. Consult a nursing diagnosis handbook.

   a. All clients have the appropriate defining characteristics: body weight 20% under ideal and total calorie intake less than RDA. For which client(s) should you use the problem label Altered Nutrition: Less Than Body Requirements?

   Mr. Jonas, who cannot swallow because of paralysis

   Ms. Petrie, who is depressed and says she is not hungry

   Bobby George, who is NPO for 2 days after surgery

b. For which child should you diagnose Risk for Poisoning?

Billy, who is 6 months old and has a babysitter

Jana, who is an active 2-year-old

Jill, whose mother keeps her cleaning supplies under the sink

c. For which client should you diagnose Impaired Skin Integrity?

Mr. A, who has a sacral decubitus ulcer

Mr. B, who has an abdominal incision

Mr. C, who has self-inflicted razor cuts on his wrists

14. Write a diagnostic statement for each set of defining characteristics and related (or risk) factors. Focus on good format. Some of the statements are collaborative problems; others are nursing diagnoses. Use P.E.S. format only when directed to do so.

a. *Use P.E.S. format*

Defining Characteristics	Overuse of laxatives and suppositories
	Expectation of a daily bowel movement
Related Factors	Impaired thought processes

b.

Defining Characteristics	Decreased frequency of bowel movement
	Dry, hard stool; abdominal distention
Related Factors	There is no apparent reason for this problem.
	Diagnostic tests are normal; diet appears normal.

c.

Defining Characteristics	Decreased frequency of bowel movement
	Dry, hard stool; abdominal distention
Related Factors	Inadequate fluid intake
	Inadequate fiber intake
	Inadequate physical activity
Medical Factors	Client is too weak to eat, drink, or exercise adequately because of advanced chronic lung disease.

d. *Use P.E.S. Format*

Defining Characteristics   Verbalizes inability to cope

Observed to be unable to solve problems

Related Factors   Related factors occupy 35 pages of history notes in the chart and show development of this problem over several years.

e. Defining Characteristics   None

Risk Factor   Intravenous therapy

f. Defining Characteristics   Possession of destructive means (gun)

Increased motor activity

(May be suicidal, but do not have adequate data to be sure)

Related Factors   Suspect toxic reaction to medications; not sure yet

g. Defining Characteristics   Expressed desire to seek higher level of wellness; has asked nurse to suggest an exercise regimen.

15. Assign high, medium, or low priorities to the following diagnoses, using a "preservation of life" criterion.

a. _____ Impaired Communication between husband and wife related to use of blaming and withdrawal

b. _____ Anxiety related to lack of knowledge of impending surgery and preoperative and postoperative routines

c. _____ Fluid Volume Deficit related to fever and vomiting secondary to gastroenteritis

d. _____ Fluid Volume Excess: Right Arm related to dependent position and effects of mastectomy

e. _____ Altered Nutrition: Less Than Body Requirements r/t refusal to eat secondary to dysfunctional grieving

f. _____ Risk for Injury (falls) related to weakness and decreased vision

g. _____ Nonadherance (to diabetic diet) related to unresolved anger

h. _____ Unrelieved Incisional Pain related to reluctance to "bother" nurses

i. _____ Altered Health Maintenance (breast self-exam) related to lack of knowledge of how to do the procedure, and of its importance

16. Use the Kalish/Maslow Hierarchy of Needs to prioritize the diagnoses in Exercise 15. Assign priorities as follows (1 being highest priority):

1—Survival   4—Love/Belonging

2—Stimulation   5—Esteem

3—Safety   6—Self-Actualization

Critical Thinking Practice: Clarifying, Comparing, and Contrasting

I. Clarifying

Refer to pages 51–52 for a discussion of clarifying: also refer to Box 2–7 on page 53 for questions to use in these exercises. People often make superficial, inaccurate statements. In order to fully understand complex ideas and situations, use the following steps to check your understanding:

1. Be sure you know the meaning of the words and phrases in the statements.
2. Analyze the clarity and accuracy of the statement itself.
3. Examine your own beliefs and perspective.
4. Examine the speaker's (or writer's) beliefs and perspective.

A. Learning the Skill of Clarifying

Situation: Steven Allis is a young adult who has been admitted to your nursing unit with seizures for the second time in 2 months. He has a history of repeated hospital admissions for seizures. He is being treated with anti-epileptic medication, which he is required to take daily. He has monthly outpatient clinic appointments, but the clinic staff reports that he has not been keeping his appointments and they suspect he has not been taking his medication. His care plan has a nursing diagnosis of "Noncompliance."

1. What words and phrases do you need to clarify? (For example, what is the name of the anti-epileptic medication he is taking?)

2. What statements do you need to be sure you understand? In this situation, you should be sure you understand what the clinic staff means by "he has not been keeping his appointments." What else do you need to know about that?

You also need to clarify the nursing diagnosis: Noncompliance. What would you need to know in order to write a clearer diagnosis? What might it be?

3. What are your beliefs about keeping appointments and taking prescribed medications?

What are your beliefs about using the nursing diagnosis, Noncompliance, for patients?

Use any other questions you need from Box 2–7, on page 53, here.

4. What do you think Mr. Allis's perspective might be?

What about the perspective of the clinic staff?

B. Applying the Skill of Clarifying

<u>Situation.</u> You receive the following change-of-shift report at an extended care facility: "Mrs. Harris is an 80-year-old woman who was admitted from home because she is no longer able to live on her own. She has impaired coordination and is occasionally confused. She needs to be watched closely to ensure her safety.

1. What words do you need to clarify? What do you need to ask about the words?

2. Clarify the statements as needed (eg, Do you understand the situation? Did the other nurse report it fairly?). What do you need to do to clarify the report?

3. What is your perspective? Which of your beliefs are relevant to this situation?

4. What beliefs do you think Mrs. Harris might have that are relevant to this situation?

5. What do you think are the beliefs and perspective of the reporting nurse?

II. Comparing and Contrasting

Questioning is one way to clarify. Another way is to compare and contrast words and ideas with other words and ideas. Still another way is to compare the "real thing" with *mental models*. Scientists make mental models to describe aspects of nature and to explain various phenomena. For example, in the Bohr model of the atom, electrons orbit the nucleus in the way that moons orbit a planet. As another example, the nursing frameworks discussed in Chapters 3 and 4 are models that describe certain aspects of nursing. In the Roy model, for instance, nursing activity is described as promoting adaptation of the individual. You might create your own model in order to understand something in your everyday life. For instance, a model for an ideal teacher might include things like the kinds of lessons the teacher designs, what he lets students do in class, how he encourages you to think about the subject, or whether the tests are based on the stated course objectives. Such a model could provide a reference point to help you describe and understand a real teacher. The following are some steps you might use when comparing real occurrences to a model.

1. List the important characteristics or behavior of the model.
2. Ask yourself if the real thing behaves like the model with regard to those same characteristics.
3. Considering the characteristics you identified in Step 2, determine what features of the real occurrence make it different from the model.

A. Learning the Skills of Comparing and Contrasting

Use the three steps outlined above to compare your model of an ideal nurse with the behavior of a real nurse.

1. *Use Step 1.* List the important characteristics you think describe the ideal nurse.

2. *Use Step 2.* Considering each of the points you listed in (1), compare the behavior of someone you consider to be a typical nurse to the ideal nurse—perhaps someone you have observed during your clinical experiences.

3. *Use Step 3.* In (1) and (2) you compared the behavior of typical and ideal nurses in a number of ways. Considering each of these points, explain why your typical nurse behaves differently from your ideal nurse.

B. Applying the Skills of Comparing and Contrasting

1. This chapter presented several models of ideal diagnostic statements. The basic format of a nursing diagnosis is **Problem r/t Etiology.** List the variations of this model.

2. The chapter section "Thinking Critically about the Content of Diagnostic Statements" on pages 218–222, provides another model of a diagnostic statement. List the qualities of an ideal diagnostic statement provided by this model.

3. Borrow a care plan from another student or copy at least six nursing diagnoses from a care plan in your clinical agency. Discuss whether or not real diagnoses are the same as the ideal diagnoses with regard to qualities listed in Steps 1 and 2 of this section.

4. If you did note a difference in Step 3, explain why a typical diagnosis might be different from the ideal diagnoses.

Case Study: Applying Nursing Process and Critical Thinking

Discuss the case with your peers. Look up unfamiliar terms, medical diagnoses, and treatments as needed. Refer to a nursing diagnosis handbook for information about specific nursing diagnoses.

Situation: Mr. Gomez, a 55-year-old man, visits his physician because of fatigue and a 7-lb weight gain. He has a history of anterior myocardial infarction a year ago. Since then, he has not changed his lifestyle. He continues to work at least 60 hours a week, consumes a high-fat diet, and has been unable to stop smoking.

Physical examination reveals: labored respirations at 34 breaths per minute; crackles (auscultated) in all lung fields; heart rate 130 bpm, with occasional irregularity and an S_3 sound noted; blood pressure 184/110 mm Hg; and 3+ pitting edema in lower extremities. He tells the physician, "I'm just working too hard. I just need some more of those water pills you gave me awhile back."

Referral is made for home health nursing visits. In preparing a report to the home health agency, the nurse is considering the following nursing diagnoses:

- Ineffective Denial r/t unknown etiology
- Noncompliance r/t lack of knowledge about treatment regimen
- Ineffective Individual Management of Therapeutic Regimen r/t failure to change lifestyle

1. Assume that the defining characteristics for Ineffective Denial are present. Evaluate the etiology of that diagnosis. Based on these data, is it correct or not? Why or why not?

2. Assume that the defining characteristics for Noncompliance are present. Evaluate the etiology of that diagnosis. Based on these data, is it correct or not? Why or why not?

3. Assume that the defining characteristics for Ineffective Individual Management of Therapeutic Regimen are present. Evaluate the etiology of that diagnosis. Based on these data, is it correct or not? Why or why not?

4. Now, make *no* assumptions about the defining characteristics of the problem. Choose the NANDA label based on the data presented in the situation. Which of the three best fits Mr. Gomez?

5. Using *only* the problems and etiologies shown in the nurse's three nursing diagnoses above, recombine them to make *one* nursing diagnosis for Mr. Gomez. Use this format: *NANDA label (specific description of problem) r/t etiology A.M.B. signs and symptoms.*

6. In addition to the psychosocial nursing diagnosis you developed in Item 5, the nurse also diagnoses (a) Fatigue and (b) Potential Complications of Congestive Heart Failure: Fluid Overload and Cardiac Decompensation. Which of these three problems would you give highest priority? Why?

7. Which of these three problems do you think is Mr. Gomez's highest priority? Explain your reasoning.

8. What biases do you have (about anything in this situation) that might affect how you interpret these data?

■ SELECTED REFERENCES

Abdellah, F. (1957). Methods of identifying covert aspects of nursing problems. *Nurs Res* 6(1):4–23.

American Medical Association. (1993). *Physician's current procedural terminology.* Chicago: AMA.

American Nurses Association. (1973). *Standards of nursing practice.* Kansas City, MO: ANA.

American Nurses Association. (1998). *Standards of clinical nursing practice.* 2nd ed. Washington, DC: ANA.

Blegen, M. A. and T. Tripp-Reimer (1997). Implications of nursing taxonomies for middle-range theory development. *Advan Nurs Sci* 19(3):37–49.

Canadian Nurses Association (1987). *Standards for nursing practice.* Ottawa, Ontario: CNA.

Clark, J. and N. Lang (1997). The International Classification for Nursing Practice (ICNP): Nursing outcomes. *Int Nurs Rev* 44(4):121–124.

Delaney, C. and S. Moorhead (1995). The Nursing Minimum Data Set, standardized language, and health care quality. *J Nurs Care Qual* 10(1):16–30.

Engebretson, J. (1996). Considerations in diagnosing in the spiritual domain. *Nurs Diag* 7(3):100–107.

Gebbie, K. (1976). Development of a taxonomy of nursing diagnosis. In: Walter, J. et al. *Dynamics of problem-oriented approaches: Patient care and documentation.* Philadelphia: J. B. Lippincott.

Geissler, E. (1992). Nursing diagnoses: a study of cultural relevance. *J Prof Nurs* 8(5):301–307.

Gordon, M. (1998). Nursing nomenclature and classification system development, *Online J Issues Nurs* 2(2). Available at *http://www.nursingworld.org/ojin/tpc7/tpc7_1.htm*. Accessed on 5/27/99.

Gordon, M. and B. Butler-Schmidt (1997). High frequency–high treatment priority nursing diagnoses in home health care nursing. In: Rantz, M. J. and P. LeMone, eds. *Classification of Nursing Diagnoses. Proceedings of the Twelfth Conference. North American Nursing Diagnosis Association.* Glendale, CA: Cinahl Information Systems.

Henderson, V. (1964). The nature of nursing. *Amer J Nurs* 64(8):62–68.

Henry, S. B. (1997). Capturing nursing's contribution to patient care: an informatics approach. *Commun Nurs Res* 30:9–21.

International Council of Nurses (1999). ICNP components. *ICNP Update* (September 13). Available at *http:/icn.ch/icnpupdate.htm.* Accessed on 5/27/99.

Johnson, M. and M. Maas, eds. (1997). *Nursing outcomes classification (NOC).* St. Louis: Mosby.

Kalish, R. (1983). *The psychology of human behavior.* 5th ed. Monterey, CA: Brooks/Cole.

Kelling, A., S. Utz, G. Shuster, 3d, et al (1993). Noncompliance revisited: A disciplinary perspective of a nursing diagnosis. *Nurs Diag* 4(3):91–98.

Keenan, G. and M. L. Aquilino (1998). Standardized nomenclatures: keys to continuity of care, nursing accountability, and nursing effectiveness. *Outcomes Manag Nurs Prac* 2(2): 81–86.

Kim, M., G. McFarland, and A. McLane (1984). *Proceedings of the Fifth National Conference. North American Nursing Diagnosis Association.* St. Louis: C. V. Mosby.

Kritek, P. (1985). Nursing diagnosis: Theoretical foundations. *Occup Health Nurs* (August): 393–96.

Leininger, M. (1990). Issues, questions, and concerns related to the nursing diagnosis cultural movement from a transcultural nursing perspective. *J Transcultural Nurs* 2:23–32.

Lesh, K. (1997). Use of nursing diagnosis in public health nursing. In: Rantz, M. J. and P. LeMone, eds. *Classification of Nursing Diagnoses. Proceedings of the Twelfth Conference. North American Nursing Diagnosis Association.* Glendale, CA: Cinahl Information Systems.

Lindell, D. G. (1997). Community assessment for the home healthcare nurse. *Home Healthcare Nurse* 15(9):618–628.

Lutzen, K. and Tishelman, C. (1996). Nursing diagnosis: A critical analysis of underlying assumptions. *Int J Nurs Studies* 33(2):190–200.

Martin, K. S. and J. Norris (1996). The Omaha System: a model for describing practice. *Holistic Nurs Prac* 11(1):75–83.

Martin, K. S. and N. J. Scheet (1992). *The Omaha system: applications for community health nursing.* Philadelphia: W. B. Saunders.

McCloskey, J. C. and G. M. Bulechek, eds. (1992). *Nursing interventions classification (NIC).* St. Louis: Mosby.

McCloskey, J. C. and G. M. Bulechek (1994). Standardizing the language for nursing treatments: an overview of the issues. *Nurs Outlook* 42(2):56–63.

McLane, A., ed. (1987). *Classification of Nursing Diagnoses: Proceedings of the Seventh Conference. North American Nursing Diagnosis Association.* St. Louis, MO: C. V. Mosby.

North American Nursing Diagnosis Association (1999). *NANDA Nursing diagnoses: definitions & classification 1999–2000.* Philadelphia, NANDA.

Nursing Information and Data Set Evaluation Center (November 4, 1999). Available at *http://www.nursingworld.org/nidsec/index.htm.* Accessed on 5/27/99.

O'Brien, M. (1982). The need for spiritual integrity. In: Yura, H., and M. Welsh, eds. *Human needs and the nursing process.* Norwalk, CT: Appleton-Century-Crofts, pp. 81–115.

Parker, L. and M. Lunney (1998). Moving beyond content validation of nursing diagnoses. *Nurs Diag* 9(4):144–150.

Pesut, D. J. and J. Herman (1999). *Clinical reasoning: the art and science of critical & creative thinking.* Albany, NY: Delmar.

Saba, V. K. (1995). Home Health Care Classifications (HHCCs): nursing diagnoses and nursing interventions. In: *An emerging framework: data system advances for clinical nursing practice.* ANA Publication #NP-94. Washington, DC: American Nurses Publishing.

Saba, V. K. (1997). Why the home health care classification is a recognized nursing nomenclature. *Computers in Nursing* 15(2):69–76.

Stolte, K. M. (1997). Wellness nursing diagnosis: accentuating the positive. *AJN* 97(7):16B, 16H, 16J, 16L, 16N.

Sumner, C. H. (1998). Recognizing and responding to spiritual distress. *AJN* 98(1):26, 28–30.

Wake, M. and A. Coenen (1998). Nursing diagnosis in the International Classification for Nursing Practice (ICNP). *Nurs Diag* 9(3):111–118.

World Health Organization (1992). *Manual of the international classification of diseases and related health problems.* 10th rev. ed. Geneva, Switzerland: WHO.

6

Planning: Overview and Outcomes

Learning Outcomes

On completing this chapter, you should be able to do the following:

- Describe the nursing activities that occur in the planning phase of the nursing process.
- Explain the relationship between planning and the other phases of the nursing process.
- Discuss the importance of initial, ongoing, and discharge planning.
- Explain how to derive measurable, observable, individualized client goals/outcomes from nursing diagnoses.
- Develop outcomes to address special needs (eg, wellness, teaching, spiritual).
- Give examples of family and community outcomes.
- Describe three standardized languages for patient outcomes.
- Explain how to use the Nursing Outcomes Classification (NOC).
- Discuss the use of computers in choosing outcomes.
- Use guidelines and critical thinking standards to evaluate the quality of your outcomes and the thinking you used.
- Discuss the ethical, cultural, and legal considerations involved in developing client goals.

■ INTRODUCTION

Planning patient care is a responsibility of professional nurses (see Box 6–1 on page 251). This chapter discusses planning as a step of the nursing process, compares various types of planning, and explains how to write individualized patient outcomes. Figure 6–1 on page 250 presents an overview of the planning phase.

■ PLANNING: THIRD PHASE OF NURSING PROCESS

In the planning phase the nurse, with patient and family input, derives desired outcomes from the diagnostic statements and identifies nursing interventions to achieve those goals. The purpose and end product of this step is a holistic plan of care tailored to the patient's problems and

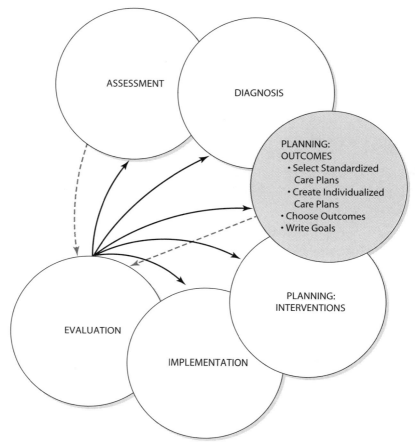

Figure 6–1
The Planning Phase: Outcomes and Goals

strengths. The planning step ends when this plan has been made. A "plan" is not always a written, individualized nursing care plan. It may be a mental plan the nurse has for achieving an outcome, or it may be a standardized set of routines (eg, vital signs every 4 hours) that meets the needs that certain patients have in common (eg, all postoperative patients on a unit).

During planning, the nurse engages in the following activities:

1. Deciding which problems need individually developed plans and which can be addressed by critical pathways, standards of care, policies and procedures, and other forms of preplanned, standardized care.
2. Choosing and adapting standardized, preprinted interventions and care plans where appropriate. (This activity is explained in detail in Chapter 10, "Creating a Care Plan.")
3. Choosing individualized outcomes and nursing orders for problems that require nursing attention beyond preplanned, routine care.

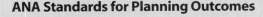

BOX 6–1

Professional Standards of Care

ANA Standards for Planning Outcomes

Standard III. Outcome Identification

The nurse identifies expected outcomes individualized to the patient.

Measurement Criteria

1. Outcomes are derived from the diagnoses.
2. Outcomes are mutually formulated with the patient, family, and other healthcare providers, when possible and appropriate.
3. Outcomes are culturally appropriate and realistic in relation to the patient's present and potential capabilities.
4. Outcomes are attainable in relation to resources available to the patient.
5. Outcomes include a time estimate for attainment.
6. Outcomes provide direction for continuity of care.
7. Outcomes are documented as measurable goals.

Source: Reprinted with permission from American Nurses Association. *Standards of Clinical Nursing Practice.* 2nd ed. © 1998 American Nurses Publishing, American Nurses Foundation/American Nurses Association, 600 Maryland Ave., SW, Suite 100 W, Washington, DC.

CNA Standards for Planning Outcomes

The nurse in any practice setting:

3.1 identifies short- and long-term objectives of nursing actions in collaboration with the client and relevant others.
3.2 indentifies short- and long-term objectives of nursing actions which are consistent and congruent with the interdisciplinary plan of care.
3.3 states these objectives in behavioural terms specifying the desired results.
3.4 states a reasonable time period for the achievement of these objectives.
3.5 considers environmental conditions that could affect achievement of these objectives.

Source: Canadian Nurses Association (1987). *Standards for Nursing Practice.* Ottawa, Ontario: CNA, pp. 4–5. Used with permission.

Remember that the nursing process phases are interdependent and overlapping. Planning is no exception. Its effectiveness depends directly on the assessment and diagnosis phases. If assessment data (assessment) are complete and accurate and the diagnostic statements are correct (diagnosis), then the goals and nursing interventions flow logically (planning) and are likely to be effective. In the same way, implementation and evaluation depend on the planning phase. The outcomes and nursing orders written during planning serve to guide the nurse's actions during implementation. Furthermore, the outcomes developed during planning are the criteria used in evaluating whether patient care has had the desired effects (more about this in Chapter 9).

The phases overlap when nurses do *informal planning* while carrying out the activities of the other steps. For example, while listening to a patient's lung sounds (assessment), the nurse may be making a mental note (planning) to notify the physician of her findings. This chapter emphasizes **formal planning**, which is a conscious, deliberate activity involving decision making, critical thinking, and creativity.

In addition to the planning involved in creating a nursing care plan, nurses use **time-sequenced planning** when they plan a patient's care for a shift or for a 24-hour period, for instance, when they

1. plan the timing and order of nursing activities for a patient (for example, giving pain medication before a painful dressing change).
2. coordinate the timing of nursing care with the actions of other healthcare team members, visits from family and friends, and the patient's circadian rhythms.
3. plan a daily work schedule. In addition to planning care for *each* patient, nurses must structure their own time so that they can give care to *all* the patients assigned for that shift.

Initial Versus Ongoing Planning

Initial planning begins with the first patient contact and continues until the nurse-patient relationship is ended, usually when the patient is discharged from the healthcare agency. The nurse who performs the admission assessment should develop the initial comprehensive care plan because she has the benefit of the client's body language and some intuitive kinds of information that are not available from the written database alone. Planning should be initiated soon after the assessment is done, especially with the trend toward short hospital stays. Even a partially developed plan can be helpful in the early nurse-client contacts. Because of time constraints or the client's condition, the initial database is sometimes incomplete. In such situations, you should develop a preliminary plan using the information available, and refine it as you are able to gather the missing data.

Ongoing planning can be done by any nurse who works with the client. It is carried out as new information is obtained and as the client's responses to care are evaluated. The initial care plan can be individualized even more as the nurses get to know the client better. Nurses who are not familiar with the client may not recognize the significance of new data, and important data could be lost.

Ongoing planning also occurs as you plan your nursing care at the beginning of each day. In your daily planning, you will use ongoing assessment data to:

1. determine whether the client's health status has changed.
2. set the day's priorities for the client's care.
3. decide which problems to focus on during this shift.
4. coordinate your activities so that you can address more than one problem at each client contact.

???

THINKING POINT

Situation: You receive the following messages almost simultaneously.

2:49 PM Mr. C. has requested pain medication: "I'm hurting real bad. Please come now."

2:50 PM Mrs. A., who is confined to bed, asks for a drink of water.

2:51 PM Mrs. B., who needs help to ambulate, says she needs to go to the bathroom right now: "Hurry, please!"

2:52 PM The nursing assistant says, "Come quick. Mr. D's dressing is all wet with blood, and it's trickling out from under it."

How will you structure your time so that you can meet all these patients' needs? You will need to look at the needs of the individuals and of the group. Try to meet the most urgent needs first. However, when needs are of equal priority, you may have to sequence your care on the basis of good time management. For example, you might deal with a simple problem first in order to free some uninterrupted time for more complex actions. What is your plan in this situation?

Discharge Planning

Discharge planning is the process of preparing the client to leave the healthcare agency. It includes preparing the client for self-care as well as providing for continuity of care between present caregivers and those who will care for the client after discharge. Because most patients are in the hospital only for a short time, it is essential to begin discharge planning on admission and continue it until the client leaves the agency. As a rule, discharge is not the end of the illness episode for the patient, but the transition to another phase of it. Research shows that discharge planning can reduce complications and readmissions (Naylor 1990; Schneider et al 1993). Tuazon (1992) has suggested using the word *MODEL* as a mnemonic device to help you concentrate on discharge planning basics:

M Make a written plan.
O Offer resources (eg, social worker).
D Devise ways to increase compliance.
E Evaluate your teaching with immediate feedback.
L Legal implications: Document.

Collaborative Discharge Planning

All patients need some degree of discharge planning, but you may not always need a separate, written discharge plan. You can sometimes include discharge assessments and teaching as nursing orders on the comprehensive care plan. For example, one nursing order for Mrs. Sanchez (in Chapters 3, 4, and 5) is to teach her to continue taking her antibiotics after discharge until they are all gone, even if she feels better. Most institutions have a standardized, preprinted discharge plan such as Figure 6–2, on page 255.

A written discharge plan is required for patients with special needs (eg, complex self-care needs, newly diagnosed chronic diseases such as diabetes). Patients are often discharged from the hospital still in need of skilled nursing care. They may be placed in a long-term care setting or sent home to continue complicated treatments and therapies (eg, apnea monitors, intravenous therapies, mechanical ventilators). Post-hospital needs are often met by members of a multidisciplinary team, which may include private-duty nurses; home care services; social services; physical therapists; housing departments; speech, occupational, and hearing therapists; physicians; and the client's family. Discharge planning must include all involved disciplines.

Discharge to Home Health Care

With the decreased length of hospital stays, transition to home and self-care has become very important. Home health nurses, too, must emphasize discharge planning as a part of their role (Cosnotti and Sprinkel 1993; Tirk 1992). Box 6–2 contains priorities to consider when discharging a client to home care. The following example illustrates the need for discharge planning:

> EXAMPLE: Anna was hospitalized for bacteremia and renal failure. After two months she went home, severely debilitated, to a one-room apartment. The diet that her nurse and dieticians had so carefully taught her in the hospital was impossible for her to follow with her low energy level and minimal cooking facilities. She could not afford to fill the prescription the physician had given her. Within 3 weeks, she was readmitted to the hospital, again with renal failure and bacteremia. (Adapted from Carr, 1990.)

■ PATIENT CARE PLANS

There are two kinds of care plans: comprehensive nursing care plans and multidisciplinary (collaborative) care plans. Both types may contain sections that are: (1) standardized, preplanned, and preprinted or (2) individualized to fit the unique needs of individual patients. The most obvious benefit of a written care plan is that it *provides continuity of care*. It is important—sometimes essential— that all caregivers use the same approach with a patient.

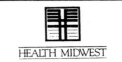

HEALTH MIDWEST

Discharge Summary Record

1. Discharge Date: _____ 2. Discharge Time: _____

Section I: DISCHARGE MODE

3. TO: ☐ Home ☐ SNU ☐ Rehab ☐ ECF ☐ Mental Health ☐ Other: _____ 4. MODE: ☐ Ambulatory ☐ WC ☐ Cart

If discharged to SNU, Rehab, ECF or other facility stop here and complete interagency transfer form.

5. TRANSPORTATION: ☐ Car ☐ Ambulance ☐ WC Van ☐ Other: _____ 6. Personal items (valuables, home meds, assist devices per NDB) returned ☐ N/A ☐ YES

Section II: CARE AT HOME

| 7. MEDICINE | DOSE | TIME | | | | | | REASON / SPECIAL INSTRUCTIONS | TIME NEXT DOSE | PRE-SCRIPTION GIVEN | USE HOME SUPPLY |
		AM	NOON	AFTERNOON	EVENING	BEDTIME	NIGHT				

☐ Addendum   ***** Medication Instructions Completed by: _____

INSTRUCTIONS

8. ☐ Call your doctor for the following _____

9. ☐ Appointment(s) with Dr. _____ Within _____ Phone _____
   Appointment made for _____ at _____

10. ☐ Appointment(s) with Dr. _____ Within _____ Phone _____
   Appointment made for _____ at _____

11. ☐ Appointment(s) with Dr. _____ Within _____ Phone _____
   Appointment made for _____ at _____

12. ☐ Outpatient appointment arranged (location/phone) _____

13. ☐ Diet (specify) _____

14. ☐ Food and your Medicine (specify food/drug interaction) _____

15. ☐ Exercise/Activity (specify) _____

16. ☐ Skin/Wound Care (Instructions) _____

17. ☐ Treatment/Therapy/Catheter/Lines/Tubes (specify) _____

18. ☐ Equipment, supplies (specify) _____
   Providing Company (name/phone) _____

19. ☐ Instructional Material (list what is given) _____

20. ☐ Home Health visits arranged (name/phone) _____

21. I have reviewed and understand the above instructions and I have also received a copy to take home for future reference.

_____ RN

_____   _____   _____
PATIENT or AGENT   DISCHARGE NURSE   REVIEWED BY

HM 10-36-605   Distribution: White - Medical Record   Yellow - Patient Copy   Pink - Physician Copy

Figure 6–2

Discharge Plan Record. *Source:* Courtesy of Research Medical Center, Kansas City, MO.

BOX 6-2

Discharge Planning Priorities

1. How will the following affect the patient's self-care ability?
   - Age
   - Medical condition
   - Financial resources
   - Disabilities/limitations (eg, secondary conditions such as poor vision)
   - Nutritional status (eg, special dietary needs)
   - Primary caregiver (eg, feelings about patient, abilities)
   - Home environment (eg, hazards, stairs, wheelchair access)
2. Is there a need for:
   - Referral to community agencies (eg, home-delivered meals)?
   - Someone to coordinate with the insurance company?
3. Home care teaching:
   - Begin when patient is receptive.
   - Include family members.
   - Notify home care agency of teaching done/needed.
4. At discharge, see that all plans are in place. For example, have arrangements been made for:
   - Transportation home (medically equipped or other)?
   - Medical supplies at home?
   - A nurse or home health aide?

Sources: Nazarko (1998), Tirk (1992), Tuazon (1992), Weissman and Jasovsky (1998), Kozier et al (2000).

EXAMPLE: Jed Goldstein is being treated on an adolescent mental health unit. The staff has been trying to modify his manipulative behavior. Val Benitez, RN, has been floated to the mental health unit from the critical care unit. She does not know Jed, but she reads an order on the nursing plan: "Do not respond to negative talk about staff on other shifts." Later, Jed begins to complain about the night nurse. Val's usual response to patients in the critical care unit is to remain neutral but encourage them to express their feelings. Instead, she remembers the nursing order and changes the subject. Val is not an experienced psychiatric nurse; without the care plan, her nurturing instincts and past experience might have prompted her to respond differently. This would not have been therapeutic for Jed, and would have undermined the work of the nurses on the other shifts.

A written care plan *promotes efficient functioning of the nursing team* by assuring that time is not wasted on ineffective approaches (as in the Jed

Goldstein example, above) and that efforts are not duplicated. By specifically outlining nursing interventions and expected client responses, written plans provide a convenient reference for organizing the nursing progress notes. They also help to assure adequate discharge planning, provide documentation for third-party reimbursement, and serve as a guide for making staff assignments.

Computerized Care Plans

Computer literacy has become another essential nursing skill. Computers are used to create both standardized and individualized care plans. The nurse can access the patient's stored care plan from a centrally located terminal at the nurses' station or from terminals in patient rooms. Computerized care plans are easy to review and update, and because they do not rely on human memory, they are likely to be thorough and accurate. Figure 6–3 is a computer screen showing an overview of the care plan for a patient with the medical condition "respiratory disorder." It includes several nursing diagnoses, as well as a section for "general patient care." Figure 6–4 is an example of a computer care plan for a single nursing diagnosis, using standardized nursing languages.

Comprehensive Nursing Care Plans

A **comprehensive nursing care plan** is made up of several different documents that integrate dependent, interdependent, and independent nursing functions. It provides a central source of patient information to guide care. The **nursing diagnosis care plan** is the section of the comprehensive plan that prescribes the interventions for the patient's nursing diagnoses and collaborative problems. This chapter focuses on nursing diagnosis care plans; comprehensive plans are discussed fully in Chapter 10.

Care plan forms differ from agency to agency. However, the format usually consists of at least three columns: nursing diagnoses, patient outcomes, and nursing orders. Some agencies add a column for evaluating patient responses to the nursing interventions. Planning usually progresses horizontally across the page. Nursing Diagnoses → Patient Outcomes → Nursing Orders → Evaluation. Figure 6–5 shows a typical format. In this format, you could write the assessment data in the same column as the nursing diagnosis if you use the *A.M.B.* format. A few agencies add a column for **rationale**, which consists of principles or scientific reasons for selecting a specific nursing action. It may also explain why the action is expected to achieve the outcome. Professional functioning requires an understanding of the rationale underlying the nursing orders, even when the rationale is not written on the care plan.

To be useful in the clinical setting, care plans must be concise and easy to use. Still, the format chosen should include adequate space to write individualized nursing orders, even when preprinted plans are used.

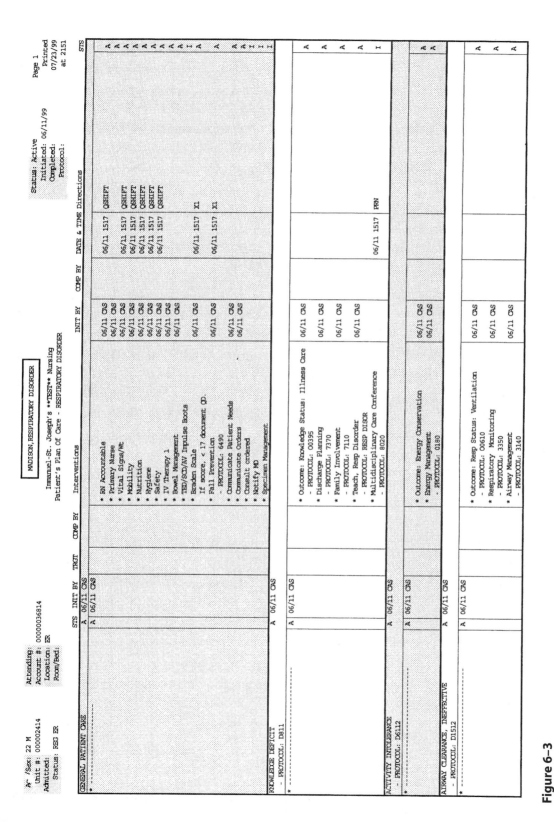

Figure 6-3

Computer Screen for Respiratory Disorder Plan of Care. *Source:* By permission of Immanuel-St. Joseph's Hospital, Albert Lea Medical Center, and Austin Medical Center of Mayo Health System, Mankato, MN.

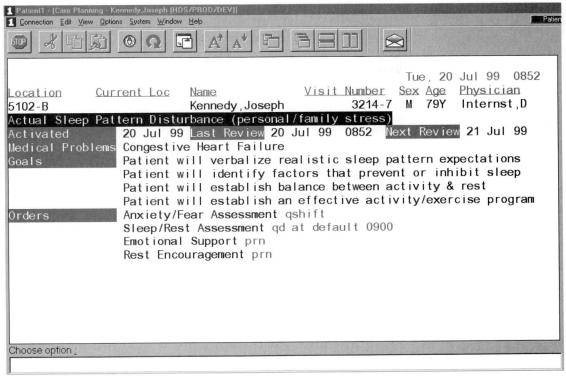

Figure 6–4
Computer Care Plan for a Single Nursing Diagnosis, Using Standardized Nursing Language. *Source:*
Courtesy of Per Se Technologies, Atlanta, GA. Used with permission.

Date	Nursing Diagnosis	Predicted Outcomes	Nursing Orders	Rationale	Evaluation
7/15/00	Decisional Conflict r/t value conflicts regarding termination of treatment A.M.B. tearfulness. Statements of inability to decide.	1. By 7/16 will discuss feelings about the situation with nurse and significant other. 2. etc.	1. Spend at least 15 minutes sitting with client during each visit. 2. Listen without making judgements. 3. etc.	1. Demonstrates support and caring. 2. Demonstrates acceptance of client's value and worth unconditionally. 3. etc.	7/16 Goal #1 Goal met. Discussed feelings of guilt with wife.

Figure 6–5
Sample Format for Nursing Care Plan

Student Care Plans

Care plans in practice settings are designed for nurses to use in delivering care. Student care plans are designed, in addition, for these purposes:

1. To help the student learn and apply the nursing process.
2. To provide a guide for giving nursing care to meet the client's needs while in the clinical setting.
3. To help the student learn about the client's pathophysiology or psychopathology and the associated nursing care.

Therefore, you may be required to write your student care plans without incorporating any preprinted plans. You may be expected to develop a list of all your patient's actual and risk (potential) nursing diagnoses and collaborative problems, not just the unusual ones, and to develop detailed nursing interventions for them. Your instructors may also ask you to provide an in-depth rationale for your nursing interventions, and perhaps to cite literature to support your rationale.

Multidisciplinary Care Plans (Critical Pathways)

A **critical pathway** (also called *interdisciplinary plan, multidisciplinary plan, collaborative plan, critical path,* and *action plan*) is a standardized, multidisciplinary care plan that sequences patient care based on diagnosis or case type. It outlines, by time (1) the crucial assessments and interventions that must be performed by nurses, physicians, and other health team members; and (2) the daily, or even hourly, patient outcomes necessary in order to achieve discharge goals within the defined length of stay. For example, for a patient undergoing an abdominal hysterectomy, part of the critical pathway might be as follows:

	Postoperative day 1	**Postoperative day 2**
Outcomes	Will verbalize pain appropriately to nurse; will state pain is < 5 on a 1–10 scale.	Will verbalize pain appropriately to RN; will state pain is < 2 on a 1–10 scale.
Interventions	Self-controlled administration of morphine per IV pump.	Tylenol #3, tabs 1, p.o. as needed.

Most critical pathways are developed for medical or surgical diagnoses, conditions, or procedures (eg, tests, treatments) and tend to emphasize biomedical problems and interventions. They work best for cases that occur frequently in an agency or that have relatively predictable outcomes. A different critical pathway is created for each case type; for example, myocardial infarction, cardiac catheterization, pneumonia, total hip replacement, etc. A critical pathway addresses the needs that *all* patients with a certain condition have in common. It does not take into account a patient's unique needs; those must be addressed by an individualized nursing diagnosis care plan, or sometimes through "variances" (refer to Chapter 4, "Using Nursing Diagnoses With Critical Pathways"). A **variance** occurs when (1) an outcome is not met in the specified time or (2) an intervention is not performed at the specified time. See Figure 10–7, on page 442, for an example of a critical pathway.

■ PATIENT OUTCOMES

Powerful market forces demand decreased healthcare costs, preferably without decreased quality. Therefore, healthcare institutions must compete for their "customers," who are not individuals but employers and businesses. This has led to outcomes-based care delivery: the use of outcomes to drive treatment planning, evaluation of care, and reimbursement by third-party payers (eg, Medicare, private insurers). The preceding discussion of critical pathways is one example of outcomes-based care. Critical pathways describe outcomes for multidisciplinary (including medical) interventions, but do not provide a way to judge *nursing* effectiveness and, therefore, do not provide a mechanism for nursing accountability. The remainder of this chapter focuses on individualized care planning and patient outcomes that are influenced by nursing care.

After determining the patient's present health status (nursing diagnosis), the next step is to set goals for changing or maintaining health status. A **goal**, or **desired outcome**, describes the patient responses you expect to achieve as a result of interventions. A **nursing-sensitive outcome** (or **goal**) is one that can be achieved or influenced by nursing interventions. The terms *goal* and *outcome* are used interchangeably by many nurses. This text will usually use the Nursing Outcomes Classification (NOC) terminology, in which the word **outcome**, when used alone, is defined as *any* patient response (good or bad) to interventions. *Goals* and *desired outcomes* are used as in the two introductory sentences of this paragraph (other terms with the same meaning are *predicted outcomes, expected outcomes,* and *outcome criteria*).

EXAMPLE:

Outcome Ambulation: walking

Goal (expected outcome, desired outcome, predicted outcome) Walks to end of hall without assistance.

You should be aware that some literature uses a slightly different scheme, defining *goals* as broad statements about the desired effects of the nursing activities, and *outcomes* (and other outcome terms) as the more specific, observable criteria used to evaluate whether the broad goal has been met.

EXAMPLE:

Broad Statements (Goals)	Specific Outcomes (Criteria)
Improve nutritional status ⟶	Will gain 5 lb by April 25.
Decrease pain ⟶	Will rate pain as less than 3 on a 1–10 scale.
Increase self-care abilities ⟶	Will be able to feed self by end of the week.

When goals are defined broadly, as in the above examples, the patient care plan must include *both* goals and outcomes. In fact, they are sometimes combined into one statement; the broad goal is stated first, followed by *as evidenced by*, and then a list of the observable responses that demonstrate achievement of the goal. Do not confuse *as evidenced by* with the phrase *as manifested by*, used in writing nursing diagnoses.

EXAMPLE:

Correct	*Incorrect*
Nutritional status will improve *as evidenced by* Weight gain of 5 lb by 4/25	Nutritional status will improve *as manifested by* Weight gain of 5 lb by 4/25

While you are learning, writing the broad, general goal first may help you to think of the specific outcomes that are needed. Remember, however, that while broad goals can be a starting point for planning, the specific, measurable outcomes *must* be written on the care plan.

Purpose of the Outcome Statement

Outcome statements guide the planning of care and the evaluation of changes in patient health status. When the outcomes state precisely and clearly what you wish to achieve, ideas for nursing actions flow logically from the outcomes, and it is relatively easy to select nursing orders to achieve the desired changes.

Outcome statements also provide a sense of achievement for both the client and the nurse and motivate them in their efforts to improve health status.

EXAMPLE: Kay Stein has essential hypertension. She has a demanding career and family life, and she needs to lose 50 lb. Even though she takes her antihypertensive medication faithfully, follows her low-calorie diet, and tries to decrease her stress, she still does not feel any better. In fact, she feels worse because the medication gives her a headache. However, she and her nurse have set measurable, achievable outcomes, such as "Loses 2 lb this week" and "B/P will be 130/80 by end of the week." When Kay's blood pressure reading is 120/80 mm Hg and the scale shows she has lost 4 lb, she has proof that her efforts are really accomplishing something. This helps motivate her to continue making lifestyle changes that she finds very difficult.

Writing Outcome Statements

Whether you use standardized language or your own wording, outcome statements must be specific and descriptive in order to be useful for planning and evaluating care. Figure 6–6 is an example of a computer screen that suggests outcomes for the nursing diagnosis entered by the nurse. Refer to Figure 6–4, on page 259, to see which outcomes were actually used for this patient.

Deriving Outcomes from Nursing Diagnoses

Except for wellness diagnoses, diagnostic statements describe human responses that are problems for the patient, family, or community. Stating a problem response suggests that the opposite response is preferred and is what you will try to achieve. The nursing diagnosis "Constipation r/t inactivity and

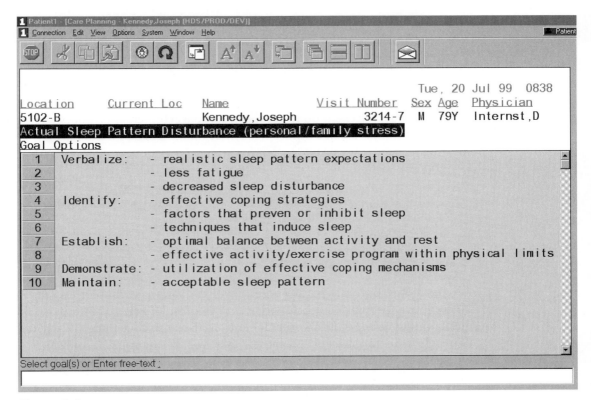

Figure 6–6

After the Nurse Enters a Nursing Diagnosis, a Computer Screen Lists Suggested Outcomes. *Source:* Courtesy of Per Se Technologies, Atlanta, GA. Used with permission.

inadequate fluid intake" indicates that the client's elimination status needs to change. An improvement in elimination status would be evidenced by an opposite (normal) response—that is, a regular, formed, soft bowel movement.

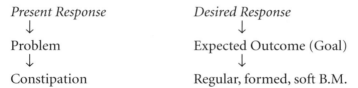

Present Response	Desired Response
↓	↓
Problem	Expected Outcome (Goal)
↓	↓
Constipation	Regular, formed, soft B.M.

When developing goal statements, look at the problem and think: What would the alternative healthy response be? To describe the response in terms of specific behaviors, ask yourself the following:

1. If the problem is solved (or prevented), how will the client look or behave? What will I be able to see, hear, palpate, smell, or otherwise observe with my senses?
2. What must the client do to show that the goal is achieved? How well must he do it?

EXAMPLE: The nursing diagnosis is "Fluid Volume Deficit r/t insufficient fluid intake." The unhealthy response is *fluid volume deficit*; the alternative healthy response would be *adequate fluid volume*.

1. If the problem is solved (fluid volume is adequate), how will the client look or behave? One observable response you could see and palpate is *elastic skin turgor*.
2. What must the client do to demonstrate goal achievement? A possible answer to this is that he must *drink more fluids than he excretes*. Also, you might specify that he would drink *a minimum amount of fluids*, perhaps 100 mL/h.

Therefore, your goal/outcome statement might be:

Will have adequate fluid volume, as evidenced by
a. elastic skin turgor
b. Intake = Output
c. drinks at least 100 mL/h

Outcomes, like nursing diagnoses, involve a variety of human responses, including appearance, body functions, symptoms, knowledge, interpersonal functioning, and emotions (see Table 6–1). Because outcomes are derived directly from the nursing diagnoses, they will be appropriate only if you have stated the nursing diagnosis correctly.

EXAMPLE: Vincent Aarusa is highly anxious about the surgery he is to undergo. He does not have a good understanding of the procedure, nor of its risks and benefits. Worse, his father died after having a similar surgery 20 years ago. His admitting nurse did not perceive the severity

Table 6–1 Examples of Alternative Healthy Responses

Nursing Diagnosis (present status)	Human Response	Desired Outcome
Ineffective Airway Clearance r/t poor cough effort 2° incisional pain & fear of "breaking stitches loose"	Appearance	Within 24 hours after surgery, will have no skin pallor or cyanosis during post-op period.
	Body functioning	Lungs clear to auscultation during entire post-op period.
	Symptoms	Within 48 hours after surgery, states having no shortness of breath when ambulating to chair.
	Knowledge	After reteaching, states rationale for turn, cough, deep breathing after surgery.
	Emotions	Within 48 hours after surgery, states he is no longer afraid to cough.

of his anxiety and wrote a nursing diagnosis of "Knowledge Deficit (Surgical Procedure) r/t no prior experience or teaching." The goal for this problem was stated as follows: "Will describe surgical procedure in general terms and discuss risks and benefits prior to surgery." When Mr. Aarusa was able to perform these behaviors, the nurse on the next shift discontinued the knowledge deficit problem, and no further discussion of his surgery was attempted by the nursing staff. Mr. Aarusa was sent to surgery with adequate information, but with no relief of his anxiety.

Essential Versus Nonessential Goals   The *essential* patient goals are derived from the problem (first) clause. The second clause sometimes suggests some goals as well.

Problem + Etiology
   ↓
Goals/Outcomes

Goals derived from the etiology are different from those derived from the problem. Their achievement may help to resolve the problem, but they could also be achieved *without* resolving the problem. In that case, the care plan might be discontinued because the goals had been met, but the client would still have the problem.

EXAMPLE:

	Problem		Etiology
Nursing Diagnosis:	Altered Nutrition: Less Than Body Requirements for Calories	r/t	Lack of appetite 2° depression
	↓		↓

Goals/Desired Outcomes:	1. Will gain 5 lb by 12/14.
	
	2. Will consume at least 2,000 calories per day.
			3. Will state his appetite is better within 3 days.
			4. Will be hungry at mealtimes by 12/1.
			5. By 12/1, will be less depressed, as evidenced by
			  a. no more than one crying spell per day.
			  b. participation in unit activities.

KEY POINT
Every nursing diagnosis must have at least one expected outcome that demonstrates resolution of the problem response.

Achieving goals 1 and 2 would actually show problem resolution. If the client gains 5 lb and consumes 2,000 calories per day, then he cannot have "less than body requirements for calories." This is not true for goals 3–5. The client's depression might lift and he might regain his appetite, but still continue to lose weight. If you discontinued the nutritional problem after measuring only objectives 3–5, you would do the client a disservice. Therefore, for every nursing diagnosis you must write at least one goal that, when achieved, shows direct resolution of the problem.

Goals for Actual, Risk, and Possible Nursing Diagnoses Outcome statements may reflect promotion, maintenance, or restoration of health, depending on the type of nursing diagnosis (see Table 6–2). For an *actual nursing diagnosis*, goals focus on restoring healthy responses and preventing further complications. They specify patient behaviors that demonstrate resolution or reduction of the problem and that patients should be able to achieve with the aid of independent nursing activities.

EXAMPLES:

Actual Nursing Diagnosis	*Outcome Statement*
Impaired Skin Integrity: Dermal Ulcer over coccyx r/t inability to move self in bed	Ulcer will not extend to deeper tissues.

Table 6–2 Goals/Desired Outcomes for Different Problem Types

Type of Problem	Patient Response Demonstrates:	Nursing Focuses on:
Actual nursing diagnosis	Resolution or reduction of problem	Resolution or reduction of problem Prevention of complication
Risk nursing diagnosis	Problem has not developed	Prevention and detection of problem
Possible nursing diagnosis	No patient responses	Confirmation or exclusion of problem
Collaborative problem	Problem has not developed	Detection and prevention of problem
Wellness diagnoses Health maintenance	Continuation of healthy functioning	Health maintenance
Health promotion	Achievement of a higher level of wellness	Health promotion

Ulcer will not become infected, as evidenced by absence of purulent exudate.

By 12/1, healing will be evidenced by decreased redness and appearance of granulation tissue in wound bed.

Goals for *risk nursing diagnoses* focus on preventing the problem; the client responses should demonstrate a problem-free level of functioning or, if that is not possible, maintenance of the present level of functioning. Achievement of these goals should mean that the problem is not present at the time the assessment is made.

EXAMPLES:

Risk Nursing Diagnosis	*Outcome Statements*
Risk for Ineffective Breast-feeding r/t breast engorgement	Infant will be observed to "latch on," suck, and swallow at each feeding.
	Mother will state satisfaction with breastfeeding.
	Infant will regain birth weight within 14 days after birth.

Possible nursing diagnoses present an exception to the rule; they are *not* written in terms of desired patient response. You use a possible diagnosis when you do not have enough data to determine whether the patient has the problem. The goal for a possible nursing diagnosis is really a *nursing* goal: that the presence of the diagnosis will be confirmed or ruled out. You do not need to write goals for possible diagnoses. However, to help assure that follow-up assessments will be done, you may wish to set a target time for confirming or ruling out the problem. If so, you could write a nursing goal. Nursing goals should *not* be written on the care plan for actual or potential problems.

EXAMPLE:

Possible Problem: Possible Hopelessness r/t abandonment by significant other after onset of chronic illness

Nursing Goal: Confirm or rule out Hopelessness by 6/12.

Goals for Collaborative Problems Outcomes for nursing diagnoses are "nurse sensitive." That is, they can be brought about primarily by nursing interventions. Nurses and physicians share accountability for achieving outcomes for *collaborative problems*. Therefore, outcomes for these problems are usually found in the agency's standardized care plans or critical pathways. Nursing care plans do not need goal statements for collaborative problems because they contain only *nursing* orders, and it is understood that the broad goal is prevention or early detection of the problem. Furthermore, it may not be legally advisable to write goals that imply nursing accountability, when accountability for the problem actually is shared with other professions.

As a student, however, it may enhance your learning to write goals for collaborative problems. This will assure that you know precisely what symptoms you are looking for and can recognize whether or not the problem is developing. When writing such outcomes, remember that a collaborative problem is a potential problem, not an actual problem. Nursing care focuses on prevention and early detection of the complication. Outcomes for collaborative problems should describe the patient responses you will observe as long as the problem has not developed. The goals may describe normal functioning or problem symptoms that you do *not* want to occur.

EXAMPLES:

Collaborative Problem	*Outcome Statements*
Potential Complication of Childbirth: Postpartum Hemorrhage	Postpartum hemorrhage will not occur, as evidenced by 1. saturating less than 1 vag. pad per hour during first 24 hours. 2. fundus firm and below umbilicus during first 24 hours. 3. pulse and B/P in normal range for patient.

Short-Term and Long-Term Goals

Short-term goals can be achieved within a few days or a few hours. Goals dealing with survival needs may even be stated in terms of minutes. For this reason, short-term goals are useful in acute-care settings, such as hospitals, where nurses often focus on the client's more immediate needs. The client may be discharged before the nurse can evaluate progress toward long-term goals. Some examples of short-term goals follow:

EXAMPLES:

Voids within 6 hours after delivery of infant.
State relief of pain within 1 hour after receiving p.o. oxycodone.
Walks to end of hall and back, unassisted, by day 2 post-op.

Short-term goals can be used to measure progress toward long-term goals. Achieving several short-term goals also provides reinforcement for the client, encouraging him to keep working on the problem.

EXAMPLE:

Long-Term Goal   Will have daily B.M. without use of laxatives *within 2 months.*

Short-Term Goals   After administration of enema will have B.M. *within 4 hours.*

Will have next B.M. *within 36 hours* without aid of p.o. laxatives.

Will use chemical or mechanical stimulation for B.M. not more than two times *this week.*

Immediately, diet changes include prune juice and oatmeal (or other high-fiber cereal) for breakfast, and substituting whole grain for white bread.

Within 1 week reports he is eating at least one good source of fiber at every meal.

As a student, you will probably care for a patient for only a few hours at a time. You should write short-term goals to measure what you can realistically accomplish while you are with the client, so that you can evaluate the results of the care you have given. In a comprehensive care plan you should also include longer-range goals that other nurses can use to evaluate patient progress when you are not there.

Long-term goals describe changes in client outcomes over a longer period—usually a week or more. The ideal long-term goal aims at restoring normal functioning in the problem area. When normal functioning cannot be restored, the long-term goal describes the maximum level of functioning that can be achieved given the client's health status and resources. Long-term goals are especially useful for clients with chronic health problems and those in home health care, rehabilitation centers, and other extended-care facilities. Some examples of long-term goals follow:

EXAMPLES:

After attending six weekly childbirth-education classes, will correctly demonstrate abdominal and shallow chest breathing.
By 12 weeks post-op, will have full range of motion of right shoulder.
Within 3 months (12/24), will feed self using fork or spoon.

Components of Goal Statement

As a rule, every goal statement (expected outcome) should contain a subject, an action verb, performance criteria, and a target time. It may sometimes be necessary to state "special conditions" as well. See Table 6–3 for examples of goal statement components.

Subject   The subject of the goal is a noun. It is the client, any part of the client, or a property or characteristic of the client.

EXAMPLES:

Client	Mucous membranes
Ms. Atwell	Anxiety
Lung sounds	

The subject is the client unless otherwise stated. Think, "Client will . . ." as you begin the goal statement, but do not write "Client will."

EXAMPLE:

Incorrect: *Client will* describe pain as < 3 on a scale of 1–10.

Correct: *Will* describe pain as < 3 on a scale of 1–10.
        Describes pain as < 3 on a scale of 1–10.

Action Verb   The verb describes the desired client action (for example, what the client is to learn or do). Using actions that can be seen, heard, smelled, felt, or measured will help make your outcomes specific and observable. Action verbs create a picture of the desired client condition or performance. Each outcome should describe only one desired client condition; therefore, each should contain only one action verb.

Table 6–3   Components of Goal/Expected Outcome Statements

Subject	Verb	Special Conditions	Performance Criteria	Target Time
Patient	will list	(after attending nutrition class)	two low-fat foods from each of the Food Guide Pyramid groups	before discharge.
Patient's lungs	will be	—	clear to auscultation	within 24 hours.
Client	will walk	(using walker)	to bathroom and back without shortness of breath	within 3 days.

EXAMPLE:

Correct: Will *describe* the food groups in the Food Guide Pyramid . . .

Incorrect: Will *describe* the food groups in the Food Guide Pyramid and *choose* a balanced diet . . .

Performance Criteria   Performance criteria are the standards used to evaluate the quality of the client's performance. They describe the *extent* to which the client is expected to perform the behavior. The performance criteria indicate what should be measured in evaluating outcomes. Performance criteria may specify amount, quality, speed, distance, accuracy, and so forth—they tell *how, what, when, or where.*

EXAMPLES:

		What	**When**
Amount	Will lose	5 lb	during the first week.

		How	**What**
Accuracy	Will draw up	correct amount	of insulin.

		What	**How**
Quality	Will inject	insulin	using sterile technique.

		Where	**When**
Distance and Amount	Will walk	to the end of the hall	three times per day.

Target Time   Each expected outcome should specify the time by which you realistically expect a change in patient response (eg, by discharge, by April 2, at all times). The target time helps to pace the patient's care, provides motivation by focusing on the future, and provides a deadline for evaluating patient progress.

EXAMPLE: Will name the food groups in the Food Guide Pyramid *within 24 hours* after receiving pamphlet.

The target time is a type of performance criterion, because it specifies the speed with which a goal is to be accomplished. In the example above, the client's progress would not be satisfactory if he took longer than 24 hours to learn the food groups.

Nursing knowledge and experience are needed for setting realistic target times. You will need to know the usual rate of progress for clients with the identified medical and nursing diagnoses and consider the client's particular capabilities and resources.

EXAMPLE: Esther Brady has just had an abdominal hysterectomy. Review of usual progress after this surgery indicates that most patients require intravenous or intramuscular narcotic analgesics for 24 hours and are then able to obtain relief from milder, oral analgesics. However, Ms. Brady is very anxious and has a history of poor pain tolerance. It would not be realistic to set a target time of 24 hours for resolution of her Pain diagnosis. A more achievable goal might be "Will obtain adequate pain relief from p.o. analgesics within 48 hours postop, as evidenced by patient's statement that pain is < 3 on a 1–10 scale."

Potential (Risk) Problems   Predicted outcomes for risk problems do not need target times. The broad goal is to prevent the problem from occurring, so in a sense the target time is *at all times*.

EXAMPLE:

Nursing Diagnosis: Risk for impaired skin integrity r/t immobility . . .

Predicted Outcome: Skin will remain intact, with no redness over bony prominences.
(Target time: At all times)
(Evaluate plan: Daily)

In the preceding example, the target time is assumed, so you would not need to write it on the care plan. However, you may wish to schedule times for evaluating the outcomes and the accompanying plan of care.

Special Conditions   If it is important to describe the conditions under which a client is to perform a behavior, you may need to add modifiers to the performance criteria. **Modifiers** describe the amount of assistance the client will need, available resources, environmental conditions, or experiences the client should have before being expected to perform the behavior. Like performance criteria, modifiers describe *how, when, where,* and *how much*.

EXAMPLES:

Type of assistance

How   Will walk to the end of the hall three times per day, using a walker, by April 8.

Prior experience

When   Will list foods high in cholesterol after consulting with dietician.

Environmental conditions

Where   In one-to-one session, will express fear of abandonment by Friday.

Not all goals need special conditions; they are included only if they are important. If the performance criteria clearly specify the expected performance, then special conditions are not necessary.

The Nursing Outcomes Classification (NOC)

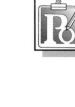

The NOC is a standardized vocabulary for describing patient outcomes. In this system, an **outcome** is "a measurable patient, family, or community state, behavior, or perception, conceptualized as a variable, largely influenced by and sensitive to nursing interventions" (Johnson, Maas, and Moorhead, 2000, p. 25). The 2000 edition of the taxonomy has 260 outcomes, organized in a taxonomy with six "domains": Functional Health, Physiological Health, Health Knowledge and Behavior, Perceived Health, Family Health, and Community Health. Each NOC outcome has a label (eg, Mobility Level), a definition, a list of indicators, and a measurement scale (see Table 6–4 below).

In the NOC taxonomy, the **outcome label** (also referred to as "the outcome"), is the broadly stated, one- to three-word, standardized name (eg, coping, mobility level, knowledge: diet). The outcome is worded as a neutral state to allow for the identification of positive, negative, or no change in a patient's status. The nurse chooses outcomes based on the nursing diagnoses that have been identified. For example, for a patient with a diagnosis of Impaired Physical Mobility, the nurse might choose mobility level, transfer performance, and balance.

Table 6–4 Example of a NOC Outcome

Mobility Level
Definition: Ability to move purposefully

Mobility Level Indicators	Dependent, does not participate	Requires assistive person and device	Requires assistive person	Independent with assistive device	Completely independent
Balance performance	1	2	3	4	5
Body positioning performance	1	2	3	4	5
Muscle movement	1	2	3	4	5
Joint movement	1	2	3	4	5
Transfer performance	1	2	3	4	5
Ambulation: walking	1	2	3	4	5
Ambulation: wheelchair	1	2	3	4	5
Other: (specify)	1	2	3	4	5

Source: Johnson M., M. Maas, and S. Moorhead, eds. (2000). *Nursing Outcomes Classification (NOC)* (2nd ed.). St. Louis: Mosby, p. 305.

Indicators are concrete, observable, behaviors and states (eg, balance performance, joint movement) that can be used to evaluate patient status. In Table 6–4, you would observe and rate the patient's balance performance and joint movement, for example, in evaluating his mobility level. Each outcome includes a list of indicators; the nurse selects the indicators that are appropriate for the patient and may add to the list. A five-point **measurement scale** is used to evaluate patient status on each indicator. Usually 1 is the least desirable and 5 is the most desirable patient condition along a continuum. Table 6–5 below provides some examples of scales.

It is not necessary to state desired outcomes (or goals) in this system. You merely rate the patient's status on each indicator (giving it a number) before and after interventions. You can, however, use the NOC outcomes to write goals (eg, on a care plan). You simply write the label, the indicators that apply to the patient, and the location on the measuring scale that is desired for each indicator. For example, using the outcome in Table 6–4, you might individualize goals for a patient as follows:

Mobility Level:

Transfer performance (5: completely independent)

Ambulation: walking (4: independent with assistive device)

Written traditionally as a goal statement, that goal would read:

> "Mobility will improve, as evidenced by the ability to: transfer independently (5) and walk with assistive device (walker) (4)."

Figure 6–3, p. 258, illustrates the use of NOC outcomes in computerized care planning.

Table 6–5   Examples of NOC Measurement Scales

1	2	3	4	5
Extremely compromised	Substantially compromised	Moderately compromised	Mildly compromised	Not compromised
Dependent, does not participate	Requires assistive person and device	Requires assistive person	Independent with assistive device	Completely independent
None	Limited	Moderate	Substantial	Extensive
Severe	Substantial	Moderate	Slight	None

Source: From Johnson M., M. Maas, and S. Moorhead, eds. (2000). *Nursing Outcomes Classification (NOC)* (2nd ed.). St. Louis: Mosby, pp. 48–61. Used with permission.

Family and Home Health Outcomes

Home health nurses use both individual and family outcomes. The NOC taxonomy includes 7 outcomes specific to the family as a group (NOC 2000). Others may be used with NANDA family diagnoses. For a diagnosis of Ineffective Family Coping, for example, an outcome of "compliance behavior" might be used. Indicators of "compliance behavior" might be that the family "relies on health professional for current information" and "keeps appointments with a health professional" (Johnson and Mass 1997, p. 132).

The Home Health Care Classification (HHCC) defines an outcome as "What really happened to the recipient of services in terms of the particular problem for which care was provided" (Head et al 1997, p. 51; Saba 1995, 1997). The HHCC system provides three modifiers: *improved*, *stabilized*, and *deteriorated*. The nurse uses these to create an outcome goal for each nursing diagnosis, as in the following example:

EXAMPLE:

Nursing Diagnosis:	Sleep pattern disturbance
Goal/Expected Outcome:	Sleep pattern disturbance, improved
Actual Status at Discharge:	Sleep pattern disturbance, stabilized

Because the resulting goals are not clearly defined and measurable, they are not useful for testing the effects of nursing interventions (Parlocha and Henry 1998). The HHCC system is designed for home health care. However, none of the HHCC nursing diagnoses is specific to families, so there are no family-specific outcomes. It seems reasonable to expect that future revisions, as NANDA has done, will include family diagnoses and outcomes. The Omaha system can also be used to describe family outcomes. Refer to Chapter 4 and the following discussion of "Community Outcomes."

Community Outcomes

Community health nurses need outcomes for individuals, families, and "aggregates" (groups of people or entire communities). NOC presently includes six outcomes specifically for use with aggregates (NOC 2000).

Using the Omaha system, the nurse creates outcomes by applying a "problem rating scale" to each nursing diagnosis. The rating scale measures what the client knows (knowledge), does (behavior), and is (status) with regard to the nursing diagnosis (see Table 6–6). An example of an expected outcome using this scale follows:

KEY POINT
NOC Family Outcomes

Family Coping

Family Environment: Internal

Family Functioning

Family Health Status

Family Integrity

Family Normalization

Family Participation in Professional Care

KEY POINT
NOC Community Outcomes

Community Competence

Community Health Status

Community Health: Immunity

Community Risk Control: Chronic Disease

Community Risk Control: Communicable Disease

Community Risk Control: Lead Exposure

Table 6–6 Omaha Problem Rating Scale for Outcomes

CONCEPT	1	2	3	4	5
Knowledge The ability of the client to remember and interpret information	No knowledge	Minimal knowledge	Basic knowledge	Adequate knowledge	Superior knowledge
Behavior The observable responses, actions, or activities of the client fitting the occasion or purpose	Never appropriate	Rarely appropriate	Inconsistently appropriate	Usually appropriate	Consistently appropriate
Status The condition of the client in relation to objective and subjective defining characteristics	Extreme signs/ symptoms	Severe signs/ symptoms	Moderate signs/ symptoms	Minimal signs/ symptoms	No signs/ symptoms

Source: Martin, K. S. and N. J. Scheet (1992). *The Omaha system: Applications for community health nursing.* Philadelphia: W. B. Saunders, p. 92. Used with permission.

EXAMPLE:

Nursing Diagnosis: Deficit in family sanitation

Rating Scale	Present Status	Expected Outcome
Knowledge:	(2) Minimal knowledge	(3) Basic knowledge
Behavior:	(3) Inconsistently appropriate	(4) Usually appropriate
Status:	(3) Moderate signs/symptoms	(4) Minimal signs/ symptoms

Because there are presently no aggregate nursing diagnoses in the Omaha system, there are no outcomes specific to groups. Table 6–7 provides a list of aggregate goals; it is the list of health promotion and disease prevention goals that the US Public Health Service has set for improving the health of the nation. The two overarching goals are:

- Increase quality and years of healthy life
- Eliminate health disparities (*Healthy People 2010*, p. 2 of Vol. I).

Outcomes for Wellness Diagnoses

Recall that wellness diagnoses describe essentially healthy responses that the client wishes to maintain or improve. Expected outcomes for these diagnoses describe client responses that demonstrate health maintenance or

Table 6–7   U.S. Public Health Service Priorities for the Year 2010

Focus Area	Goal
1. Access to Quality Health Services	Improve access to comprehensive, high-quality health care services
2. Arthritis, Osteoporosis, and Chronic Back Conditions	Prevent illness and disability related to arthritis and other rheumatic conditions, osteoporosis, and chronic back conditions
3. Cancer	Reduce the number of new cancer cases as well as the illness, disability, and death caused by cancer
4. Chronic Kidney Disease	Reduce new cases of chronic kidney disease and its complications, disability, death, and economic costs
5. Diabetes	Through prevention programs, reduce the disease and economic burden of diabetes, and improve the quality of life for all persons who have or are at risk for diabetes
6. Disability and Secondary Conditions	Promote the health of people with disabilities, pervent secondary conditions, and eliminate disparities between people with and without disabilities in the U.S. population
7. Educational and Community-Based Programs	Increase the quality, availability, and effectiveness of educational and community-based programs designed to prevent disease and improve health and quality of life
8. Environmental Health	Promote health for all through a healthy environment
9. Family Planning	Improve pregnancy planning and spacing and prevent unintended pregnancy
10. Food Safety	Reduce foodborne illnesses
11. Health Communication	Use communication strategically to improve health
12. Heart Disease and Stroke	Improve cardiovascular health and quality of life through the prevention, detection, and treatment of risk factors; early identification and treatment of heart attacks and strokes; and prevention of recurrent cardiovascular events
13. HIV	Prevent HIV infection and its related illness and death
14. Immunization and Infectious Diseases	Prevent disease, disability, and death from infectious diseases, including vaccine-preventable diseases
15. Injury and Violence Prevention	Reduce injuries, disabilities, and deaths due to unintentional injuries and violence
16. Maternal, Infant, and Child Health	Improve the health and well-being of women, infants, children, and families
17. Medical Product Safety	Ensure the safe and effective use of medical products
18. Mental Health and Mental Disorders	Improve mental health and ensure access to appropriate, quality mental health services
19. Nutrition and Overweight	Promote health and reduce chronic disease associated with diet and weight
20. Occupational Safety and Health	Promote the health and safety of people at work through prevention and early intervention
21. Oral Health	Prevent and control oral and craniofacial diseases, conditions, and injuries and improve access to related services
22. Physical Activity and Fitness	Improve health, fitness, and quality of life through daily physical activity
23. Public Health Infrastructure	Ensure that federal, tribal, state, and local health agencies have the infrastructure to provide essential public health service effectively
24. Respiratory Diseases	Promote respiratory health through better prevention, detection, treatment, and education
25. Sexually Transmitted Diseases	Promote responsible sexual behaviors, strengthen community capacity, and increase access to quality services to prevent sexually transmitted diseases (STDs) and their complications
26. Substance Abuse	Reduce substance abuse to protect the health, safety, and quality of life for all, especially children
27. Tobacco Use	Reduce illness, disability, and death related to tobacco use and exposure to secondhand smoke
28. Vision and Hearing	Improve the visual and hearing health of the Nation through prevention, early detection, treatment, and rehabilitation

Source: From *Healthy People 2010*. U.S. Department of Health and Human Services, Washington, DC. For more information, visit www.health.gov/healthy people or call 1-800-367-4725.

achievement of a higher level of healthy functioning (eg, "Over the next year, Mrs. Jacobs will continue participating in religious activities that provide spiritual support.") The goals in Table 6–7, on page 277, are examples of wellness outcomes for groups. By using the highest number on the rating scale (5), both the NOC and Omaha systems can be used to write wellness outcomes.

EXAMPLES:

NOC: *Nursing Diagnosis*: Health-Seeking Behaviors
Expected Outcomes: (5) Very strong health orientation

Omaha: *Nursing Diagnosis*: Health Promotion: Physical Activity
Expected Behavior: (5) Superior knowledge, (5) consistently appropriate behavior with regard to physical activity

Nurses who use a wellness framework focus on the client potentials rather than on client problems. They lead clients to envisioning change and action rather than prescribing for the client. Nevertheless, goals are important. If the client commits to a plan of action (ie, sets a goal), that is a good predictor of actual behavior change. Research suggests that nurses set goals with clients to begin their intended behaviors within a 2-month time frame (Frenn and Malin 1998).

Patient Teaching Outcomes

Some patients need a special teaching plan to address their learning needs (see Chapter 10). **Teaching objectives** are patient outcomes that describe what the patient is to learn or how he will demonstrate learning. Objectives should reflect whether the learning is to take place in the cognitive, psychomotor, or affective domain. **Cognitive learning** involves perception, understanding, and the storing and recall of new information. **Psychomotor learning** involves physical skills. **Affective learning** involves changes in feelings, attitudes, and values.

EXAMPLES:

Cognitive domain   Learner will *explain* the effect of weight on B/P.

Psychomotor domain   Learner will *apply* B/P cuff correctly.

Affective domain   Learner will state that he *feels* confident with his ability to obtain correct B/P readings.

As with all goals, choose active verbs for learning objectives; they will help you to think of teaching strategies and make it easier to evaluate whether learning takes place. Table 6–8 provides a few suggestions for active verbs in each of the learning domains.

When writing objectives for the affective domain, keep in mind that you cannot directly observe a feeling or an attitude. Therefore, you could not write a goal such as "Learner will feel happier by May 2." You can, however,

Table 6–8   Active Verbs for Learning Objectives

Cognitive Domain	Psychomotor Domain	Affective Domain
Compare	Arrange	Choose
Define	Assemble	Defend
Describe	Construct	Discuss
Differentiate	Manipulate	Express
Explain	Organize	Help
Identify	Show	Justify
List	Start	Select
Name	Take	Share
State		

observe behaviors that *indicate* the client's feelings or moods. The following examples allow you to infer that the client is happy:

EXAMPLES: By May 2, will state that he feels happier than before.
By May 2, will be observed smiling at least twice a day.
By May 2, will resume past habit of singing in the shower.

■ CRITICAL THINKING: REFLECTING ON PLANNING

You will use critical thinking to decide which of the patient's problems can be addressed by standards of care, critical pathways, or other standardized approaches, and to develop outcomes for the nursing diagnoses that require an individualized approach. Outcome projection is an aspect of therapeutic judgment, in which the nurse predicts what is possible to achieve based on available human, material, and economic resources (Gordon et al 1994). Core questions for reflecting on the planning phase are:

- Is this a useful and usable care plan?
- Do these outcomes provide a good picture of the changes desired in the patient's health status?
- Are these outcomes stated in a way that makes them useful for planning and evaluating care?

Table 6–9, on page 280, provides a summary of questions to help you think about your thinking in the planning phase. The remainder of this chapter discusses guidelines to help you think critically about your outcome statements and about the legal, ethical, spiritual, and cultural implications of outcome statements.

Table 6–9 Planning Outcomes: Think About Your Thinking

Standard of Reasoning	Questions for Reflection
Refer to Chapter 2 for a review of standards of reasoning, as needed.	
Clarity	■ Are the goals/expected outcomes stated clearly, so that any nurse could use them to measure patient progress? ■ Are the outcomes stated concisely?
Accuracy	■ Would goal achievement indicate problem resolution? ■ Is the outcome appropriate to and derived from the nursing diagnosis? ■ Are outcomes revised to reflect changes in patient status?
Precision	■ Are the goals/outcomes stated precisely and in detail, rather than vaguely? ■ Are the outcomes observable or measurable?
Relevance, Significance, Depth	■ What are the most important goals to accomplish? ■ Overall, what is the primary focus of the care for this patient? ■ Am I qualified to make this plan, or do I need help? ■ Are there enough outcomes to completely address each nursing diagnosis? ■ Does each goal statement have the necessary components?
Breadth	■ Does the standardized plan or critical pathway address all the important patient needs, or do I need an individualized plan? ■ Did I make sure the patient and family agree with the goals? ■ Are the goals congruent with the total treatment plan? ■ Are the goals realistic and achievable?
Logic	■ Are the goals/outcomes derived from the patient problem? ■ Is each outcome derived from only *one* nursing diagnosis? ■ Is the outcome stated as a patient response, not a nurse activity?

Guidelines for Judging the Quality of Outcome Statements

1. (Standards: Accuracy, Logic) The outcome is appropriate to and derived from the nursing diagnosis. For each diagnosis, at least one outcome demonstrates resolution of the problem clause. Outcomes *b* and *c* in Figure 6–7 demonstrate this guideline.

2. (Standard: Logic) Each outcome is derived from only *one* nursing diagnosis. An outcome should have only one patient behavior; otherwise evaluation is difficult. In Outcome *a*, Figure 6–7, suppose the patient had no urge incontinence but was still having pain when voiding. Would you conclude that the outcome was met or not met?

3. (Standard: Logic) The outcome is stated in terms of patient responses rather than nurse activities. Thinking "Patient will . . ." at the beginning of each goal can help you focus on patient behaviors, rather than on your own actions; but do not write "patient will."

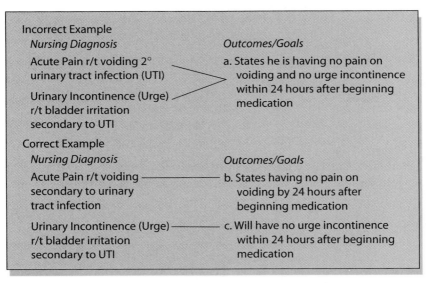

Incorrect Example

Nursing Diagnosis   *Outcomes/Goals*

Acute Pain r/t voiding 2°   a. States he is having no pain on
urinary tract infection (UTI)   voiding and no urge incontinence
                                               within 24 hours after beginning
Urinary Incontinence (Urge)   medication
r/t bladder irritation
secondary to UTI

Correct Example

Nursing Diagnosis   *Outcomes/Goals*

Acute Pain r/t voiding ——————— b. States having no pain on
secondary to urinary   voiding by 24 hours after
tract infection   beginning medication

Urinary Incontinence (Urge) ——————— c. Will have no urge incontinence
r/t bladder irritation   within 24 hours after beginning
secondary to UTI   medication

Figure 6–7
Example for Guidelines 1 and 3

EXAMPLE:

Nurse Activity (Incorrect)   Prevent infection of incision.

Patient Response (Correct)   Incision will not become infected, as
                                evidenced by:
                                1. absence of redness
                                2. no drainage
                                3. edges approximated

**4. (Standard: Accuracy) The outcomes are revised to reflect changes in pa-
tient status.** As you work with a patient you will gain a clearer idea of her
health status and abilities. You will then be able to write more accurate, individualized outcomes. The following example shows how outcomes can be individualized and revised for a patient with a nursing diagnosis of Activity
Intolerance r/t prolonged immobility.

EXAMPLE:

Initial Goal/Outcome: Ability to tolerate activity will improve, as
                           evidenced by:
(General)   1. walking progressively farther each day.
                           2. increased ability to perform self-care
                              (hygiene, etc.)

Revised Goal/Outcome: Ability to tolerate activity will improve, as
                           evidenced by:
(More specific)   1. by 5/12, walks to chair (8 ft.) without
                              shortness of breath

	2. by 5/12, assists with bath by washing own hands, face, and torso
Revised Goal/Outcome:	Ability to tolerate activity will improve, as evidenced by:
(After condition deteriorates)	1. by 5/18, sits on side of bed with no change in vital signs.
	2. by 5/18, assists with bath by washing own face.

5. (Standard: Clarity) Predicted outcomes are phrased in positive terms— that is, in terms of what you hope will occur, rather than what you hope will *not* occur.

EXAMPLE:

Negative wording: Skin will not become broken or ulcerated.

Positive wording: Skill will remain intact.

For potential problems, it may be difficult to think of positive terms. It is easier, for example, to write "No redness" than to describe exactly the color of normal skin. You cannot just write "Skin color will be normal," because *normal* is too vague. In such instances, you may use negative terms. A measurable, negatively worded outcome is actually a list of the signs and symptoms you are trying to prevent. In Item 3, preceding, outcomes 1 and 2 are negatively worded; outcome 3 is positively worded. The nurse would try to prevent outcomes 1 and 2, and achieve outcome 3.

6. (Standard: Clarity) The outcome is concise. Outcomes should be stated in as few words as possible without sacrificing clarity.

EXAMPLE:

Wordy: By April 15, the patient will demonstrate adequate knowledge of an appropriate low-calorie diet by listing foods to avoid and foods allowed in each of the Food Guide Pyramid groups.

More Concise: By 4/15, lists for each food group foods to avoid and foods allowed on low-calorie diet.

As a rule, do not write "patient will." Specify who is to perform the behavior only when it is *not* the patient. You might write, for example, "By dismissal, *Ms. Rauh* will demonstrate ability to change Mr. Rauh's dressing according to printed guidelines she received."

7. (Standard: Precision) The outcome is directly observable or measurable. Use action verbs to describe what the client will be able to do, and to what extent. This assures that others can make observations to determine whether the goal has been met and the problem resolved. In the following example, you cannot observe what the patient knows. However, you could observe whether she can name the high-sodium foods.

EXAMPLE:

Incorrect: By 11/30 will *know* which foods to avoid

Correct: By 11/30 will *name* the high-sodium foods to avoid in each food group

You cannot observe actions such as *understands*, *knows*, *feels*, or *appreciates*. If you cannot avoid using such verbs, make them more precise by adding the phrase "as evidenced by," followed by the responses you wish to see.

8. (Standard: Precision) The outcome is specific and concrete. Other nurses should have no doubt about the focus for nursing care when reading an outcome. Vague, general words can be interpreted in several ways and lead to disagreement about whether the outcome has been met. Avoid performance criteria such as *normal*, *adequate*, *sufficient*, *more*, *less*, and *increased*. Does "increased activity tolerance" mean that the patient can run a mile, or does it mean that he can walk from the chair to the bed with no shortness of breath?

When possible, individualize outcomes to describe the patient's normal baseline measurements. The upper limit of "normal" blood pressure is 140/90 mm Hg, and a goal of "B/P within normal limits" would imply this number. However, for a patient whose B/P is usually 90/50 mm Hg, the "normal" limit is too high.

9. (Standard: Depth). Each goal statement has all the necessary components: subject, action verb, performance criteria, special conditions (when needed) and target time (usually).

10. (Standard: Depth). Outcomes are adequate (eg, in number) to address each nursing diagnosis. This is related to Guideline No. 1. Ask, "If these predicted outcomes are achieved, will the problem be resolved?" If they are written in very specific terms, several outcomes may be needed for each diagnosis in order to meet this guideline. For the diagnosis of Anxiety, none of the following outcomes by itself would show that anxiety was resolved.

EXAMPLE:

Nursing Diagnosis: Severe Anxiety r/t unresolved role conflicts (mother/wife/attorney)

Outcomes: After one-on-one interaction, will be less anxious, as evidenced by:
1. statements that she feels better
2. fewer than two episodes of tearfulness in the next 24 hours
3. smoking no more than one cigarette per hour

11. (Standard: Breadth) The outcome is valued by the client, family, or community. The plan of care is more likely to be effective if it is designed to help clients achieve goals that they value. For example, knowing that obesity aggravates hypertension, your goal may be that a client will lose 40 lb. However, if eating is the client's only pleasure, he may not share your goal; he may prefer to accept the risks of hypertension rather than lose his only pleasure. If his goals do not include losing weight, then no matter how good your plan is, it will probably fail.

When nurse and patient goals conflict, it may help to explore the patient's reasoning with him, provide a rationale for your goals, and look for alternative approaches. This will involve the patient in decisions about his care and keep communication open. Involve patients and families to the extent of their interests and abilities. Be sure they agree that the problem is one that requires change and that the outcome is worth achieving. This ensures that your time and energy are spent on plans that meet patient needs and are likely to succeed.

12. (Standard: Breadth) The outcome is congruent with the total treatment plan. For example, the outcome "Will demonstrate correct technique for bathing baby by postpartum day 2" would not be compatible with the medical treatment plan for a mother whose newborn is too ill to be bathed.

13. (Standard: Breadth) Remember that outcomes can be written for families and communities, as well as individuals. Refer to discussions of "Family and Home Health Outcomes" and "Community Outcomes" on pages 275– 276.

14. (Standards: Breadth and Depth) The predicted outcomes are realistic and achievable in terms of the client's internal and external resources. Be sure you have considered physical and mental status, coping mechanisms, support system, financial status, and available community services. The outcome "Will demonstrate desire to comply with treatment by keeping all clinic appointments," is not realistic for a client with no car and no money for cab fare. Clients are not motivated to achieve outcomes they believe to be impossible.

Consider also whether the capabilities of the staff and the resources of the agency are adequate to achieve the outcomes. For example, "Uses relaxation techniques to achieve pain relief" is not achievable unless staffing is adequate to allow time for teaching and supervised practice.

Ethical Considerations in Planning

The planning process raises issues about the extent to which patients should be involved in planning their own care and about whether they are truly able to make free and informed decisions about their care. Goals are not value-neutral—not even the goals that nurses and patients set together. Merely by stating a goal in the direction of health, we declare that health is something we value. Most people probably do value health, but the situation is not so clear with all goals.

Obligation to Inform

The ANA *Code for Nurses* (1985) states that "The nurse provides services with respect for human dignity and the uniqueness of the client . . ." Respect for human dignity derives from the moral principle of autonomy. An autonomous person is one who is both free and able to choose. This suggests that after determining that a client is physically and mentally capable, you should provide the client with information necessary to make informed choices about his care—that is, about the goals for improving health and the means for achieving those goals (interventions and treatments).

Obligation to Respect Choices

It is practical to involve clients in goal setting because it increases their motivation to achieve healthy outcomes. Client motivation is also a moral obligation. Mutual goal setting and care planning demonstrate respect for clients' values and their dignity and worth. Ill persons are vulnerable and dependent. They often feel that health professionals are more capable than they are to make decisions about their care, and their decision-making abilities may be diminished by their illness. When clients are experiencing conflict about choices or when they are too ill to choose, it is appropriate to propose alternatives. In your eagerness to help, however, you can without even realizing it, impose your own values on the client. Unless you are very sensitive, clients may defer to what they believe you want them to do, without making their true preferences known. Be aware of your power to influence patient decisions and make sure the choices are truly the patient's.

Managed Care and Nursing Values

The prevailing view now is that healthcare is a business. Treating healthcare as an item to be bought and sold like furniture is far different from the concept of healthcare as a human service created by society to meet the needs of the ill. The underlying values in business are economic: cost, efficiency, and effectiveness. Traditional nursing ethical values are respect for persons, advocacy, holistic care, and concerns of justice and fairness (Aroskar 1995). Managed care and multidisciplinary critical pathways for the most common and most costly illnesses attempt to balance the business values of cost and quality. Although they may guarantee the best care for the majority of patients, they can cause hardship for individuals. Consider the following example:

> EXAMPLE: Mrs. Ex, a 65-year-old patient who has diabetes, underwent a quadruple coronary bypass 4 days ago. Before her surgery, she controlled her diabetes with oral hypoglycemic agents, but she now needs insulin injections. She has been discharged home today (Friday), as dictated by the critical path for quadruple bypass. The discharge

plan is for a home health nurse to teach her how to administer her insulin. However, the home health nurse does not work on weekends, and is not scheduled to see Mrs. Ex until Monday. Who is supposed to administer the insulin twice a day between Friday and Monday? What ethical judgment was used when this patient was assigned to this critical path? A more appropriate hospital stay could have prevented this situation. Or if the family had been involved in the discharge planning, perhaps the husband or one of the children could have been taught (during the hospital stay) to administer the insulin. (Adapted from McGinty 1997, pp. 267–268.)

When the only outcomes measured in an institution are cost and length of stay, nurses' ethical obligations to care for patients may be compromised (refer to the example of Anna, on page 254). It is up to nurses to challenge "cookbook" treatment when it is not appropriate or safe. You should understand the need to vary critical pathways in some situations, educate patients, and speak up when this does not happen. If it is not possible to do this where you work, then do so away from work—in churches, schools and other organizations, or by political action. Patients depend on nurses, whether they know it or not, to balance considerations of cost with considerations of care. Nurses know that each intervention is done to a person, not a "case." They must remind the healthcare industry that this is so.

Legal Issues in Planning

Writing an outcome and target time on a nursing care plan implies that you accept accountability for helping the patient achieve the outcome. Consider this outcome: "Will be able to walk to the bathroom without help by discharge on 8/15." If the patient goes home without achieving this goal and falls while walking to the bathroom, you could be found negligent unless you have documented good reasons why the desired outcome was not achieved. For this reason, you may wish to write goals for collaborative problems on multidisciplinary care plans only. Recall that for each patient problem you identify, you must decide whether to refer the problem to another discipline or make a nursing plan of care. To help you decide, ask: "Is nursing responsible for initiating the plan to achieve this outcome? Can nursing care produce the outcome (or contribute to it in a major way)?" If not, refer the problem to the professional who is accountable. If you are unsure, consult a more experienced nurse.

Spiritual Planning and Outcomes

Nurses taking a holistic approach ensure that care plans reflect spiritual needs and outcomes. Spiritual care is usually missing from care plans, sometimes because of the nurse's own spiritual uncertainty and sometimes because the nurse fears imposing her own spirituality on the patient. If you have carefully assessed and diagnosed the patient's spiritual needs (see Chapters 3, 4, and 5), you will have a good idea of whether, and what, spiritual care is needed.

Planning should be directed toward helping patients achieve the overall goals of spiritual strength, serenity, and satisfaction. The specific goals you write will, of course, depend on the nursing diagnoses you have made. NOC suggests the following outcomes for a nursing diagnosis of Spiritual Distress (1997, p. 266):

Dignified Dying: Maintaining personal control and comfort with the approaching end of life (p. 139).

Hope: Presence of internal state of optimism that is personally satisfying and life-supporting (p. 162).

Spiritual Well-Being: Personal expressions of connectedness with self, others, higher power, all life, nature, and the universe that transcend and empower the self (p. 282).

Using the Omaha system (Martin and Scheet 1992), you would apply the Problem Rating Scale for Outcomes to the diagnosis of Spiritual Distress to create desired outcomes. Examples might be:

Spiritual Distress—Goal: Superior Knowledge (5)

Spiritual Distress—Goal: Status: Minimal signs/symptoms (4)

Using the HHCC (Saba 1995), you would apply the modifiers, *improved*, *stabilized*, and *deteriorated* to the HHCC diagnoses of Spiritual State Alteration or Spiritual Distress (eg, Spiritual Distress, Improved). Other, nonstandardized, desired outcomes might include that the patient will:

- fulfill religious obligations
- draw on and use inner resources to meet present situation
- maintain or establish a dynamic, personal relationship with a supreme being in the face of unpleasant circumstances
- find meaning in existence and the present situation
- acquire a sense of hope
- access spiritual resources

Cultural Considerations in Planning

The focus for culturally competent planning is to support a client's practices and incorporate them into the plan of care whenever possible and when they are not contraindicated for health reasons. This requires you to be open to learning about different beliefs and values, and to not be threatened when they differ from your own. When patients are "noncompliant," it may be because they are complying with their valued cultural beliefs, rather than the caregiver's valued plan of care. Clients are more likely to adhere to an agreed upon plan that incorporates their cultural perspective.

Specific outcomes, whether you use standardized language or create your own, depend on the nursing diagnoses you have identified for the patient. For example, for a diagnosis of Impaired Communication r/t foreign language barrier, you might have a goal that the patient "will be able to communicate basic needs to the staff."

■ SUMMARY

Planning

- begins when the patient is admitted and continues until dismissal.
- can provide a written framework necessary for individualizing care and obtaining third-party reimbursement.
- helps assure continuity of care when the patient is discharged.

Care Plans

- can be standardized or individualized.
- can be multidisciplinary or primarily for nursing care.

Goals/Expected Outcomes

- are guides to planning and evaluation that motivate the patient and the nurse by providing a sense of achievement.
- are stated in terms of specific, observable, achievable patient behaviors.
- should consist of subject, action verb, performance criteria, target time, and special conditions.
- may be short-term or long-term.
- can be written for individuals, families, and groups.
- should be culturally sensitive.

Standardized Language for Nursing-Sensitive Outcomes

- have been developed by NOC, the Omaha system, and the HHCC.
- can be used to write goals in acute-care, home, and community settings.

Ethical and Legal Considerations in Planning

- are based on the principle of autonomy, imply a moral obligation to inform and involve clients in their own care.
- require the nurse to be accountable for outcomes written on the nursing care plan.
- require the nurse to carefully balance the values of cost and care.

❑ Is the outcome possible for this patient?
❑ Is the patient motivated to do it?
❑ Is the goal stated in concrete, observable terms?

Nursing Process Practice

1. Place a check mark beside the measurable, observable outcomes (for brevity, none of the outcomes has a target time).

_____ **a.** Will be progressively less anxious.

_____ **b.** Eats fruit at least 3 times/day.

_____ **c.** Skin warm and dry to touch.

_____ **d.** Temp. will be < 100.1°F.

_____ **e.** Explains importance of exercise.

_____ **f.** Normal skin color.

_____ **g.** States he feels more confident.

_____ **h.** Rates pain as < 3 on a 1–10 scale.

_____ **i.** States less anxious than before exercise.

_____ **j.** Will not have foul-smelling lochia.

_____ **k.** B/P will be normal.

_____ **l.** Tolerates increased activity.

_____ **m.** Experiences increased confidence.

_____ **n.** Verbalizes understanding of home-care instructions.

2. The problem responses are given for you. Write an opposite, normal response that might be used in an outcome statement. The first one is done for you.

	Problem Response	Desired (Opposite) Response
a.	Constipation	Regular, formed, soft bowel movement
b.	Impaired Skin Integrity: Pressure Sore	
c.	Hypothermia	
d.	Dressing Self-Care Deficit	
e.	Altered Oral Mucous Membrane	

3. Use the normal responses you wrote in Exercise 2 to create expected outcomes. Fill in the boxes with the necessary components. Because there is no actual client, target times have been omitted. The first one has been done for you.

Subject	Action Verb	Special Conditions	Performance Criteria
a. (Client)	will have	(none)	regular, soft, formed B.M.
b.			
c.			
d.			
e.			

4. Write expected outcomes for the following nursing diagnosis:

   Back Pain r/t incision of recent spinal fusion and muscle stiffness from decreased mobility

   a. An outcome derived from the *problem*:

   b. An outcome derived from the *etiology*:

5. Write goals for the nursing diagnosis in Exercise 4, using the following NOC labels, indicators, and scales.

   Outcome: Pain Level
   Indicators: *Reported* pain; oral expressions of pain, restlessness
   Measurement Scale: (1) severe, (2) substantial, (3) moderate, (4) slight, (5) none

6. One of Ms. Jackson's nursing diagnoses is "Risk for Impaired Skin Integrity (Pressure Ulcers) r/t long periods of lying in bed." Write goals/expected outcomes for this diagnosis.

7. Circle the letter of the correctly written goals. If a goal is incorrectly written, state what is wrong with it (refer to Table 6–3 and "Guidelines for Judging the Quality of Outcome Statements" on pages 280–284). Some of the predicted outcomes address potential problems, so it is not an error if no time frame is given.

		Predicted Outcome	Errors (Guideline Violated)
a.		Client will develop adequate leg strength by 9/1.	
b.		Will have no signs of hemorrhage: VS-WNL, Hct and Hbg WNL, uses < 1 vag. pad per hour.	
c.		Will state the signs and symptoms of angina by 9/1.	
d.		Will feel better by morning.	
e.		Improved appetite.	
f.		Will be able to feed self by 9/1.	
g.		(On a 30-bed unit with only 2 wheelchairs) Will spend 4 hours each day in a wheelchair.	
h.		Client will discuss expectations of hospitalization and will relate the effects of a high-carbohydrate diet on blood sugar levels with a basic knowledge of exchange diet for diabetes.	
i.		After second teaching session, will demonstrate correct technique for testing blood glucose.	
j.		Injects self with insulin.	

	Predicted Outcome	Errors (Guideline Violated)
k.	Will state adequate pain relief from analgesics and will take at least 100 mL of p.o. fluids per hour.	
l.	IV will remain patent and run at 125 mL/hr.	
m.	By 7/15, expresses a desire for social contact and interaction with others.	
n.	Reports no numbness or tingling in left hand.	
o.	Voids at least 150 mL within 4 hr after removal of catheter.	

CASE STUDY: Exercises 8–10 pertain to this case.

Ms. Nancy Atwell is a 32-year-old, unmarried teacher who has had rheumatoid arthritis for 4 years. This change has made her knees painful and has limited the motion and weight-bearing ability of the knee joints themselves. Ms. Atwell's knee inflammation is aggravated by the fact that she is 75-lb overweight. Her diet history reveals that she eats when feeling depressed or stressed and that she snacks frequently on potato chips and colas.

She has recently been diagnosed with endometriosis, and now enters the hospital to have a hysterectomy. On her previous admission for treatment of her arthritis, she had been quiet, withdrawn, and extremely concerned for her privacy. Now she seems more outgoing and less overtly concerned about privacy. When questioned, Ms. Atwell states that she has had no previous surgical experience, but denies feeling nervous about the operation.

Her preoperative orders follow:

1. NPO
2. Shower before surgery
3. Pre-op med: Demerol 50 mg and Vistaril 25 mg IM at 0700

The nurse has identified the following nursing diagnoses for Ms. Atwell (*Note:* There are other appropriate nursing diagnoses; for simplicity, we consider only these four.)

a. Risk for Situational Low Self-esteem r/t unresolved feeling about inability to bear children after hysterectomy
b. Chronic Pain r/t inflammation of knees 2° rheumatoid arthritis
c. Altered Nutrition: More than Body Requirements for calories r/t excess calorie intake from "emotional eating"

d. Risk for Noncompliance with NPO order r/t lack of understanding of its importance for anesthesia

8. Underline the portion of each of the nursing diagnoses for which you *must* write a goal.

9. Prioritize the nursing diagnoses. Number them in order, with 1 being the highest priority. Put an asterisk beside the ones that the nurse *must* address today.

10. Using one of the frameworks in Chapter 5, explain how you prioritized the nursing diagnoses in Exercise 9.

11. Write goals/expected outcomes for the two top-priority diagnoses in Exercise 9.

12. Refer to Figure 3–2 (Luisa Sanchez's database in Chapter 3, page 86), and to the problem list for Luisa in Chapter 4, pages 165–166. One of Ms. Sanchez's collaborative problems is Potential Complications of Intravenous Therapy: Inflammation, phlebitis, infiltration. Write outcomes for this problem.

(1) List the signs and symptoms of each of the complications:

Inflammation:_____

Phlebitis:_____

Infiltration:_____

(2) In the columns below, using the signs and symptoms you listed, write goals/outcomes for each of the complications. The first one is started for you.

For inflammation	Will not develop inflammation at IV site, as evidenced by:
For phlebitis	
For infiltration	

Critical Thinking Practice: Classifying

Refer to "Classifying" in Chapter 2 as needed. Also refer to the discussion of "Nursing Models" and Tables 3–10 through 3–14 in Chapter 3.

When gathering patient data, nurses classify it according to their chosen theoretical framework (eg, Gordon, NANDA, Maslow). Unclassified data about a patient might look something like the following:

Harold Sims is a 35-year-old carpenter. He is married and has three children. There is a 2-in. scar on his forearm. He states that he has been "short of breath" on exertion and is coughing frequently. Scattered wheezes are auscultated throughout his lungs. He is able to read newsprint without glasses. Active bowel sounds are auscultated in all four quadrants of his abdomen.

Now look at the same data, in list format, with the related cues in bold print:

Age 35

Works as a carpenter

2-in. scar on forearm

States he has been "**short of breath**" on exertion.

States having **frequent cough**.

Able to read newsprint without glasses.

Scattered wheezes auscultated throughout lungs

Married; 3 children

Active bowel sounds auscultated in all 4 quadrants of abdomen.

Even though this is only a small part of the total data you would collect for a patient, notice how difficult it is to find the related items, even when they are in bold print. Using a framework to group the data makes it more meaningful and makes the patterns more obvious. A framework also helps prevent omission of data, since categories with scant or no data will be obvious when you have finished your assessment.

A. Learning the Skill of Classification

1. Start with a simple example. Classify the various jobs in your community into the following categories. List some local jobs that fit each classification.

   Agricultural:_____

   Technical: _____

   Healthcare: _____

   Clerical: _____

   Other: _____

   - Compare your answers with those of your peers and discuss any differences in your classifications. Explain why each job fits in its category.
   - Why do you think a classification should include a category called "Other"?

2. Put the following items into groups on the basis of characteristics they have in common. You may not think these items have anything in common at first, but if you continue comparing and contrasting them, you should discover some common characteristics.

   A grapefruit   A yellow marble   Grass in the Spring
   A white envelope   Snow   Sheet of blue paper
   A white tennis ball   A one-dollar bill

3. Did you try classifying the items in Exercise 3 based on their color? What other characteristics might you have used?

4. Choose one of those characteristics and group the items again based on that characteristic. Did you need an "Other" category?

5. Although the two classification systems you used were different, both allowed you to group the items. The criteria, or characteristics, you choose give meaning to the groups. Discuss this exercise with other students. What other classification systems did they use?

Applying the Skill of Classification

Classify the following patient data using two different frameworks: Gordon's and one other. Review the discussion in Chapter 3 about these frameworks and refer to Tables 3–10 and 3–13 as needed.

Discuss your answers with your classmates individually or in class. There is no answer key for this exercise because the emphasis is not on whether your answers are *correct*, but on the thinking process you used to arrive at the answers—this is, the skill of *classifying*. The only way to evaluate your thinking process is to discuss it with others and get feedback from them.

Patient Data

Age 37

States having continual vaginal bleeding for the past 6 months

States has never been pregnant

Skin warm and dry

Hears normal speech at 10 feet

Takes iron supplements

Weighs 130 lb

States she is "light social drinker"

States she has asthma

States she is not concerned about effect of hysterectomy on her sexuality

Works as a hairdresser

"I sleep a lot" when under stress

Blood sugar 124 mg/dL

Chest x-ray normal

Manages all activities of daily living independently

Takes a bulk-forming laxative daily

Blood pressure 120/80 mm Hg

Oriented to time, place, and person

Wants to see hospital chaplain before surgery

States vision is 20/20 with glasses

Good skin turgor

Full range of motion of neck

Hemoglobin 9.5

Height 5 ft, 5 in.

Has smoked 1/2 pack per day for 16 years

Lungs clear to auscultation

Allergic to penicillin

States eats 3 meals a day, but snacks often

States mother had cervical cancer

Has frequent headaches, takes aspirin to relieve

Unmarried

Urinates 5–6 times per day, "No difficulty"

Temperature 100° F

Drinks "lots of water"

Hospitalized in 1980 for appendectomy

One formed stool per day; occasional constipation

1. **Classify the data using Gordon's framework.** Refer to Table 3–10 on pages 105–106 as needed. (A few items have been classified for you. Notice that some of the data appear in more than one pattern.)

Patterns	Data
Health Perception/ Health Management	Takes iron supplements
Nutritional/Metabolic	Takes iron supplements

Patterns	Data
Elimination	
Activity/Exercise	States she has asthma
Cognitive/Perceptual	
Sleep/Rest	
Self-Perception/ Self-Concept	
Role/Relationship	
Sexuality/Reproductive	
Coping/Stress-Tolerance	
Value/Belief	
Other	Age 37

Notice that in some categories (or patterns) you may have entered no data. If you have classified the data correctly, this would indicate to you, as a practicing nurse, that your data collection is incomplete.

2. **Classify the same data using one of the following frameworks.** Make your own table using the categories of the model you choose.

- Orem's Self-Care Model, Table 3–11 on page 107
- Roy's Adaptation Model, Table 3–12 on page 107
- NANDA Human Response Patterns, Table 3–13 on pages 108–109
- Maslow's Basic Needs, Table 3–14 on page 110
- The body systems model, on page 110

Case Study: Applying Nursing Process and Critical Thinking

Your patient is a 69-year-old African American man who has had hypertension and diabetes for 15 years. This is his fourth postoperative day after undergoing partial amputation of his foot because of poor circulation. His diabetes is under control, and before hospitalization, he was injecting his own insulin. He is being discharged with a referral to a home health agency. A nurse will be assigned to administer IV antibiotics, change his foot dressings, and monitor his blood glucose levels. (Look up diabetes and peripheral vascular insufficiency in a medical/surgical textbook, as needed, to answer the questions for this case.)

1. Does this patient actually need a nurse to monitor his blood glucose levels when he returns home? Explain your reasoning, considering the following:
   a. What is the effect of stress (eg, surgery) on diabetes and blood glucose levels?
   b. What is the relationship between activity and diabetes? What can you say about this patient's activity level?
   c. How predictable is the course of his wound healing?
   d. What is the relationship between food intake and diabetes? How might this patient's intake differ from pre-surgery days?
   e. Given all that, do you think his insulin needs will decrease, increase, fluctuate, or remain the same?

2. The discharge care plan contains a nursing diagnosis, "Risk for Delayed Wound Healing related to impaired peripheral circulation." What risk factors are present to support this diagnosis?

3. State a goal that is the opposite, healthy response of delayed wound healing. How will you be able to tell if the goal is being met? What would you assess for?

4. Would you write "delayed wound healing" as a potential nursing diagnosis or as a collaborative problem? Why?

5. Because of the potential for infection of his wound, you need to teach the patient the signs and symptoms of infection, as well as actions to take if symptoms occur. How will you know that he has mastered this knowledge? Write outcomes you could use on a care plan.

6. Should the home health agency try to assign an African American nurse to his case? Why or why not? If a male nurse is available, should he be assigned? Why or why not?

7. After returning home, do you think this patient will be able to provide for his:

   ■ nutritional needs?
   ■ self-care needs (eg, bathing, hygiene, toileting, dressing)?

   Explain your reasoning.

8. Write goals/expected outcomes that would demonstrate that the patient's nutritional and self-care needs are being met.

9. This is postoperative day 4, the patient is being discharged tomorrow. What is your highest priority for care today? Explain your reasoning.

10. What is the home health nurse's highest priority for care during the first week of visits to the patient's home? Explain your reasoning.

Remember that answers will vary based on knowledge, experience, and values. The most meaningful learning comes from discussing the case with others.

■ SELECTED REFERENCES

American Nurses Association (1985). *Code for nurses with interpretive statements.* Kansas City, MO: ANA.

Aroskar, M. A. (1995). Managed care and nursing values: a reflection. *J Nurs Law* 24(4):63–70.

Carr, P. (1990). Two halves don't make a whole. *RN* 53(7):96.

Cosnotti, J. and L. Sprinkel (1993). Roanoke Memorial Hospitals' Home Health Services discharge planning process. *Caring* 12(8):70–77.

Frenn, M. and S. Malin (1998). Health promotion: theoretical perspectives and clinical applications. *Holistic Nurs Prac* 12(2):1–7.

Gordon, M., C. Murphy, D. Candee (1994). Clinical judgment: an integrated model. *Advan in Nurs Sci* 16(4):55–70.

Head, B., M. Maas, and M. Johnson (1997). Outcomes for home and community nursing in integrated delivery systems. *Caring* 16(1):50–56.

Healthy People 2010. (2000). Volumes I and II. U.S. Department of Health and Human Services, Washington, DC.

Ireson, C. L. (1997). Critical pathways: effectiveness in achieving patient outcomes. *J Nurs Admin* 27(6):16–23.

Johnson, M. (1998). Overview of the Nursing Outcomes Classification (NOC). *Online J Nurs Informat* 2(2):1–3. Available at: *http://cac.psu.edu/~dxm12/johnart.html.* Accessed on 8/6/99.

Johnson, M. and M. Maas (eds.) (1997). *Nursing Outcomes Classification (NOC).* St. Louis: Mosby.

Johnson, M., M. Maas, and S. Moorhead (eds.) (2000). *Nursing Outcomes Classification (NOC)* (2nd ed.). St. Louis: Mosby.

Kozier, B., G. Erb, A. Berman (2000). *Fundamentals of nursing.* Upper Saddle River, NJ: Prentice Hall Health.

Lamb-Havard, J. (1997). Nurses at the bedside: influencing outcomes. *Outcomes Measure Manage Nurs Clin North Amer* 32(3):579–587.

Maas, M. (1998). Nursing outcomes accountability: nursing's role in interdisciplinary accountability for patient outcomes. *Outcomes Manage Nurs Prac* 2(3):92–94.

Martin, K. S. and N. J. Scheet (1992). *The Omaha system: applications for community health nursing.* Philadelphia: W. B. Saunders.

McCloskey, J. C. and M. Maas (1998). Interdisciplinary team: the nursing perspective is essential. *Nurs Outlook* 46(4):157–163.

McGinty, J. (1997). Issues and interventions. Look at cost savings and care paths with an ethical eye. *Nurs Case Manage* 2(6):267–268.

Moorhead, S. (1999). Health care terminology: Nursing Outcomes Classification (NOC). NCVHS Hearings on Medical Terminology and Code Development. May 18, 1999. Rockville, MD.

Naylor, M. (1990). Comprehensive discharge planning for hospital elderly: a pilot study. *Nursing Research* 39(3):156–161.

Nazarko, L. (1998). Improving discharge: the role of the discharge co-ordinator. *Nurs Standard* 12(49):35–37.

Oermann, M. H. (1999). Patient outcomes: a measure of nursing's value. *AJN* 99(9):40–47.

Parlocha, P. K. and S. B. Henry (1998). The usefulness of the Georgetown Home Health Care Classification system for coding patient problems and nursing interventions in psychiatric home care. *Computers in Nursing* 16(1):45–52.

Reed, J. (1992). Individualized nursing care: some implications. *J Clin Nurs* 1:7–12.

Rosswurm, M. and D. Lanham (1998). Discharge planning for elderly patients. *J Gerontol Nurs* 24(5):14–21, 56–57.

Saba, V. K. (1995). Home Health Care Classifications (HHCCs): Nursing diagnoses and nursing interventions. In: *An emerging framework: data system advances for clinical nursing practice.* ANA Publication #NP-94. Washington, DC: American Nurses Publishing.

Saba, V. K. (1997). Why the home health care classification is a recognized nursing nomenclature. *Computers in Nursing* 15(2):69–76.

Schneider, J., S. Hornberger, J. Booker, et al (1993). A medication discharge planning program. Measuring the effect on readmissions. *Clin Nurs Res* 2(1):41–53.

The Status of NANDA, NIC and NOC. Panel presentation at the 2nd Conference on Nursing Diagnoses, Interventions & Outcomes: April 1999. New Orleans, LA.

Tirk, J. (1992). Determining discharge priorities. *Nursing92* 22(7):55.

Tuazon, N. (1992). Discharge teaching: Use this MODEL. *RN* 55(4):19–22.

Walsh, M. (1997). Will critical pathways replace the nursing process? *Nurs Standard* 11(52):39–42.

Webster, J. (1998). The effect of care planning on quality of patient care. *Pro Nurse* 14(2):85–87.

Weissman, M. A. and D. A. Jasovsky (1998). Discharge teaching for today's times. *RN* 61(6): 38–40.

Zander, K. (1997). Rethinking discharge planning. *New Definition* 12(3):1–2.

Zander, K. (1998). Historical development of outcomes-based care delivery. *Crit Care Nurs Clin North Amer* 10(1):1–11.

7

Planning: Interventions

Learning Outcomes

After completing this chapter, you should be able to do the following:

- Define the terms "nursing interventions," "nursing activities," and "nursing orders."
- Recognize nursing interventions for observation, prevention, treatment, and health promotion.
- Given a nursing diagnosis or patient outcome, generate alternatives for nursing interventions.
- Name the components of a nursing order.
- Follow specified guidelines for writing nursing orders.
- Use critical thinking standards to evaluate the quality of nursing interventions and orders.
- Describe the use of standardized terminology for nursing interventions (eg, NIC).
- Discuss interventions specific to family, home, and community health.
- Describe the ethical, legal, and cultural factors to consider in planning interventions.

■ INTRODUCTION

In the nursing process, the nurse identifies (1) the patient's nursing diagnoses (present health status) and (2) goals/expected outcomes (the desired health status). The next logical step is to choose the interventions that are most likely to bring about the desired changes. This chapter focuses on choosing nursing interventions and writing nursing orders. Box 7–1, on page 305, contains professional standards of care for planning interventions.

■ NURSING INTERVENTIONS

A **nursing intervention** is "any treatment based upon clinical judgment and knowledge, that a nurse performs to enhance patient/client outcomes" (McCloskey and Bulechek 2000, p. 3). Nursing interventions are also

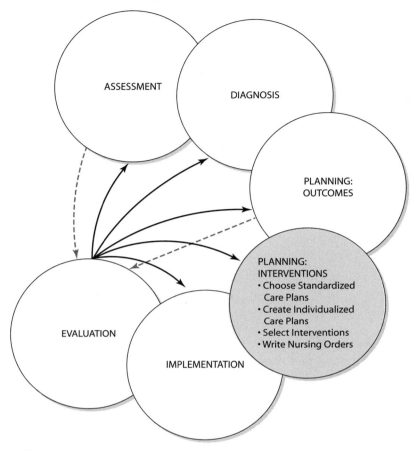

Figure 7–1
The Planning Phase: Interventions and Nursing Orders

referred to as *nursing actions*, *activities*, *measures*, and *strategies*. As a rule, this text will use *interventions* and the other terms interchangeably, except when referring specifically to the Nursing Interventions Classification (NIC) standardized labels, which are called *interventions*.

Types of Interventions

Nursing interventions and activities are identified and ordered during the planning phase; however, they are actually performed during the implementation phase. They may be independent, dependent, or interdependent.

Independent interventions are those that nurses are licensed to prescribe, perform, or delegate based on their knowledge and skills. NIC refers to these as *nurse-initiated treatments* (McCloskey and Bulechek 2000, p. 20). Mundinger uses the term *autonomous nursing practice*: "Knowing why, when, and how to position clients and doing it skillfully makes the function

BOX 7–1

Professional Standards of Care for Planning Interventions

American Nurses Association

Standard IV. Planning

The nurse develops a plan of care that prescribes interventions to attain expected outcomes.

Measurement Criteria

1. The plan is individualized to the patient (eg, age-appropriate, culturally sensitive) and the patient's condition or needs.
2. The plan is developed with the patient, family, and other healthcare providers, as appropriate.
3. The plan reflects current nursing practice.
4. The plan provides for continuity of care.
5. Priorities for care are established.
6. The plan is documented.

Source: Reprinted with permission from American Nurses Association, *Standards of Clinical Nursing Practice*. 2nd ed, © 1998 American Nurses Publishing, American Nurses Foundation/American Nurses Association, 600 Maryland Ave, SW, Suite 100 W, Washington, DC, pp 8–9.

Canadian Nurses Association

Standard II. Nursing practice requires the effective use of the nursing process.
3. Nurses are required to **plan** their nursing actions based upon the identified actual and potential client problems, in accordance with their conception of the focus and modes of intervention
   The nurse in any practice setting:
   3.6 identifies required resources
   3.7 considers a number of nursing actions in accordance with the specified focus and modes of intervention
   3.8 selects nursing actions based on the highest probability of their effectiveness
   3.9 communicates with appropriate others regarding the planned actions

Source: Canadian Nurses Association (1987). *Standards for Nursing Practice*. Ottawa, Ontario: CNA, pp. 4–5. Used with permission.

an autonomous therapy" (1980, p. 4). Nurses are accountable, or answerable, for their decisions and actions with regard to independent activities. For example, a nurse may diagnose Impaired Oral Mucous Membranes and plan and provide special mouth care for a patient. The nurse is then accountable for the effects of that action.

Dependent interventions are prescribed by the physician and carried out by the nurse. Medical orders commonly include orders for medications, intravenous (IV) therapy, diagnostic tests, treatments, diet, and activity. Nurses are responsible for explaining, assessing the need for, and administering the medical orders. Nurses may write orders to individualize the medical order, based on the patient's status.

EXAMPLE:

Medical Order	Progressive ambulation, as tolerated
Nursing Orders	1. Dangle for 5 min, 12 hr post-op
	2. Stand at bedside 24 hr post-op; observe for pallor, dizziness, and weakness
	3. Check pulse before and after amb. Do not progress if P >110.

Interdependent interventions (also called *collaborative interventions*) are carried out in collaboration with other health team members, such as physical therapists, social workers, dietitians, and physicians. Collaborative activities reflect the overlapping responsibilities of, and collegial relationships among, health personnel. For example, the physician might order physical therapy to teach the client crutch-walking. The nurse would be responsible for informing the physical therapy department and for coordinating the client's care to include the physical therapy sessions. When the client returns to the nursing unit, the nurse would assist with crutch-walking and collaborate with the physical therapist to evaluate the client's progress.

Theory-Based Planning

Recall from Chapter 3 that theories are used to organize assessment data; and from Chapter 4, that theories provide the perspective for what is likely to count as a problem. This idea carries through to planning, when goals and nursing actions are generated to address the identified problem. For example, if an infant has Pain (Colic), a nurse taking a "gastrointestinal" (GI) perspective might say that the etiology is ineffective peristalsis propulsion of intestinal gas, with overdistention of the GI tract. A logical nursing action, then, might be to decrease gas by burping the infant frequently. A nurse using a "parental anxiety/tension" theory might say that the etiology is overstimulation or unmet needs because of parental anxiety/tension. That nurse might write a nursing order to decrease parental tension by encouraging the parents to relax and spend some time away from the baby (Ziegler 1993).

Nursing Interventions and Problem Status

Depending on the status of the nursing diagnosis, you will choose nursing interventions for observation, prevention, treatment, and health promotion (see Table 7–1).

1. *Observation.* This includes observations to determine whether a complication is developing, as well as observations of the client's responses to nursing, medical, and other therapies. Observation interventions are needed for every problem: actual, risk, and possible nursing diagnoses and collaborative problems.

   EXAMPLES:

   Auscultate lungs q8h.
   Observe for redness over sacrum q2h.
   Assess for urinary frequency.
   Intake and output, hourly.

2. *Prevention.* Prevention activities are those that prevent complications or reduce risk factors. They are used mainly for risk nursing diagnoses and collaborative problems, but they can also be appropriate for actual nursing diagnoses.

   EXAMPLES:

   Turn, cough, and deep breathe q2h.   (Prevents respiratory complication)

Table 7–1   Types of Nursing Orders in Relation to Diagnoses

Actual Nursing Diagnoses	Risk Nursing Diagnosis	Possible Nursing Diagnosis	Collaborative Problems
Observation for improvement or complications	**Observation** for change to "actual" status	**Observation** to confirm or rule out diagnosis	**Observation** for onset of complication
			Physician notification of problem onset
Prevention of further complications	**Prevention** Remove or reduce risk factors		**Prevention** Includes physician orders, nursing policies and procedures
Treatment Remove causal and contributing factors Relieve symptoms			**Collaborative treatments** to relieve or eliminate problem

| If fundus is boggy, massage until firm. | (Prevents postpartum hemorrhage) |
| Refer to county health department for measles immunizations. | (Prevents specific disease: measles) |

3. *Treatment.* This includes teaching, referrals, physical, and other care needed to treat an existing problem. Treatment measures are appropriate for actual nursing diagnoses. Notice that the same nursing activity may accomplish either prevention or treatment of a problem (compare examples below to the preceding examples).

EXAMPLES:

Turn, cough, deep breathe q2h.	(Treat respiratory problem)
If fundus is boggy, massage until firm.	(Treat actual pospartum hemorrhage)
Help client plan exercise regimen.	(Treat actual activity intolerance)

4. *Health Promotion.* When there are no health problems, the nurse helps the client to identify areas for improvement that will lead to a higher level of wellness. Health-promotion strategies help the client promote positive outcomes, rather than avoid negative outcomes. Health promotion is not specific to any disease or problem, but aims to encourage activities that will actualize the client's general health potential.

EXAMPLES:

Discuss the importance of daily exercise.
Teach components of a healthy diet.
Explore infant-stimulation techniques.

Specific nursing activities for each of the preceding categories might include physical care, teaching, counseling, emotional support, making referrals, and managing the environment.

Teaching Not all teaching requires a separate, formal teaching plan. Informal teaching is an intervention for many, if not most, nursing diagnoses. You will find that you are teaching almost constantly as you explain to clients what you are doing for them and why. Informal teaching may include such activities as explaining the expected effects and side effects of a medication, explaining why the client should not ambulate without help, clarifying the need for fluid restrictions, or teaching patients for self-care (eg, to use a blood glucose meter).

Counseling and Emotional Support Counseling includes the use of therapeutic communication techniques to help clients make decisions about their healthcare and perhaps make lifestyle changes. It also involves techniques for helping clients recognize, express, and cope with feelings such as anxiety, anger, and fear. Counseling includes emotional support—but emotional support may occur on a less complex level: it may be given simply by the nurse's touch, presence, or apparent understanding of the patient's situation. An example of a counseling strategy would be to help a client to recognize when she is anxious by pointing out symptoms as you observe them.

Referral You should make referrals when the client needs in-depth interventions for which other professionals are specifically prepared. For instance, while the nurse may counsel an anxious patient, long-term treatment of severe anxiety would be referred to a psychotherapist or counselor. Nurses often make referrals for follow-up care after discharge. An example of a referral activity is referring a patient to the Social Service Department for transportation to a clinic.

Environmental Management Nursing activities are often intended to provide for a safe, clean, therapeutic environment. Environmental management includes removing hazards for clients who are particularly at risk for injury—for instance, children, the elderly, and those with a decreased level of consciousness.

EXAMPLES:

Teach mother to check temperature of formula with back of hand.
Remain at bedside while client is smoking.
Keep crib rails up at all times.

Selection Grid Figure 7–2 is a grid you might use to be sure you have considered all the various types of nursing interventions for a patient. First think of the observations that apply to the problem. For example, if one of your interventions is to auscultate the patient's lungs, place an X in the box under "Observation" and beside "Physical Care." You might wish to teach a patient to assess her own blood glucose levels; if so, place an X in the box under "Observation" and beside "Teaching." Probably none of the other actions in

	Observation	Prevention	Treatment	Health Promotion
Physical Care	X			
Teaching	X			
Counseling				
Emotional Support				
Activities of Daily Living				
Environmental Management				
Referrals				

Figure 7–2
Grid for Identifying Nursing Interventions

the vertical column would fit under "Observation." Next consider what kind of physical care, teaching, and so on would be involved in preventive nursing orders. Continue to move across the top of the grid in this manner.

???

THINKING POINT

When deciding whether to make a referral or deal with a patient's problem yourself, ask (1) What are my knowledge and experience in this area? (2) Does this require in-depth or specialized knowledge that I lack? (3) Do I have any values, beliefs, or biases that could interfere with the quality of care I give for this problem? Which of the following situations would you refer? Why?

1. Mary has come to the clinic for a prenatal visit. When you comment on some bruises, she tells you that her husband beats her. She says, "I'm even afraid for my kids. We need to get out of there, but I don't know where to go or how I'd support the kids."
2. Elaine has just given birth and plans to breastfeed the baby. She is about 25 lb overweight now and asks you how she can lose the weight and still maintain her milk supply.
3. A patient's care plan has a nursing diagnosis of "Impaired Gas Exchange r/t changes in alveolar-capillary membranes secondary to chronic lung disease."
4. Would an experienced community health nurse or psychiatric nurse practitioner have answered No. 1 the same as you did?

How to Generate and Select Nursing Activities/Interventions

For any given problem, several nursing interventions might be effective. Select the ones that are most likely to achieve the desired goal, taking into consideration the patient's abilities and preferences, the capabilities of the nursing staff, the available resources, and the policies and procedures of the institution. You need creativity for generating new and effective interventions. Even if an intervention has been useful in the past, always rethink it to be sure it is the best way for the patient with whom you are working. The following decision-making process will guide you in selecting the best interventions.

Review the Nursing Diagnosis

Choose nursing strategies that elminate or reduce the etiology (cause) of the nursing diagnosis. When it is not possible to change the etiologic factors, choose interventions/activities to treat the signs and symptoms, or the defining characteristics in NANDA terminology. Review the nursing diagnosis to be sure you understand the problem and etiology. Be sure you are familiar with the factors causing or contributing to actual problems, and the risk factors that predispose the client to potential problems. You should also know the signs and symptoms associated with any risk diagnoses or collaborative problems. In the following example, the nursing actions should reduce the contributing factor, breast engorgement.

EXAMPLE:

Nursing Diagnosis: Ineffective breastfeeding r/t breast engorgement

Nursing Actions: 1. Teach to massage breast before feeding.
2. Use hot packs or hot shower before nursing infant.

Nursing interventions are individualized primarily from the second clause (etiology) of a nursing diagnosis. The etiology describes the factors that cause or contribute to the unhealthy response, and the nursing activities would specifically target these causal and contributing factors.

Problem + Etiology

Nursing activities

Any number of factors may contribute to a problem, but it would be inefficient and probably ineffective to address them all. Nursing orders should address the etiological factors specific to a given client. For example, many factors could contribute to Chronic Constipation: lack of knowledge, lack of exercise, eating habits, long-term laxative use, or a schedule that causes the client to ignore the urge to defecate. A well-written nursing diagnosis states which factors are causing the client's problem, suggesting nursing interventions that deal directly with those factors. The following example illustrates how different etiologies suggest different nursing actions. Notice that in both cases, the *problem* is the same.

EXAMPLE:

Nursing Diagnosis		*Nursing Orders/Activities*
Chronic Constipation r/t *long-term laxative use*	→	1. Work with the client to develop a plan for gradual withdrawal of the laxatives.
Chronic Constipation r/t *inactivity and insufficient fluid intake*	→	1. Help client to develop an exercise regimen he can follow at home. 2. Help client plan for including sufficient fluids in his diet.

You may also need to select interventions for the problem clause of the nursing diagnosis. For a diagnosis of chronic pain related to joint inflammation, nursing orders might include some pain-relief interventions that have nothing to do with relieving joint inflammation; for example:

Observe level of pain before and after activity.

Give back rub (to promote general relaxation of tension).

Instruct client to take analgesic before pain becomes too severe.

Teach slow, rhythmic breathing as a pain control method.

Review the Patient Outcomes

You should also review the patient outcomes you wish to produce. They will help you to choose nursing interventions that are specific to the individual patient.

EXAMPLE: *Nursing Diagnosis*: Risk for Ineffective Breastfeeding r/t breast engorgement

Goals:	*Nursing orders suggested by goals*:
1. Infant will be observed to "latch on," suck, and swallow.	**1a.** Observe infant at breast for effective latching on, sucking, and swallowing.
	1b. Teach mother to make these observations.
	1c. When sucking is not long and rhythmic, institute massage of alternate areas of breast without removing infant from breast.
2. Infant will regain birth weight of 8 lb 6 oz within 14 days after birth.	**2a.** Weigh infant daily at 0600.

Identify Alternative Interventions/Actions

Keeping goals and etiology in mind, think of all the nursing activities that might bring about the desired responses. Include unusual or original ideas. Don't try to predict at this point which ones would be best.

Perhaps you are wondering, "How will I be able to think of interventions to address the etiology? How will I know which actions will achieve the goals?" Principles and theories from nursing and related courses (eg, anatomy, physiology, psychology) are good sources of ideas for nursing actions. You may also wish to consult resources such as standardized taxonomies (eg, NIC), model care plans, agency procedure manuals, nursing texts, journal articles, instructors, and practicing nurses. Remember to consult the patient and his family about the care they find to be most helpful.

Ask yourself two broad questions: (1) What should I watch for? and (2) What should I do? Then branch out to consider all the possible activities that might address the etiology or achieve the goals. Depending upon the type of problem, include both independent and collaborative activities from the categories in the Selection Grid, Figure 7–2 on p. 309.

Select the Best Options

Selecting the *best* of the alternative interventions is a matter of hypothesizing that certain actions will bring about the desired outcome. The best options are those you expect to be most effective in helping the client to achieve the goals. To determine this, ask yourself the following questions:

1. What do I know about this patient (health status, knowledge, abilities, resources)?
2. What do I know about the patient outside the hospital (eg, beliefs, behaviors, feelings)?
3. How would I feel, what would I think, if I were in this situation?
4. What have I done in the past for patients in similar situations?
5. Do I have any personal discomfort with this intervention?
6. What does the patient want or request?
7. What potential ill effects might this intervention have on the patient, and how can we manage them?

Your knowledge, experience, and intuition will help you make these judgments, as will the guidelines for writing nursing orders in the section, "Reflecting on Interventions" (see pages 327–328).

Even carefully selected nursing orders do not guarantee success in meeting client goals. A successful intervention for one client may not work at all for another. In fact, for the same client, an intervention may be effective at one time and not at another. Use interventions based on scientific principles and sound research, when possible, to improve the likelihood of success. For example, research indicates that axillary temperatures for newborns are accurate and safer than rectal temperatures.

Computerized Planning

When you use a computerized care planning system, the computer will generate a list of suggested interventions when you enter either a nursing diagnosis or an outcome (see Figures 7–3 and 7–4, on pages 314 and 319, respectively). You can then choose appropriate interventions from the list or enter strategies of your own. Use of computer prompts helps to assure that a wide range of interventions is considered. However, one danger in using computerized (and standardized) care plans is the temptation to plug in ready-made solutions, rather than look for different, more effective approaches for a particular patient. Always think, "What else might work" and "How should this be adapted for *this* patient?"

■ WRITING NURSING ORDERS

After selecting the appropriate nursing interventions, write them on the care plan in the form of nursing orders. With computerized care planning, the computer records the interventions as you choose them. You may, however, need to

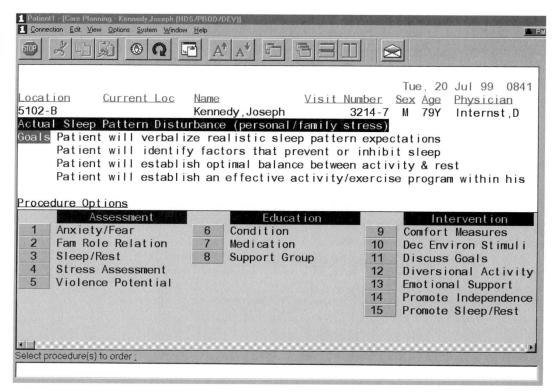

Figure 7–3
Computer-Generated List of Options for Nursing Interventions. *Source:* Courtesy of Per Se Technologies, Atlanta, GA. Used with permission.

add details specific to your patient. **Nursing orders** are written, detailed instructions for performing nursing interventions. They prescribe the activities and behaviors performed to change present client responses to the desired responses (outcomes). Nursing orders may be something you do for the client or something you help her to do for herself. Nursing orders contain more specific, detailed instructions than physician's orders. A physician's order regarding a client's nutritional status might read "Diet as tolerated." Related nursing orders would specify how the diet is to progress, as well as assessments that need to be made.

EXAMPLES:

1. Auscultate bowel sounds q4h.
2. Observe for abdominal distention, nausea, or vomiting.
3. Limit ice chips to 1 cup per hour until bowel sounds are auscultated; then give clear liquids as tolerated, for 8 hrs.
4. If no nausea or vomiting, progress to full liquids . . .

Purpose

Nursing orders provide specific direction and a consistent, individualized approach to the patient's care. They are written as instructions for others to follow, and other nurses are held responsible and accountable for their implementation. Because many different nurses may be involved in caring for a patient, nursing orders must be detailed enough to be interpreted correctly by all caregivers. An order to "force fluids" could be interpreted in many ways. A nurse accustomed to working with young adults might expect this to mean 200 mL/hour; a gerontology nurse might think it means 50 mL/hour; another nurse might focus on total volume, rather than a consistent hourly intake. A better nursing order would be "Give fluids hourly: Day shift = 1,000 mL total; Evening shift = 1,000 mL; Night shift = 400 mL."

Components of a Nursing Order

A well-written nursing order contains the following components (see Table 7–2 for examples):

1. *Date the order was written.* The date will be changed to reflect review or revisions.
2. *Subject.* The subject is implied, not written. Nursing orders are written in terms of *nurse* behaviors; so the subject of the order is *the nurse*. As you learn to write nursing orders, think "The nurse will . . ." or "The nurse should . . ." at the beginning of the statement, but do not write it.

   EXAMPLE:

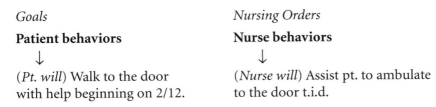

Goals	Nursing Orders
Patient behaviors	**Nurse behaviors**
↓	↓
(*Pt. will*) Walk to the door with help beginning on 2/12.	(*Nurse will*) Assist pt. to ambulate to the door t.i.d.

Table 7–2 Examples of Nursing Orders

Subject	Action Verb	Descriptive Phrase	Time Frame	Date and Signature
(Nurse)	(will) Monitor	for verbalization of interest in group activities	With each patient contact	4-14-00 J. Jonas, RN
(Nurse)	(will) Instruct	to avoid drinking liquids with meals if nausea occurs	Evening shift 4/14	4-14-00 J. Jonas, RN
(Nurse)	(will) Pad	side rails	During periods of restlessness and confusion	4-14-00 J. Jonas, RN

3. *Action verb that directs what the nurse is to do.* Examples of action verbs are *offer, assist, instruct, refer, assess, auscultate, change, give, listen, demonstrate,* and *turn.*

> EXAMPLES: *Auscultate* lungs at 0800 and 1600 daily.
> *Assist* to chair for 30 min. t.i.d.

4. *Descriptive qualifiers.* This is the phrase that tells the nurse how, when, and where to perform the action. It may also describe the action in more detail (*what*). When one activity depends on another, the descriptive qualifier also includes the sequence in which actions are to be done.

> EXAMPLES: **What**   **When**
>
> Give   written instructions for incision care   before discharge.
>
>   **What**   **Sequence/When**
>
> Take   B/P   before and after ambulating.

5. *Specific times.* State when, how often, and how long the activity is to be done.

> EXAMPLE: Assist to chair *for 30 minutes b.i.d.*
> Change dressing at *0800 and 1400 daily.*

When scheduling times for the nursing actions, consider the patient's usual rest time, visiting hours, mealtimes, and other activities of daily living. Also coordinate the times with collaborative tests and treatments (eg, physical therapy).

6. *Signature.* The nurse who writes the order should sign it, indicating acceptance of legal and ethical accountability. A signature also allows other nurses to contact the writer for questions or feedback about the order.

■ STANDARDIZED LANGUAGE FOR NURSING INTERVENTIONS

Chapter 5 discussed efforts to standardize nursing language and presented vocabularies for describing problems that require nursing care. Chapter 6 presented information about standardized languages for describing patient outcomes. The following is a discussion of standardized terminology for *nursing interventions.* Standardized vocabularies provide a means for nurses to communicate their contributions and participate fully in the multidisciplinary team.

The Nursing Interventions Classification (NIC)

The NIC system was developed by a nursing research team at the University of Iowa. It includes 486 interventions that nurses perform on behalf of patients. NIC classifies nursing interventions into seven *domains*: basic physiological, complex physiological, behavioral, safety, family, health system, and community (McCloskey and Bulechek 2000).

Each NIC intervention has a label, a definition, and a list of *activities* that outline the key actions of nurses in carrying out the intervention (see Box 7–2). NIC interventions are linked to NANDA nursing diagnosis labels and NOC outcome labels. The nurse can look up either a client's nursing diagnosis or

---

BOX 7–2

NIC Intervention: Touch

Definition: Providing comfort and communciation through purposeful tactile contact.

Activities:

Observe cultural taboos regarding touch

Give a reassuring hug as appropriate

Put arm around patient's shoulders as appropriate

Hold patient's hand to provide emotional support

Apply gentle pressure at wrist, hand, or shoulder of seriously ill patient

Rub back in synchrony with patient's breathing as appropriate

Stroke body part in slow, rhythmic fashion as appropriate

Massage around painful area as appropriate

Elicit from parents common actions used to soothe and calm their child

Hold infant or child firmly and snugly

Encourage parents to touch newborn or ill child

Surround premature infant with blanket rolls (nesting)

Swaddle infant snugly in a blanket to keep arms and legs close to the body

Place infant on mother's body immediately after birth

Encourage mother to hold, touch, and examine the infant while umbilical cord is being severed

Encourage parents to hold infant

Encourage parents to massage infant

Demonstrate quieting techniques for infants

Provide appropriate pacifier for nonnutritional sucking in newborns

Provide oral stimulation exercises prior to tube feedings in premature infants

Source: Iowa Intervention Project. (2000). McCloskey, J., and G. Bulechek, eds. *Nursing Interventions Classification (NIC)* (3rd ed). Philadelphia: Mosby, p. 669.

Table 7–3   NIC Suggested Interventions for Sleep Pattern Disturbance

Sleep pattern disturbance: Time-limited disruption of sleep (natural, periodic suspension of consciousness) amount and quality.

Suggested Nursing Interventions for Problem Resolution

Dementia Management	Medication Prescribing
Environmental Management	Security Enhancement
Environmental Management, Comfort	Simple Relaxation Therapy
Medication Administration	Sleep Enhancement
Medication Management	Touch

Additional Optional Interventions

Anxiety Reduction	Meditation Facilitation
Autogenic Training	Music Therapy
Bathing	Nutrition Management
Calming Technique	Pain Management
Coping Enhancement	Positioning
Energy Management	Progressive Muscle Relaxation
Exercise Promotion	Self-Care Assistance: Toileting
Exercise Therapy: Ambulation	Simple Massage
Kangaroo Care	Urinary Incontinence Care: Enuresis

Source: Nursing Interventions Classification (NIC), 3rd ed. McCloskey, J. C., and G. M. Bulechek, eds. 2000. Philadelphia: Mosby, p. 781. Used with permission.

desired outcomes to see which nursing interventions are suggested. Each diagnosis and outcome contains suggestions for several interventions, so nurses must select appropriate interventions based on their judgment and knowledge of the client. For example, the NIC link to Sleep Pattern Disturbance (see Table 7–3) has 10 "suggested interventions" and 18 "additional optional" interventions from which to choose. The shaded intervention is a "priority intervention" (the intervention most likely to resolve the diagnosis).

The NIC *label* is the standardized terminology used in planning and documenting care. As evident from Box 7–2, not all activities would be needed for a particular client, so the nurse chooses the appropriate activities and individualizes them to fit the supplies, equipment, and other resources available in the agency.

Standardized languages are especially useful in computerized care planning systems. Figure 7–4 shows a computer screen of NIC interventions suggested for the NANDA diagnosis, Ineffective Management of Therapeutic Regimen. Figure 7–5 shows the NIC intervention, Values Clarification; the nurse chooses from the list of activities provided. Use of standardized terminology and computerized planning does not mean that the nurse gives routine, "cookbook"

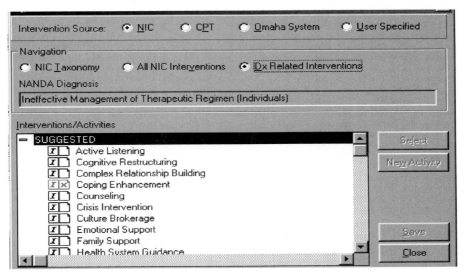

Figure 7–4

Computer Screen Listing Standardized (NIC) Interventions for a NANDA Diagnosis. *Source:* Copyright © Ergo Partners, L.C. All rights reserved. Used with permission.

care. The nurse using NIC chooses which interventions to use for a particular patient (as in Figure 7–5), when to use them, and which activities to adapt to the patient's needs and preferences. Figure 7–6 shows how the nurse can individualize a nursing activity chosen from a computer list. Box 7–3 summarizes the benefits of standardized language for interventions.

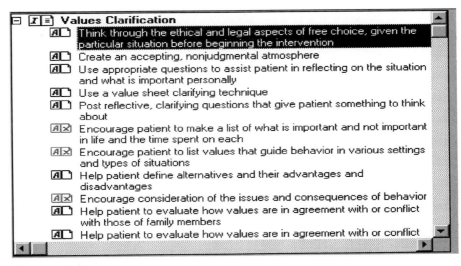

Figure 7–5

Computer Screen Showing Suggested Nursing Activities for the NIC Intervention, Values Clarification. *Source:* Copyright © Ergo Partners, L.C. All rights reserved. Used with permission.

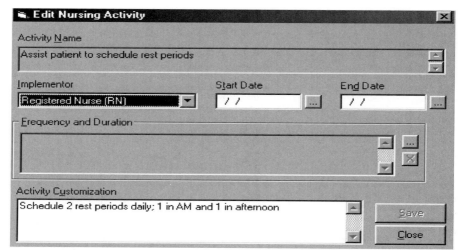

Figure 7–6
Screen Illustrating the Customization of an Activity Chosen from a Computer List.
Source: Copyright © Ergo Partners, L.C. All rights reserved. Used with permission.

Community Nursing Interventions

Community health nurses need terms to describe interventions for individuals, families, and "aggregates" (groups of people or entire communities). An example of a nonstandardized community intervention would be to establish a nurse-managed foot clinic.

BOX 7–3

Benefits of Standardized Interventions

Standardized language:

- Enhances communication among nurses and between nurses and non-nurses.
- Makes it possible for researchers to determine the effectiveness and cost of nursing treatments.
- Helps communicate the nature of nursing to the public.
- Helps demonstrate the impact that nurses have on healthcare.
- Makes it easier for nurses to select appropriate interventions by reducing the need for memorization and recall.
- Facilitates the teaching of clinical decision making.
- Contributes to the development and use of computerized clinical records.
- Assists in effective planning for staff and equipment needs.
- Aids in development of a system of payment for nursing services.
- Promotes full and meaningful participation of nurses in the multidisciplinary team.

The NIC is presently being used in community settings such as schools (Redes and Lunney 1997) and public health departments (Parris 1999). "A **community (or public health) intervention** is targeted to promote and preserve the health of populations. Community interventions emphasize health promotion, health maintenance, and disease prevention of populations and include strategies to address the social and political climate in which the population resides" (McCloskey and Bulechek 2000, p. xix). The NIC includes 16 interventions to support the health of the community (see Table 7–4).

The Omaha System has four categories of interventions: (1) health teaching, guidance, and counseling; (2) treatments and procedures; (3) case management; and (4) surveillance. These are used in combination with 63 *targets* (objects of nursing interventions or activities). In addition to physical targets such as bowel care, cardiac care, and nutrition, examples of public health targets are: caretaking/parenting skills, day-care/respite, durable medical equipment, employment, environment, finances, housing, legal system, and transportation. The following are examples of intervention statements (the italicized portions of the interventions are nonstandardized, client-specific words, added by the nurse to individualize the interventions):

"Surveillance: Safety: *basics in home*"
"Health Teaching, Guidance, and Counseling: Nutrition: *normal patterns*"

Despite the fact that it was developed specifically for community health nursing, the Omaha System does not have any diagnoses or interventions specifically identified for entire communities or aggregates.

Table 7–4 NIC Community Health Interventions

Community Health Promotion: Interventions that promote the health of the whole community	*Community Risk Management*: Interventions that assist in detecting or preventing health risks to the whole community.
Case Management	Community Disaster Preparedness
Community Health Development	Communicable Disease Management
Fiscal Resource Management	Environmental Management: Community
Health Education	Environmental Management: Worker Safety
Health Policy Monitoring	Environmental Risk Protection
Immunization/Vaccination Management	Health Screening
Program Development	Risk Identification
	Surveillance: Community
	Vehicle Safety Promotion

Source: McCloskey, J. C. and G. M. Bulechek, eds. (2000). *Nursing Interventions Classification (NIC)* (3rd ed). Philadelphia: Mosby, p. 103. Used with permission.

Table 7–5   NIC Family Interventions Classes

Classes	Examples
Childbearing Care: Interventions to assist in the preparation for childbirth and management of the psychological changes before, during, and immediately following childbirth.	Birthing Family Planning: Contraception Newborn Care Preconception Counseling
Childrearing Care: Interventions to assist in raising children.	Attachment Promotion Developmental Enhancement: Adolescent Lactation Counseling Teaching: Toddler Nutrition
Life Span Care: Interventions to facilitate family unit functioning and promote the health and welfare of family members throughout the life span.	Caregiver Support Family Therapy Home Maintenance Assistance Respite care

Source: McCloskey, J. C. and G. M. Bulechek, eds. (2000). *Nursing Interventions Classification (NIC)* (3rd ed). Philadelphia: Mosby, p. 101. Used with permission.

Family and Home Health Interventions

Home health nurses use both individual and family interventions. The NIC taxonomy (see Table 7–5) includes three classes of 74 interventions that support the family (McCloskey and Bulechek 2000). Other NIC interventions can be used with NANDA family diagnoses as well. For example, for Ineffective Family Coping, an intervention of "Developmental Enhancement: Adolescent" might be used, although it is not found in the family classes. The NIC is particularly useful because it can be used in all healthcare settings. This helps to bridge the gap between inpatient and home care.

The Home Health Care Classification (HHCC) defines a *nursing intervention* as "a single nursing service—treatment, procedure, or activity—designed in response to a diagnosis to achieve an outcome—medical or nursing—for which the nurse is accountable" (Saba 1995, p. 63). It includes 160 nursing interventions, each consisting of a label (eg, Denture Care) and a definition. For each intervention the nurse must specify the *type of intervention action*—one or more of the following: assess/monitor, care/perform, teach/instruct, or manage/coordinate. For example, a complete intervention statement might be: Denture Care: Assess and Teach. Interventions are linked to the nursing diagnoses they address. Although none are specifically designated as family interventions, some are useful for families (eg, Terminal Care: Bereavement Support, Terminal Care: Funeral Arrangements, and Stress Control). See Box 7–4 for examples of HHCC nursing components and interventions.

The Omaha System can also be used to describe home health interventions for individuals and families. In this system, problems are designated as

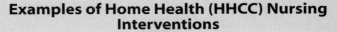

Examples of Home Health (HHCC) Nursing Interventions

M. Role Relationship Component
    38. Communication Care
    39. Psychosocial Analysis
        39.1 Home Situation Analysis
        39.2 Interpersonal Dynamics Analysis

N. Safety Component
    40. Abuse Control
    41. Emergency Care
    42. Safety Precautions
        42.1. Environmental Safety
        42.2. Equipment Safety
        42.3. Individual Safety

Specify Type of Intervention Action: Assess/Monitor, Care/Perform, Teach/Instruct, Manage/Coordinate.

Source: Saba, V. K. (1995). Home Health Care Classifications (HHCCs): Nursing diagnoses and nursing interventions. In: *An emerging framework: Data system advances for clinical Nsg practice.* ANA Pub. #NP-94. Washington, DC: American Nurses Publishing, pp. 85–86. Used with permission.

"family" or "individual," which determines whether the intervention is for the family or an individual.

■ FORMAL TEACHING PLANS

Nurses provide a great deal of informal teaching. In fact, at least some teaching interventions may be needed for every one of a patient's nursing diagnoses. Patients with complex teaching needs (eg, a patient with newly diagnosed diabetes) may need separate, formal teaching plans.

Teaching plans should include the teaching strategies to use in presenting the new information or skill. The appropriate strategy depends on the client's needs and the learning outcome you are working toward. Cognitive content is usually taught through discussion, lecture, printed materials, and audiovisuals. Psychomotor skills need to be demonstrated and discussed, and then reinforced with practice. Affective goals generally require role-modeling, discussion, and counseling to help the client gain insight. Nursing orders for teaching plans are written in the same format as other orders. They contain the content to be covered, the teaching strategy to be used, and the learner activities assigned or used in the session. An example of a teaching order would be "Demonstrate technique for drawing up insulin."

Teaching orders and strategies should be based on principles of teaching and learning. You may wish to refer to a basic nursing text for more information about teaching strategies, such as role modeling, discussion, demonstration, and use of audiovisual materials. To improve the effectiveness of your teaching plan, keep the following principles in mind:

1. *Assess the learner's knowledge and abilities.* Many factors affect a client's ability to learn, including existing knowledge, previous experience, education, age, and health status. Misconceptions and misinformation may interfere with learning new facts. Illness or sensory-perceptual deficits may make it difficult for the client to process or remember information.
2. *Teaching should proceed from simple to complex.* This makes the content easier to understand. Learning is a sequential process, in which new information builds on previous knowledge and experience.
3. *Use repetition and reinforcement.* Continued practice helps the client to retain new information. Rewards may be internal (personal) or external (praise). Pride in accomplishment can be a good learning incentive.

???

THINKING POINT

> As a home health nurse, you are adding a new family to your caseload. The chart indicates that the 3-year-old toddler has many dental caries and has already had two extractions and two root canals with crowns. The children eat mostly "junk food," including candy and colas, and the mother is lax about helping them brush their teeth. The care plan says, "Teach mother about nutrition and dental hygiene" in order to achieve a general goal of "Improve Jimmy's dental health."
>
> 1. The nurse tells you that the mother has a low IQ and that she is not interested in changing the family's eating patterns. How would you individualize the teaching intervention? What strategies would you use?
> 2. Suppose, instead, that the nurse tells you the mother has been going through some rough times, but is intelligent and strongly motivated to make whatever changes are needed to prevent further dental problems for her little boy. How would you individualize the teaching intervention? What strategies would you use?

■ WELLNESS INTERVENTIONS

Wellness interventions stress self-responsibility and active client involvement. The nurse may suggest health-promotion strategies, considering the client's age, sex, lifestyle, education, sociocultural background, and other variables. However, the client is the primary decision maker; the nurse functions mainly as teacher and health counselor. Activities needed for goal achievement may be written in terms of what the nurse is to do or what the client is to do.

Nursing orders on wellness care plans may take the form of specific behavioral changes the client wishes to make (eg, "I would like to stop smoking") and strategies for reinforcing the new behaviors. The most effective rewards are self-rewards rather than reinforcement from the nurse.

EXAMPLE: A moderately overweight client wishes to lose weight.

Specific Behavioral Changes	*Rewards*
I will walk for 45 minutes every day for the next 2 weeks.	I will buy myself a new jogging suit.
I will not eat between meals for 1 week.	I will treat myself to dinner out at my favorite seafood restaurant.

Most disease-prevention/health-promotion strategies involve lifestyle modifications such as diet changes, regular exercise, stress reduction, or smoking cessation. Motivation for change is sometimes difficult when no actual problem exists. A number of behavior-change strategies are available for helping clients to modify health behaviors; for example, self-reevaluation, cognitive restructuring, modeling, consciousnesss raising, and reward management. Pender (1996, Chapter 8) and Frenn and Malin (1998) may be useful if you wish to develop detailed nursing strategies to promote high-level wellness.

Standardized Wellness Interventions

Nurses will find the NIC useful in health promotion. It contains all of the interventions nurses use to promote wellness, although they are not all grouped together in one class (McCloskey and Bulechek 2000). A few HHCC interventions also have specific wellness applications.

The Omaha System also works well in health promotion. One of the Omaha intervention *targets* is "Wellness." It is defined as "Practices that promote health, including immunization, exercise, nutrition, and birth control" (Martin and Scheet 1992, p. 83). Using the Omaha System, the nurse would combine a *target* (eg, Wellness, Screening, Stimulation/Nurturance, and Support System) and the *intervention categories*, "Health Teaching, Guidance, and Counseling; and Surveillance" to create wellness interventions for health promotion diagnoses. Examples of such interventions might be: "Health Teaching, Guidance, and Counseling: Nutrition" and "Wellness: Surveillance."

■ SPIRITUAL INTERVENTIONS

Planning should be directed toward helping clients achieve the overall goals of spiritual strength, serenity, and satisfaction. A common intervention is to arrange a visit from a clergy member. Some clients may directly ask to see the hospital chaplain or their own clergyman. Others may discuss their concerns

KEY POINT

Examples of NIC Wellness Interventions

Decision-Making Support

Exercise Promotion

Health Education

Weight Management

Oral Health Promotion

Parent Education

Substance Use Prevention

KEY POINT

HHCC Wellness Interventions

Health Promotion

Nutrition Care: Regular Diet

Safety Precautions

Mental Health Promotion

Mental Health Screening (Saba 1995)

with the nurse and ask about the nurse's beliefs as a way of seeking an empathic listener. However, it is important to ask the client before arranging such assistance. Some people may profess no religious beliefs and may not wish to see a chaplain. The nurse should respect the clients' wishes in this area and not make judgments about whether they are right or wrong.

Spiritual care includes anything that touches a patient's spirit—comforting the family of a dying patient, a late-night conversation with a patient before surgery, or simply sitting quietly at the bedside. If you choose to provide spiritual care, and the patient wishes it, interventions can include talking, listening, prayer, reading scripture, fostering hope, and talking to patients about the role of religion in their life (Davis 1994; Laukhuf and Werner 1998). In a recent study, nurses were asked which interventions they used most often to support client spirituality. Box 7–5 contains their responses.

NIC priority interventions for Spiritual Distress are Spiritual Growth Facilitation and Spiritual Support. The other NIC suggested interventions for Spiritual Distress are found in Box 7–6. The Omaha System includes an intervention *target* of Spiritual Care, defined as "activities directed toward management of religious concerns" (Martin and Scheet 1992, p. 84). Although not categorized as "spiritual," other standardized interventions could also be used (eg, Support System: Case Management in the Omaha System; Meditation Facilitation in the NIC).

BOX 7–5

Spiritual Interventions Implemented Most Frequently

As reported by 208 oncology, parish, and hospice nurses in the Midwest, in order of frequency.

1. Active listening
2. Conducting a spiritual history and assessment
3. Conveying acceptance, true regard, respect, and a nonjudgmental attitude
4. Therapeutically communicating with clients to facilitate and validate clients' feelings and thoughts
5. Affirming the value of being part of a religious community
6. Touch
7. Conducting self-assessment of own spirituality
8. Presence
9. Prayer
10. Health education

Source: Sellers, S. C. and B. A. Haag (1998). Spiritual Nursing Interventions. *J Holistic Nurs* 16(3):338–354.

■ THINKING CRITICALLY ABOUT PLANNING

Generating interventions is similar to generating hypotheses in the scientific method. Nurses use therapeutic judgment to determine which interventions are most likely to achieve the desired outcomes. This requires critical thinking skills such as generalizing, explaining, and predicting, making interdisciplinary connections, and using insights from subjects such as physiology and psychology.

Reflecting on Interventions

Use the following questions to think critically about the interventions you have chosen. The critical thinking standards are in parentheses (review Table 2–3, on page 65, as needed).

1. **(Accuracy and Relevance) Is there research to support the intervention?** If not, do scientific principles or expert opinions provide rationale for the intervention (eg, ANA or agency standards of care)?
2. **(Clarity) Are the nursing orders concise?** Complex statements may be unclear. Do not include complex, routine procedures on the care plan. Instead write, for example, "See Unit 6 Procedure Manual for tracheal suctioning procedure." If the procedure needs to be modified for a client, the procedural changes should be noted in the nursing order (eg, "Use alcohol; client allergic to Betadine").
3. **(Clarity) Are the nursing orders clearly stated?** Would they be interpreted in the same way by other nurses?
4. **(Precision) Do the nursing orders give specific directions,** including "when," "how often," and so forth? Instead of "Ambulate with help of

KEY POINT
Professional Standard VII (1):

"The nurse utilizes best available evidence, preferably research data, to develop the plan of care and interventions" (ANA 1998, p. 15).

one person," the orders should specify, "Ambulate length of hall twice a day, with help of one person." A clear, complete order (see Questions 3 and 6) will probably be precise.

5. **(Precision) Is the intervention individualized for the patient's unique needs?** For example, "Encourage fluids" is not individualized. A better nursing order would be "Offer fluids every hour; patient likes orange juice."

6. **(Depth) Is each nursing order complete—does it contain all the components:** date, signature, action verb, descriptive qualifiers, and specific times?

7. **(Depth) Does the plan include a variety of interventions and activities? Have I overlooked any approaches?** Does it include (as appropriate) interventions/activities:
    - that are dependent, independent, and collaborative?
    - for monitoring/assessment, prevention, treatment, and health promotion?
    - For physical care, emotional support, teaching, counseling, activities of daily living, environmental management, and referrals?

8. **(Breadth) Is the intervention realistic:**
    - **in terms of patient abilities and resources?** For example, it would be unrealistic to order "Refer to home health agency for aide" if the patient could not afford this service.
    - **in terms of institution resources?** For example, "Turn hourly" may not be a realistic order on a unit that is short-staffed.

9. **(Breadth) Is the intervention safe?** An example would be a nursing order for range-of-motion exercises that specifies "Do not force beyond the point of resistance."

10. **(Breadth) Is the intervention acceptable to the patient?** Was the patient given an informed choice? Were the patient's values and culture taken into consideration? For example, even if a vegetarian client were protein-deficient, you would not write an order to add meat to the diet.

11. **(Breadth) Are the nurses (including myself) capable/competent to carry out the intervention?** An intervention should be used only if the nurse knows the scientific rationale for the intervention and has the necessary interpersonal and psychomotor skills.

12. **(Breadth) Is the intervention compatible with medical and other therapies?** For example, when there is a medical order for bed rest, you would not write an order to assist the patient with ambulation to prevent constipation.

13. **(Logic, Depth) Do the interventions address all aspects of the problem etiology?** If the etiology cannot be changed, do the interventions address the symptoms of the problem?

14. **(Significance) Which nursing orders must be carried out first, or immediately?**

Reflecting on Ethical Factors

The ANA *Code for Nurses* (1985), in Appendix A, emphasizes the role of nurses as patient advocates. An **advocate** is one who defends the rights of another. The healthcare system is complex and patients may be too uninformed or too ill to deal with it. Many need an advocate to cut through the layers of bureaucracy and help them get what they require. In addition to informing and supporting patients (see Chapter 6), nurses can advocate by mediating—by intervening on the patient's behalf, often by influencing others (Leddy and Pepper 1993).

> EXAMPLE: Ms. Alberghetti is undergoing combined radiation therapy and chemotherapy for cancer. She tells the nurse she wonders what these treatments are supposed to accomplish and how long she must take them. "I keep forgetting to ask the doctor. He asks me how I'm feeling, and by the time I finish telling him, I just forget." The nurse intervenes by asking the physician to review with Ms. Alberghetti the reasons for the therapies and their expected duration.

Although the nurse's input is important, many people are involved in making ethical (and other) decisions about interventions (eg, patient, family, other caregivers). Therefore, collaboration, communication, and compromise are important skills for nurses. When nurses do not have the autonomy to advocate for patients, compromise becomes essential. Integrity-producing compromises are most likely to be produced by collaborative decision making. The following mnemonic, LEARN, may remind you how to mediate and collaborate regarding interventions for patients (Berlin and Fowkes 1983):

L isten to others
E xplain your perceptions
A cknowledge and discuss differences
R ecommend alternatives
N egotiate agreement

Refer to Box 7–7 for your professional responsibilities for providing care in an ethical manner.

Reflecting on Cultural Factors

During planning, the nurse uses information about the client's and family's cultural values, beliefs, and practices to identify interventions that will support client practices and incorporate them into care as much as possible. For example, the nurse considers the client's food preferences and practices; identifies the person responsible for selecting and preparing foods; and then works with the family to teach them how to select and prepare cultural foods that will comply with therapeutic diet prescriptions (eg, a low-fat diet).

When planning care activities, you should assess language barriers and consider the need for an interpreter. Sometimes culturally diverse clients require information to avoid confusion or embarassment. For example, the position for bowel evacuation or the norm for the frequency of bowel movements may differ; or the client who is very modest may need much preparation and support before having an enema. When planning client education for clients whose primary language is not English, try to have written materials translated, use pictures to reinforce the written instructions, and have an interpreter give verbal instructions in the client's primary language.

Identify community resources available to assist clients of different cultures. And finally, try to learn from each transcultural nursing situation you encounter in order to improve the delivery of culture-specific care to future clients.

■ SUMMARY

Nursing Interventions

- are treatments based on clinical judgment and knowledge that a nurse performs to achieve patient goals/outcomes.

- may be independent, dependent, or interdependent.
- may involve observation, prevention, treatment, or health promotion, depending on the patient's health status.
- include the activities of physical care, teaching, counseling, emotional support, managing the environment, and making referrals.

When selecting nursing interventions, the nurse should choose those that

- eliminate or reduce the etiology of the nursing diagnosis; or if that is not possible, treat the signs and symptoms of the nursing diagnosis.
- are most likely to achieve desired outcomes.
- are based on research, principles, or expert opinion.

Nursing orders

- provide specific direction and a consistent, individualized approach to patient care.
- are stated as nurse behaviors—describe what the nurse is to do.
- are composed of date, subject, action verb, descriptive qualifiers, specific times, and signature.
- are concise and clearly stated.

Standardized vocabularies for nursing interventions

- provide a means for nurses to communicate their contributions to patient outcomes and the multidisciplinary team.
- include NIC, the Omaha System, and the HHCC.
- can be used to describe the individual, family, and community interventions.

A formal teaching plan

- may be needed for patients with complex teaching needs.
- should be based on principles of teaching and learning (eg, proceed from simple to complex; use repetition and reinforcement).

PLANNING INTERVENTIONS—THINKING QUICK-CHECK

- ❏ Have I considered all the possible approaches?
- ❏ Is there reason to believe this will work?
- ❏ Are the interventions realistic and acceptable to the patient?
- ❏ Have I chosen the best interventions?

Nursing Process Practice

1. A patient has a nursing diagnosis of "Risk for Impaired Skin Integrity (Pressure Ulcers) r/t long periods of lying in bed and inability to turn independently."

   A. Write nursing orders to decrease the etiological factors (risk factors, in this case).

   B. Write nursing orders for the problem side of the nursing diagnosis.

2. The collaborative problem is Potential Complications of Intravenous Therapy: Inflammation, Phlebitis, Infiltration. Refer to the outcomes you wrote for the Chapter 6 "Nursing Process Practice," item 12, on page 293.

   A. Write nursing orders for *observations* to make for this collaborative problem.

   B. Write *prevention* orders for this problem.

   For inflammation:

   For phlebitis:

   For infiltration:

   C. Write *patient teaching* orders for this problem.

3. The client has a nursing diagnosis of "Activity Intolerance: Level III r/t sedentary lifestyle and obesity." The nurse plans to (1) involve the patient in an exercise program to increase his muscle strength and (2) teach and promote a weight-loss diet. Which of the following NIC interventions seem the most likely ones to describe:
Intervention no. 1 (choose two): _____.

Intervention no. 2 (choose one): _____.

   a. Art Therapy

   b. Energy Management

   c. Exercise Promotion: Strength Training

   d. Exercise Therapy: Joint Mobility

   e. Teaching: Prescribe Activity/Exercise

   f. Nutrition Management

   g. Weight Management

   h. Sleep Enhancement

You would, of course, need to look these up in the NIC (2000) book to be sure they really do describe what the nurse intends.

4. Place an *N* by the nursing orders (stated as nursing behaviors).

   a. _____ Will verbalize anxieties about his surgery by 12/16.

   b. _____ Will rate pain as < 3 on a scale of 1–10.

   c. _____ Keep head of bed elevated to 45°.

   d. _____ Turn patient every 2 hours.

   e. _____ Force fluids up to 250 mL/hr.

   f. _____ Circulation to left foot will be improved, as evidenced by pink color, warm skin.

   g. _____ Infection will be prevented, as evidenced by temp < 100.1° F.

   h. _____ Wear sterile gloves for dressing change.

   i. _____ Take temperature hourly if elevated.

   j. _____ Will list foods allowed on low-fat diet by 12/16.

5. Fill in the blanks. For what kind of content are the following teaching orders designed? (A = Affective, C = Cognitive, P = Psychomotor)

a. _____ Demonstrate how to draw up the correct amount of insulin.

b. _____ Explain the syringe markings.

c. _____ Encourage patient to discuss and explore his fear of needles.

d. _____ Give patient pamphlet on food exchange groups.

e. _____ Counsel patient regarding appropriate expressions of anger.

f. _____ Demonstrate and explain to patient how to inject himself, maintaining sterile technique.

g. _____ Explain the relationship between exercise and insulin requirements.

h. _____ Demonstrate and have patient pratice an injection angle of 45°.

6. Read the following list of nursing actions. Classify them (eg, Dependent/Independent) by writing the letters beside the appropriate category in the chart. Interventions can be classified in several ways, so most will belong in more than one category. (The first one has been done for you.)

Nursing Orders

a. Review booklet on postmastectomy exercises with Ms. Petrie on evening of 7/13.

b. Spend at least 10 minutes per shift sitting with Ms. Adkins; encourage her to express her feelings about her husband's death.

c. Give acetaminophen 500 mg, p.o. q3h if temp >101.2° F.

d. Remove staples from abdominal incision today.

e. Minimize environmental stimuli: dim lights, restrict visitors, speak and move slowly and quietly.

f. DO NOT take rectal temperatures.

g. Cut food for patient. Allow at least an hour for meals. Reheat food as needed.

h. Palpate uterine fundus for firmness q hr until saturating <1 pad/hr.

i. B/P q4h unless elevated. If >150/94, take q hr.

j. Pad side rails with blankets or rubber pads.

k. Teach patient to wash hands carefully before handling infant.

l. Refer to Public Health Dept. for rubella immunization.

m. Give pamphlets on "The Food Guide Pyramid" and "Foods for Healthy Living."

Independent: *a*   Dependent:
Observation: Treatment: *a*   Prevention: Health promotion:
Physical care: Teaching: *a*   Counseling: Referral: Environmental management:

7. Use the critical thinking questions on pages 327–328 (Reflecting on Interventions) to evaluate the following nursing orders. Write the number of the question/standard violated by the intervention; or write "OK" if it is satisfactory. Rewrite orders to correct them. (To save space, the orders are not dated or signed. Do not count that as an error.)

_____ **a.** Monitor intake and output hourly.

_____ **b.** Force fluids to tolerance.

_____ **c.** Monitor serum potassium levels and report levels < 3.5.

_____ **d.** Change dressing daily. Remove soiled dressing with protective gloves. Cleanse around wound with betadine. Pack with sterile gauze, cover with nonstick dressing, and finally with 4 × 6 bandage. Tape all 4 sides.

_____ **e.** Collect midstream urine specimen in AM on 11/10. See unit procedure manual. Pt. will need help holding specimen cup.

_____ **f.** Encourage patient to ambulate more.

8. Your patient is hospitalized with a severe coagulation problem. He is very ill, sometimes confused, and confined to bed. He has no family or significant other. His care plan contains the NIC intervention: "Bleeding Precautions." All of the following are NIC activities for that intervention. Circle the letters of the ones that are appropriate for *this* patient.

   a. Monitor the patient closely for hemorrhage.

   b. Maintain bed rest during active bleeding.

   c. Do not take rectal temperature.

   d. Instruct patient to avoid aspirin or other anticoagulants.

   e. Monitor orthostatic vital signs, including blood pressure.

   f. Instruct the ambulating patient to wear shoes.

   g. Instruct the patient or family on signs of bleeding and appropriate actions (eg, notify the nurse) if bleeding occurs.

Critical Thinking Practice: Recognizing Relevant Information

In everyday life you often analyze complex situations. You might watch a football game and try to understand the plays. Analyzing football plays is easy for some people because they have learned to see the relevant information. They know, for instance, that watching the quarterback just after the play starts can help them understand whether the play is a run or a pass. If you want to learn to analyze football plays you must learn how to find the relevant information. (Refer to "Distinguishing Between Relevant and Irrelevant Data," in Chapter 2, as needed.)

Learning the Skill

Example A. Recognizing football plays is a two-step process.

   Step 1. Learn the names used to identify the various plays. The meanings of these names help you to remember what the plays are. For instance, there are *running* plays and *passing* plays; during a running play, what is the player doing?

   Step 2. Learn to focus your attention on the relevant aspects of the play—the people involved and the situation at hand. At the beginning of a football play, which player should you watch most carefully?

Example B. Recognizing the presence of a client's nursing diagnosis uses the same two-step process. Use a nursing diagnosis handbook (eg, Wilkinson 2000, *Nursing Diagnosis Handbook*) for the remainder of this exercise.

   Step 1. Learn the names and definitions of the various NANDA labels.

In the nursing diagnosis handbook you will find lables like Anxiety, Fear, and Personal Identity Disturbance. These names may be familiar to you. Which one means inability to distinguish between self and nonself?

Which one means a vague, uneasy feeling with a nonspecific source?

Step 2. Learn to focus your attention on important aspects of the nursing diagnosis—the definitions and defining characteristics or risk factors. If you do not know which signs and symptoms are associated with a particular label, you may not realize the significance of the client's signs and symptoms. In fact, if you do not know what signs and symptoms to look for, you may not even be aware of the cues, much less the existence of a problem.

Nurses often misdiagnose Fear and Anxiety because some of the physical and emotional manifestations may be the same. If you focus only on the relevant cues, however, you can make the distinction. Use your nursing diagnosis handbook as needed.

1. For which label is the feeling *apprehension and fright*?
   For which label is the feeling *vague and uneasy discomfort*?
   Write a rule you could use to tell these two labels apart.

2. In which label is the source of the feeling known to the client?
   In which label is the source of the feeling nonspecific or unknown to the client?

   Write another rule you could use to tell these two labels apart.

3. Which of these labels has *poor eye contact* as a defining characteristic?
   Which label has *wide-eyed* as a defining characteristic?
   Write another rule you could use to differentiate between anxiety and fear.

4. In the following case study, your client is exhibiting physical and emotional signs of distress. Circle the cues that are *relevant* to a diagnosis of fear.

   Mr. Cheng has pneumonia. His intake and outflow record shows he has not been drinking fluids. When you auscultate his lungs, you hear bilateral crackles and rales. His temperature is 100° F and his B/P is 140/90. He says he is very weak. He states, "I just feel like something awful is going to happen to me." He is perspiring and his hands are shaking. He has just been started on oxygen therapy, and he tells you the mask makes him feel that he is suffocating. You check his database and find he has a history of claustrophobia.

Applying the Skill

The same process is used in identifying collaborative problems. You must know the complications that may occur with medical diagnoses and therapies and the signs and symptoms of the complications.

1. Read the following case study. Refer to a basic nursing text or a medical-surgical nursing text if necessary.

   Katie O'Hara has severe vomiting and diarrhea due to gastroenteritis. Because she needs fluids and antibiotics, her physician has prescribed IV therapy, which she will need for several days.

   a. What are two obvious potential complications of IV therapy?

   b. What are the symptoms of those complications?

      (1)

      (2)

   c. If you are assessing Katie for Complications of Intravenous Therapy: Infiltration and Phlebitis, which data would be relevant? (Circle the relevant data.)

      B/P 110/80, pulse 80, temperature 100° F. Katie states that she feels afraid, but "just can't put my finger on what it is." She remains NPO. Her output for the shift is 350 mL emesis, 150 mL of urine, and six unmeasured liquid stools. Her hands are warm and dry; the skin turgor is good on her forearms. Her IV is infusing at 100 mL/hr, but it is positional (ie, it sometimes stops running when she changes the position of her arm). You have opened the roller clamp completely, but it will not run at the prescribed rate of 150 mL/hr. There is no redness at or above the insertion site. The area around the insertion site is pale and cool to touch. Katie states that it is a little tender to touch. When you hang her piggyback antibiotic, she complains that it burns her arm. Katie's database shows no allergy to any medications.

2. Suppose you were assessing a patient for Impaired Tissue Integrity (Decubitus Ulcer). List the relevant data (ie, what signs, symptoms, and risk factors would you look for?).

3. Think of two assessments that would *not* be relevant in Exercise 2.

Adapted from Wilbraham et al (1990). *Critical Thinking Worksheets*, a Supplement of *Addison-Wesley Chemistry*. Menlo Park, CA: Addison-Wesley.

Case Study: Applying Nursing Process and Critical Thinking

Dorothy Evans, an obese 40-year-old woman, is recovering from abdominal surgery, performed yesterday. Her care plan includes orders for incentive spirometry and regular turning, coughing, and deep breathing. When you prepare to help her with these activities, she says, "You can help me turn, but I'm not doing that breathing stuff. It hurts too much. I'm just so tired. I need rest more than anything."

1. What complication is the breathing exercises designed to prevent?

2. What factors place Ms. Evans at risk for this complication? Explain.

3. What do you need to know before you can decide what to do first? How will you get that information?

4. What is the most important goal in this situation?

5. What will you say and do to respond to Ms. Evans' concerns about pain and rest? Explain your reasoning.

6. What will you say and do to get her to comply with the treatment plan? Why do you think that will help?

7. How will you know if the plan is successful? What specific assessments must you make?

■ SELECTED REFERENCES

American Nurses Association (1998). *Standards of Clinical Nursing Practice*. 2nd ed. Washington, DC: American Nurses Publishing.

American Nurses Association (1985). *Code for Nurses with Interpretive Statements*. Kansas City, MO: ANA.

Berlin, E. A., and W. C. Fowkes (1983). A teaching framework for cross-cultural health care. *West J Med* 139(b):934–938.

Button, P. S. (1997). Computers in practice: Challenges and uses—using standardized nursing nomenclature in an automated careplanning and documentation system. In: Rantz M. J. and P. LeMone, eds. *Classification of Nursing Diagnoses: Proceedings of the Twelfth Conference. North American Nursing Diagnosis Association*. Glendale, CA: Cinahl, pp. 327–331.

Canadian Nurses Association (1987). *Standards for Nursing Practice*. Ottawa, Ontario: CNA.

Davis, M. C. (1994). The rehabilitation nurse's role in spiritual care. *Rehab Nurs* 19(5): 298–301.

Frenn, M. and S. Malin (1998). Health promotion: theoretical perspectives and clinical applications. *Hol Nurs Pract* 12(2):1–7.

Henry, S. B., W. L. Holzemer, C. Randell, et al (1997). Comparison of Nursing Interventions Classification and Current Procedural Terminology codes for categorizing nursing activities. *Image: J Nurs Scholar* 29(2):133–138.

Iowa Intervention Project (1997). Proposal to bring nursing into the information age. *Image: J Nurs Scholar* 29(3):275–281.

King, C. and P. Harber (1998). Community environmental health concerns and the nursing process. *AAOHNJ* 46(1):20–27.

Laukhuf, G. and H. Werner (1998). Spirituality: the missing link. *J Neurosci Nurs* 30(1):60–67.

Leddy, S. and J. M. Pepper (1993). *Conceptual bases of professional nursing.* 3rd ed. Philadelphia: Lippincott.

Lindsey, E. and G. Hartrick (1996). Health-promoting nursing practice: the demise of the nursing process? *J Advan Nurs* 23:106–112.

Martin, K. S. and N. J. Scheet (1991). *The Omaha System: applications for community health nursing.* Philadelphia: W. B. Saunders.

McCloskey, J. C. and G. M. Bulechek, eds. (2000). *Nursing Interventions Classification (NIC).* 3rd ed. Philadelphia: Mosby.

Mundinger, M. O. (1980). *Autonomy in nursing.* Gaithersburg, MD: Aspen Systems.

Parris, K. M., P. J. Place, and E. Orellana (1999). Integrating nursing diagnoses, interventions, and outcomes in public health nursing practice. *Nurs Diag* 10(2):49–56.

Pender, N. J. (1996). *Health promotion in nursing practice.* 3rd ed. Stamford, CT: Appleton & Lange.

Radwin, L. E. (1995). Knowing the patient: a process model for individualized interventions. *Nurs Res* 44(6):364–370.

Redes, S. and M. Lunney (1997). Validation by school nurses of the Nursing Intervention Classification for computer software. *Computers in Nursing* 15(6):333–338.

Saba, V. K. (1997). Why the Home Health Care Classification is a recognized nursing nomenclature. *Computers in Nursing* 15(2):S69–76.

Saba, V. K. (1995). Home Health Care Classifications (HHCCs): nursing diagnoses and nursing interventions. In: *An emerging framework: Data system advances for clinical nursing practice.* ANA Publication No. NP-94. Washington, DC: American Nurses Publishing.

Sellers, S. C. and B. A. Haag (1998). Spiritual nursing interventions. *J Hol Nurs* 16(3): 338–354.

Ziegler, S. M. (1993). *Theory-directed nursing practice.* New York: Springer Publishing.

8

Implementation

Learning Outcomes

On completing this chapter, you should be able to do the following:

- Discuss the relationship of implementation to the other phases of the nursing process.
- Compare and contrast managed care and case management.
- State ways to enhance patient learning and compliance.
- State guidelines for implementing and delegating safe, effective, and efficient care.
- Explain how to provide ethically, culturally, and spiritually competent care.
- Compare and contrast seven methods of writing nursing progress notes: narrative, SOAP, PIE, PART, Focus® Charting, charting by exception, and integrated plans of care.
- Discuss the pros and cons of computerized documentation.
- Observe guidelines for documenting and reporting patient care and status.
- Explain how documentation in home health and long-term care settings is different from that in institutional settings.
- Describe four common legal pitfalls for nurses and what should be included when documenting them.

■ INTRODUCTION

Implementation is the phase in which the nurse performs or delegates the activities necessary for achieving the client's health goals. Described broadly, the activities in this step are (1) doing, (2) delegating, and (3) recording (see Figure 8–1). Implementation ends when nursing actions and the resulting client responses have been recorded in the client's chart.

Professional standards for nursing practice support client participation in implementation, as in all phases of the nursing process (see Box 8–1). The degree of participation may vary. For example, an infant or an unconscious person cannot participate at all in implementation strategies; all interventions for such patients are carried out by nurses, significant

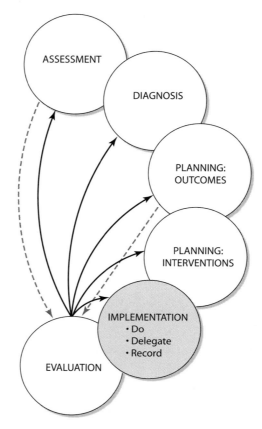

Figure 8–1
The Implementation Phase.

others, or other caregivers. In the case of health-promotion stages, the client alone might carry out the strategies.

EXAMPLE: With the help of his nurse, David Mikos devised a plan for lowering his cholesterol intake. The plan is to follow a low-fat diet at home and reward himself with concert or theater tickets for each month of successful dieting. In this case, the nurse is not involved at all in the implementation phase.

Relationship of Implementation to Other Nursing Process Phases

Implementation depends on the first three phases of the nursing process: assessment, diagnosis, and planning. Those steps provide the basis for the autonomous nursing actions performed during implementation. Without them, implementation (and nursing) would reflect only dependent functions—

BOX 8–1

Nusing Standards of Care

ANA Standard V: Implementation

The nurse implements the interventions identified in the plan of care.

Measurement Criteria

1. Interventions are consistent with the established plan of care.
2. Interventions are implemented in a safe, timely, and appropriate manner.
3. Interventions are documented.

Source: Reprinted with permission from American Nurses Association, *Standards of Clinical Nursing Practice* (2nd ed.) © 1998 American Nurses Publishing, American Nurses Foundation/American Nurses Association, 600 Maryland Avenue, SW, Suite 100W, Washington, DC 20024-2571, p. 9.

CNA Standard II (Nursing Process)

Implementation of the Intervention

4. Nurses are required to perform nursing actions which implement the plan.

The nurse in any practice setting:

4.1 encourages client participation whenever possible in carrying out nursing actions to meet objectives

4.2 carries out nursing actions demonstrating required knowledge, attitudes, and skills

4.3 exercises judgment in carrying out nursing responsibilities within the interdisciplinary plan of care

4.4 delegates activities to auxiliary personnel as required

4.5 supervises auxiliary personnel in carrying out delegated activities

4.6 utilizes appropriate resources

4.7 manipulates the environment to meet the objectives

4.8 communicates with appropriate others regarding nursing actions

Source: Canadian Nurses Association (1987). *Standards for Nursing Practice*. Ottawa: Ontario, p. 5.

carrying out medical orders and institutional policies. In turn, the implementation step provides the actual interventions and client responses that are evaluated in the evaluation phase.

Implementation overlaps with the other phases. Using data acquired during assessment, the nurse can individualize the care given during implementation, tailoring interventions to fit a specific client, rather than applying them routinely to categories of patients (eg, "All pneumonia patients . . .").

While implementing, you will continue to assess the patient at every contact, gathering data about responses to the nursing actions and about any new problems that may develop. Ongoing assessment is not the *same* as implementation; it occurs *during* implementation.

EXAMPLES:

Implementation	*Assessment*
While bathing an elderly patient,	the nurse observes a reddened area on the patient's sacrum.
When emptying the catheter bag,	the nurse measures 200 mL and notices a strong odor.

The nurse also implements nursing orders that specifically *direct* ongoing assessment. For example, a nursing order might read, "Auscultate lungs q4h." When performing this activity, the nurse is both carrying out the nursing order and performing ongoing, focused assessment.

Data obtained during implementation activities are used to identify new diagnoses or to revise existing diagnoses (diagnosis step). These data also enable the nurse to revise and adapt the original goals and nursing orders (evaluation and planning) as the patient's unique needs become more apparent.

Healthcare Delivery Systems

Organizations influence implementation by creating the environment within which nurses provide care. Responding to the demand for healthcare reform, organizations have developed client care approaches that are intended to be cost-effective and to provide continuity of care. Two such systems are managed care and case management.

Managed Care

Managed care is used to standardize practice for the most common case types in an agency. For example, case types in a cardiac care unit might be myocardial infarction and cardiac catheterization. The care of a patient is carefully planned from the initial contact to the conclusion of the health problem. Managed care emphasizes cost control, cilent ("customer") satisfaction, health promotion, and preventive services. Health maintenance organizations (HMOs) and preferred provider organizations (PPOs) are examples of managed care systems. Some hospitals also use managed care approaches.

Third-party payers (eg, insurance companies, Medicare) usually pay healthcare agencies according to a client's diagnosis or *diagnosis-related group (DRG)*; or they pay a fixed amount for each patient treated, regardless of the time and resources a client consumes. Therefore, it is essential to achieve specified client outcomes within the length of stay allowed by the client's payer. To this end, managed care systems use standardized multidisciplinary care plans called **critical pathways** for high volume case types or situations that have relatively predictable outcomes. The critical pathway (1) specifies the time by which each client outcome is to be achieved and (2) outlines crucial activities to be performed by all health team members at designated times. Refer to Chapter 6, "Multidisciplinary Care Plans (Critical Pathways)," on pages 260 and 261, for a discussion of critical pathways. See Figure 10–7, on page 442, for an example of a critical pathway.

Case Management

Case management is used to coordinate care for high-risk, complex populations who may use a disproportionate share of healthcare resources (eg, patients with AIDs or chronic obstructive pulmonary disease). Case managers deal with the unusual cases—patients whose condition changes frequently and unpredictably or whose complex needs cannot be addressed by a standardized critical pathway. A case manager—usually a nurse, a nurse-physician team, or a social worker—assumes responsibility for a group of patients from preadmission to discharge or transfer and recuperation. Caseloads may be organized geographically (eg, clients from all surgical units in a hospital), by diagnosis (eg, a group of cardiac rehabilitation clients), or by physician. Case managers link patients and families to services (eg, home health nurse, physical therapy, transportation) in all settings in which the patient receives care. They plan and evaluate the most cost-effective services to meet specified patient outcomes. They also help patients to develop the skills they need to care for themselves and to obtain what they need from the healthcare system.

■ PREPARING TO ACT

Preparation for patient-care activities actually begins in the planning phase of the nursing process. When you use time-sequenced planning to set your work priorities and make your daily work schedule, you are actually taking the first step in delivering care to your assigned patients. Box 8–2 is a guide you may wish to use in organizing your nursing care for a clinical day.

Most institutions are focusing on cost and efficiency, so it is important that each nurse-patient encounter be fully utilized. When possible, implement care for several goals simultaneously. For instance, while at the bedside taking vital signs and making physical assessments, you might use the time to talk with the patient, show interest and concern, or do patient teaching.

Preparing the Nurse

Before beginning an intervention, be sure that both you and the patient are prepared. Always review the care plan to clarify any details and determine if you need help in performing any of the interventions. You may require assistance under the following conditions:

BOX 8-2

Student Guide for Organizing Clinical Activities

Client profile: Name _____ Age _____

Admitting diagnosis_____ Admit date _____

Name client wishes to be called _____

Significant other(s) _____

Current health status (today):

Has the client's physical or emotional status changed since you received your assignment?

Do you need to modify your care plan?

Basic Care Needs:

Hygiene _____

Elimination _____

Feeding _____

Dressing _____

Other _____

Special safety precautions _____

Medications and IVs:

Collaborative tests and treatments (for scheduling and observation)—eg, physical therapy, x-ray.

Prioritized nursing diagnoses and strategies (that you can realistically address today):

New medical orders that need to be implemented (eg, discontinue IV, ambulate):

Special teaching or counseling needs:

1. *You lack the skill or knowledge to implement a nursing order.* For example, if you have never taught a patient to crutch-walk, you should ask a colleague for help or review the written procedure before attempting the intervention.
2. *You cannot safely perform the action alone.* For example, you should obtain help when moving a large, immobile patient from a bed to a chair.
3. *Assistance would reduce the client's stress.* For example, having help in repositioning a patient who experiences pain when being moved will minimize her pain.

You are legally and ethically responsible for questioning nursing or medical orders that you believe to be inappropriate or potentially harmful. This should also be done as a part of your preparation.

Preparation includes identifying points in the activity where you need to pause for feedback. The immediate feedback you obtain during an activity guides you in making on-the-spot alterations in the action. For example, when preparing to help a patient ambulate, you might plan to look for responses (feedback) after he sits on the side of the bed for a minute, after standing, after walking to a chair, and again after he has been sitting in the chair for 15 minutes.

Preparing the Patient

Just before implementing, you should *reassess whether the intervention is still needed.* Never assume that an order is still necessary simply because it is written on the care plan; the situation or the client's condition may have changed. For example, Gayle Fischer has a nursing diagnosis of Sleep Pattern Disturbance related to anxiety and unfamiliar surroundings. When the nurse makes rounds, she discovers that Gayle is sleeping, so she omits the back rub that was planned as a relaxation strategy.

Also *assess the client's readiness.* The client's behavioral cues will help you to choose a time when the activity will benefit her most. Much time can be wasted in performing interventions when a client is not psychologically ready. For example, when the nurse goes to Ms. Fischer's room to teach her about diabetic foot care, she notices that Ms. Fischer has been crying. Realizing that the patient would probably not be receptive to new information at this time, the nurse decides to postpone the teaching. Do not assume that the patient is ready to progress just because the critical pathway says so.

On the critical pathway for Ms. Fischer, one of the nursing orders for today (postoperative day 2) is "Discontinue IV fluids." However, Ms. Fischer's bowel sounds are infrequent and she is taking only scant amounts of oral fluids. As her nurse, what would you do?

???
THINKING POINT

Finally, *explain to the client what is to take place.* The client is entitled to an explanation of the action, the sensations he can expect, what he is expected to do, and the results the therapy or procedure is expected to produce. Preparation also includes provision for privacy, as well as any physical preparation, such as positioning.

EXAMPLE: Before administering an enema to Jo Slevin, the nurse explains that this will prevent contamination of the surgical area during her bowel surgery. She shuts the door, pulls the curtain around the bed, helps Jo to assume a side-lying position, and drapes her with a bath blanket. She tells Jo she will feel pressure and perhaps some cramping as the fluid is instilled, and that she should retain the solution for 5 or 10 minutes, until she feels a strong urge to defecate.

Preparing Supplies and Equipment

KEY POINT
Is the Patient Prepared?

- Determine whether the action is still needed.
- Assess the patient's readiness.
- Explain what is to be done and what results to expect.
- Tell the client what sensations to expect.
- Tell the client what he is expected to do.
- Provide for privacy.

Assemble all necessary equipment and materials before entering the room, so that you can proceed efficiently and with a minimum amount of stress to the patient. You may need supplies for dressing changes, equipment for removing staples from an incision, linen for a bath and bed change, or pamphlets for a teaching session. The following example demonstrates how inefficient and ineffective it is to stop in midprocedure because the necessary supplies are not at hand.

EXAMPLE: A nurse is inserting a urinary catheter. After draping the patient, opening the sterile kit, and donning sterile gloves, one of the nurse's gloves brushes against the patient's leg. Because she did not think to bring an extra pair of sterile gloves into the room, she is faced with the choice of leaving the patient draped and positioned while she goes for another pair, continuing the procedure with an unsterile glove, or going for new gloves, opening a new cath kit, and redraping the patient to be sure sterility is maintained.

■ ACTION: DOING OR DELEGATING

After preparations are complete, action begins. The nurse applies a wide range of knowledge and skills in performing or delegating planned nursing strategies. The number and kind of specific nursing activities is almost unlimited. They consist of every skill, process, and procedure you have learned as a student and as a practitioner. Cognitive, interpersonal, and technical skills are discussed individually in Chapter 1 in order to facilitate understanding; in practice, however, you will use them in various combinations and with different emphasis, depending upon the activity. For instance, when inserting a urinary catheter, you need cognitive knowledge of the principles and steps of the procedure, technical skills in draping the patient and manipulating the equipment, and interpersonal skills to inform and reassure the patient. See Table 8–1 for examples.

Table 8–1   Nursing Skills Used in Implementation

Skill	Examples
Cognitive Skills	When helping a patient walk, the nurse notices that the IV flow rate is too slow. He quickly checks to see that the tubing is not kinked and that the IV has not infiltrated. When no mechanical problems are noted, he opens the roller clamp to increase the flow. When it is still slow, he raises the bag higher to make use of gravity.
Interpersonal Skills	Interpersonal skills are used with patients, families, and other health team members. The nurse listens actively; conveys interest; gives clear explanations; comforts; makes referrals; delegates activities; and shares attitudes, feelings, and knowledge.
Psychomotor (Technical) Skills	Performing hands-on skills, such as changing dressings, giving injections, turning and positioning patients, attaching a monitor to a patient, and suctioning a tracheostomy.

The nursing process enables nurses to identify, evaluate, and emphasize their independent activities. However, the full nursing role encompasses dependent and collaborative functions as well. Most nurses provide care for ill clients, whose comprehensive health needs include attention to their medical condition. In the implementation step, you will implement both (1) the nursing orders on the patient's care plan and (2) physician's orders for the medical care plan.

Recall that **dependent interventions** are those performed when following physician orders or agency policies. Usually they relate directly to the client's medical diagnosis or disease processes.

Collaborative (interdependent) interventions are performed either with other health professionals (eg, physician, dietitian) or as a result of decisions made jointly with them. **Coordination** of the patient's care is an important nursing activity that is related to, but not the same as, collaboration. This activity involves scheduling the client's contacts with other hospital departments (eg, laboratory and x-ray technicians, physical and respiratory therapists) and serving as a liaison among the members of the healthcare team. As the professionals who are in touch with the patient 24 hours a day, nurses are in the best position to receive all the fragments of information and synthesize a holistic view of the patient. By making rounds with other professionals, reading their reports, and interpreting their findings to patients and families, the nurses assure that everyone gets the "big picture" as well as the specialized one.

Independent (autonomous) interventions are performed when carrying out the nursing orders, and often in conjunction with medical orders.

In addition to legally conferred autonomy, the nurse's knowledge and critical thinking determine the degree to which an action can be considered autonomous; the same activity can be independent in one situation and dependent in another.

> EXAMPLE: Mr. Rauh has a temperature of 100.1° F. The nurse realizes that many things can affect body temperature, and asks Mr. Rauh if he had anything to eat or drink before his vital signs were taken. The medical order reads, "V.S. t.i.d"; but because the temperature represents an unusual reading for Mr. Rauh, and because the nurse knows he is at risk for infection, she retakes his temperature an hour later to establish whether this is a pattern or an isolated cue.

This nurse's actions are independent. If she had been functioning dependently, she would have recorded Mr. Rauh's vital signs without validating their accuracy or questioning their meaning. She might have telephoned the physician for instructions, or simply passed the data on to the next shift without checking to see if Mr. Rauh's temperature remained the same, continued to rise, or returned to normal.

Accountability is an aspect of autonomy. **Autonomy** implies that the nurse is answerable for her actions and can define, explain, and evaluate the results of her decisions. The nurse in the preceding example is answerable (accountable) for the decisions she made (ie, to wait an hour and retake Mr. Rauh's temperature before calling the physician) and would have been able to provide a rationale for her actions.

Teaching for Self-Care

In this era of early discharge and self-care, patient teaching is an important nursing activity. However, you cannot assume that teaching leads to learning. *Learning* is more likely to occur under the following conditions:

1. The learner has no unmet physical or emotional needs that interfere with learning (eg, pain, fatigue, hunger).
2. The learner is ready and motivated to learn.
3. The learner is actively involved (eg, supervised practice with feedback).
4. The environment is conducive to learning (eg, quiet, appropriately lighted).
5. The emotional climate is favorable (eg, the client is not angry or anxious).
6. Rapport exists between patient and nurse.

Even when learning occurs, you cannot assume that the patient will use the information he learns. Patients have many reasons for failing to follow treatment instructions, for example:

- lack of education for understanding the concepts
- cultural differences that create a barrier
- lack of a support system (eg, lack of money to buy medications)
- lack of confidence because of past failures (eg, "I've tried to quit smoking before.")
- reluctance to "bother the doctor (or nurse)" with questions
- a lifestyle that makes adherence difficult (eg, a salesperson who frequently entertains customers may find it difficult to follow a low-fat, low-salt diet).

You can encourage by assessing the patient's understanding of his illness or injury. This will help you to clear up any knowledge deficits or misinformation. Ask questions and try to discover the patient's viewpoint, priorities, and needs so that you can personalize your teaching. For more tips on enhancing adherence, refer to Box 8–3.

BOX 8–3

Tips for Enhancing Adherence

- **Accept the patient as he is**. Respect his values and beliefs. Accept that some attitudes cannot be changed. For example, if a patient does not *want* to quit smoking, encourage him to reduce the number of cigarettes he smokes each day.
- **Ask the patient what *he* wants to know and what *his* concerns are.** Most patients won't voice their fears unless you ask them. After teaching, ask the patient if there is anything he wants to know that you haven't covered.
- **Be realistic**. Patients may reject big lifestyle or behavioral changes outright. You may need to aim for small changes. No matter how badly he needs to exercise, a patient with overwhelming demands on his time will not be able to exercise every day. It might be better for that person to set a goal to exercise three times a week.
- **Do not assume**. Every patient's situation is different. Don't make the mistake of assuming that the patient understands his disease; that the family is supportive; that there is money to buy food or medicine; or that the patient can read, owns a car, or has a phone. Assess carefully.
- **Promote patient confidence**, especially if he has failed in the past. If you can, give examples of other patients who were in similar circumstances and tell how they were able to succeed.
- **Remind the patient that change takes time**. Refer him to a local support or self-help group for ongoing encouragement.

Source: Adapted from London, F. (1998). Improving compliance. What you can do. *RN* 61(1):43–46.

Recall a time when you did not follow a doctor's or other health professional's advice. For example, you may have not taken all of the antibiotic capsules, even though the instructions clearly said to do so. (1) List all the reasons you had for not complying. (2) What, if anything, could a nurse have done that would have changed what you did in that situation?

KEY POINT
Registered nurses *cannot* delegate decision-making authority to LPNs or UAPs; they *can* delegate the responsibility for performing defined tasks or activities.

KEY POINT
You can delegate data gathering duties, such as vital signs or intake and output—but do not confuse these activities with assessment. The RN must be sure the data are accurate, and know what the data mean.

Delegation and Supervision

Assignment is the transfer of both the responsibility and accountability of an activity from one person to another. For example, when a unit leader assigns a group of patients to an RN for a shift, the RN is both responsible for the care and accountable for the results of that care. **Delegation** is the transfer of responsibility for the performance of a task or activity from one person to another while retaining accountability for the outcome (ANA 1996). For example, the RN can assign an LPN or UAP to take a patient's blood pressure; but if it is inaccurate and the patient becomes seriously hypertensive, it is the RN who must answer for not recognizing that a problem was developing. Because many healthcare institutions use RN extenders (LPNs, UAPs), delegating patient care and assigning tasks is a vital skill. Delegating includes three responsibilities: (1) *appropriate delegation* of duties, (2) *appropriate communication*, and (3) *adequate supervision* of the RN extender (RNE).

Appropriate Delegation

Appropriate delegation means assigning the right activities to the right person. As an RN, when you delegate a task to an RNE, you are essentially guaranteeing that that person is motivated and able to perform the task. This means you must know the RNE's background, experience, knowledge, skills, strengths, and legal scope of practice. You must assess the patient and family in order to match their needs with the abilities of the various RNEs. Box 8–4 provides suggestions for appropriate delegation, taking into consideration the task, the caregiver, and the patient.

Appropriate Communication

Communication may be oral or written, depending on the circumstances. However, you should leave no room for misinterpretation when giving instructions. For successful delegation, refer to the following guidelines:

1. Set clear boundaries about what to do and what not to do.
2. Be specific in your request (eg, "Tell me if he seems pale" or "Come get me if he has trouble breathing.")
3. Indicate priorities. Explain what must be done immediately and what can be done later.

BOX 8-4

What Can I Delegate?

ACTIVITIES: *You can usually delegate activities which:*

- are within your scope of practice and the nurse extender's job description and training.
- reoccur frequently in the daily care of a group of patients.
- require minimal problem solving.
- have predictable results.
- have low potential for harm to the patient.
- are performed according to a standard procedure and require little innovation.
- do not require the RNE to use nursing judgment.
- do not require repeated nursing assessments.

PATIENTS: *You can usually delegate care for patients who:*

- do not need extensive assistance for self-care activities.
- are relatively stable (ie, who have a chronic/predictable condition rather than one that has a strong potential for change).

PERSONNEL: *You can usually delegate activities to a caregiver who:*

- has demonstrated skill in the activity.
- has performed the activity often.
- has worked with patients with similar diagnoses.
- is motivated to perform the activities.
- has a workload that allows time to do the task properly.

4. Verify comprehension. Be sure the RNE understands what you want done.
5. Identify and address any of the RNE's concerns.
6. Check your attitude. Be courteous and show respect for each person and the job she does.

Adequate Supervision

The RN is responsible for seeing that delegated tasks are performed adequately. This may mean that you spot-check the RNE's work (eg, retake a blood pressure, check to be sure a patient has been bathed well). How often you need to monitor the RNE's performance will depend on the complexity of the task and how well you know the RNE. You or another RN should be available to observe, facilitate, coach, answer questions, and help as needed.

Be sure to speak with the patients after care is given, and evaluate both the physical response and the relationship between the patient and the RNE.

Give frequent, positive feedback for good performance. When necessary, communicate privately the specific mistakes that were made and listen to the RNE's view of the situation. Perhaps there were too many tasks to complete in the allotted time; or there were unforeseen situations that took priority; or the task took longer than expected. Many RNEs receive minimal training, so be prepared to role model and demonstrate caregiving activities as needed.

■ THINKING CRITICALLY ABOUT IMPLEMENTATION

In the implementation phase, nurses must use knowledge, experience, and critical thinking as they simultaneously "think and do." As you are giving patient care, you should constantly reassess the patient's responses to care. If the patient does not respond as you expected, try to find out why, and then modify what you are doing "on the spot." Box 8–5 provides guidelines to use as you prepare to implement safe, effective, and efficient care. After caring for the patient, use the questions in Box 8–6 to reflect on what you have done.

■ RECORDING

After doing or delegating, the nurse completes the implementation step by recording the nursing interventions and client responses. These nursing progress notes are a part of the agency's permanent record for the client. The **client record (or chart)** is a permanent, comprehensive account of information about the client's healthcare. It consists of various forms on which information is recorded about all aspects of the client's care (eg, physician's orders, results of laboratory and diagnostic tests, and progress notes written by physicians, nurses, and other caregivers). *Nursing* documentation in the permanent record is found on the following forms:

1. The initial, comprehensive nursing assessment (admission database)
2. The individualized nursing care plan
3. Nursing progress notes
4. Flowsheets (eg, graphic sheets, medication records)
5. The client discharge summary

Functions of Client Records

Client records are kept for a number of purposes. The record provides for *communication* among health professionals who interact with a client, helping to prevent fragmentation, repetition, and delays in client care. Health team members also refer to the client record when *planning care*. For example, a

BOX 8–5

Guidelines for Successful Implementation

Prepare the Nurse

1. Determine whether you need help to perform the action safely and minimize stress to the client.
2. Be sure you know the rationale for the action, as well as any potential side effects or complications. When actions are based on practice wisdom, examine them critically.
3. Question any actions you do not understand or that seem inappropriate or potentially unsafe.
4. Determine feedback points and assess the client's response during the activity.
5. Schedule activities to allow adequate time for completion.
6. Delegate tasks to other team members in order to use your time efficiently.
7. Improve your knowledge base by continually seeking new knowledge.

Prepare the Client

8. Reassess for changes in patient status.
9. Determine that the action is still needed and appropriate.
10. Assess client readiness.
11. Inform the client of what to expect and what is expected of him.
12. Provide for privacy and comfort.

Prepare Supplies and Equipment

13. Gather and organize all necessary supplies.

During Implementation:

14. Observe the patient's initial response to the intervention.
15. Continue to observe responses as you implement.
16. Adapt activities to the client's age, values, culture, and health status. Remain flexible and make creative modifications as you work.
17. Encourage the client to participate actively.
18. Perform actions according to professional standards of care and agency policies and procedures.
19. Perform actions carefully and accurately.
20. Supervise and evaluate delegated activities.

BOX 8–6

Critical Reflection: Implementation

The critical thinking standards are in parentheses. Review Table 2–3, on page 65, and Chapter 2, as needed.

1. (*Clarity*) Did I explain clearly to the patient what to expect? Did he understand?
2. (*Clarity; Accuracy*) Did I communicate what I intended? Could my facial expressions or body language have communicated something different than what I intended?
3. (*Accuracy*) Did I perform the activities/skills accurately (eg, Did I maintain sterile technique when inserting the catheter)?
4. (*Precision*) Did I follow recommended procedures carefully and exactly (eg, Did I perform a full 3-minute scrub instead of hurriedly washing my hands)?
5. (*Relevance/Significance*) Did I prioritize my care in order to carry out the most important interventions, or did I waste time on trivial activities?
6. (*Depth*) Did I forget to do anything?
7. (*Breadth*) Have I assessed responses from the patient's point of view as well as my own? Did I ask for feedback from the patient?
8. (*Breadth*) Did I convey respect for the patient and the family's cultural and spiritual values, beliefs, and practices?
9. (*Logic*) If the patient's responses to the intervention were not as expected, did I recognize that and make adjustments?

---

nurse may use the social worker's data about the client's home environment when developing the discharge teaching plan.

Client records provide information used by healthcare agencies to *evaluate and improve client care* within an institution (see Chapter 9). In addition to internal monitoring, accrediting bodies, such as the Joint Commission on Accreditation of Healthcare Organizations (JCAHO), review clinical records to ensure that the institution is meeting their standards. Documentation is also needed in order for a facility to receive *reimbursement* from Medicare, Medicaid, and insurance companies.

The client's record is a *legal document* and is usually admissible in court as evidence. The chart may be the only evidence that competent care was given. A record is usually considered the property of the agency, but as a rule, clients have a right to the information in the record on request.

Finally, client records provide data for *research*, information for *educating students* in health disciplines, and *statistics* for local, national, and international data banks.

Documenting Nursing Process

The client record should describe the client's ongoing status and reflect the full range of the nursing process. Regardless of the records system used, nurses document evidence of the nursing process on a variety of forms throughout the clinical record (see Table 8–2). This section describes flowsheets, progress notes, and discharge/transfer notes, which reflect various aspects of the nursing process.

Flowsheets

Nurses use **flowsheets** to record assessments and interventions that they perform routinely (eg, daily hygiene care) or frequently (eg, hourly position changes). For numerical data (eg, vital signs), **graphic flowsheets** may be used, for example, the top of Figure 8–2. At the bottom of Figure 8–2, a computer-generated flowsheet, is a section for nurses to record routine interventions. Flowsheets provide a quick, accurate method of recording and make it easy to keep data current and track changes in a client's condition. Intervals for recording data may vary from minutes to months. In a hospital intensive care unit, the nurse may monitor a client's blood pressure by the minute; in

Table 8–2   Documenting Nursing Process

Nursing Process Components	Documentation Forms	Comments
Assessment	Initial comprehensive database (nursing history and physical assessment), graphic sheets, flowsheets, nursing progress notes, discharge and referral summaries	Document initial and ongoing assessments. Frequency is determined by organization policy and client condition.
Diagnosis and Planning	Individualized and standardized care plans and critical pathways, protocols, Kardex, teaching plans, discharge plans, problem lists, SOAP (see Table 8–3 on p. 362) and other progress notes containing nursing diagnoses and intervention plans	Document client problems, nursing diagnoses, and strengths. Plans include desired outcomes and interventions. Care plans may be separate or a part of the chart.
Implementation and Evaluation	Nursing interventions and patient responses recorded in progress notes, flowsheets, graphics, and critical pathways	■ Document observations, interventions performed, and teaching. ■ Document client and family responses to nursing and medical interventions and important events; progress toward goals; and questions, comments, or complaints. ■ Document communication with other disciplines (eg, physician) and results of the communication.

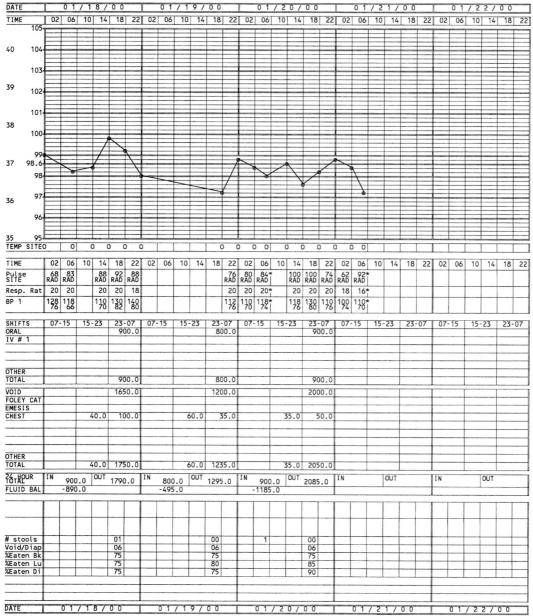

DATE		01/18/00					01/19/00						01/20/00						01/21/00						01/22/00					
TIME		02	06	10	14	18	22	02	06	10	14	18	22	02	06	10	14	18	22	02	06	10	14	18	22	02	06	10	14	18	22

	40 104					
	39 102					
	38 100					
	37 98.6					
	36 97					
	35 95					

| TEMP SITE | | O | 0 | 0 | 0 | 0 | | | | | | | O | 0 | 0 | 0 | | O | 0 | 0 | 0 | 0 | 0 | 0 | | | | | | |

TIME		02	06	10	14	18	22	02	06	10	14	18	22	02	06	10	14	18	22	02	06	10	14	18	22	02	06	10	14	18	22
Pulse SITE		68 RAD	83 RAD		88 RAD	92 RAD	88 RAD						76 RAD	80 RAD	84* RAD		100 RAD	100 RAD	74 RAD	62 RAD	92* RAD									
Resp. Rat		20	20		20	20	18						20	20	20*		20	20	20	18	16*									
BP 1		128 76	118 66		110 70	130 82	140 80						112 76	110 70	118* 74		118 76	130 80	110 76	100 74	110* 70									

SHIFTS	07-15	15-23	23-07	07-15	15-23	23-07	07-15	15-23	23-07	07-15	15-23	23-07	07-15	15-23	23-07
ORAL			900.0			800.0			900.0						
IV # 1															
OTHER TOTAL			900.0			800.0			900.0						
VOID			1650.0			1200.0			2000.0						
FOLEY CAT															
EMESIS															
CHEST		40.0	100.0		60.0	35.0		35.0	50.0						
OTHER TOTAL		40.0	1750.0		60.0	1235.0		35.0	2050.0						
24 HOUR TOTAL	IN 900.0	OUT 1790.0		IN 800.0	OUT 1295.0		IN 900.0	OUT 2085.0		IN	OUT		IN	OUT	
FLUID BAL	-890.0			-495.0			-1185.0								

# stools			01			00	1		00						
Void/Diap			06			06			06						
%Eaten Bk			75			75			75						
%Eaten Lu			75			80			85						
%Eaten Di			75			75			90						

| DATE | | 01/18/00 | | 01/19/00 | | 01/20/00 | | 01/21/00 | | 01/22/00 | |

* ADDITIONAL INFORMATION AVAILABLE ONLINE IN OPIS

Shawnee Mission Medical Center
9100 West 74th Street
Shawnee Mission, KS 66204

11:05 01/21/00 FROM *07L,VSPOGSF1

Figure 8–2
Graphic Flow Sheet. *Source*: Courtesy of St. Luke's Shawnee Mission Medical Center, 9100 W. 74th St, Shawnee Mission, KS 66204.

an ambulatory clinic, nurses may check a client's blood glucose levels only once a month.

Progress Notes

Progress notes (also called *nurses' notes*) provide information about the client's progress toward outcome achievement. They should augment but not duplicate flowsheet data. Progress notes should include (1) assessments of the patient's mental and physical condition, (2) patient activities, (3) both nurse-initiated and physician-initiated treatments and interventions, with patient responses, and (4) visits by other caregivers or family members, if relevant. Various kinds of progress notes are discussed in "Documentation Methods" below. For examples, refer to Figure 8–3, on page 361, and Figure 8–4, on page 363. Some progress notes (eg, Table 8–3 on page 362) also include nursing diagnoses or patient needs.

Discharge and Referral Summaries

A **discharge summary** is a special nursing progress note written at the time a client is discharged from the agency. It should include services provided to the client, status of client outcomes at discharge, and recommendations for further care. Many institutions have a special discharge summary form, which is sometimes combined with the discharge planning form (see Figure 6–2 on page 255). If the client is being transferred to another institution or requires a visit by a home health nurse, the discharge note takes the form of a referral summary. Regardless of format, discharge and referral summaries usually include some or all of the following information:

- Description of client's condition at discharge (including current status of each client problem)
- Current medications and treatments that are to be continued
- Teaching and counseling that was done to prepare the client for discharge
- Instructions for follow-up care given to the client at discharge
- Activity level and self-care abilities
- Support system, significant others
- Mode of discharge (eg, walking, wheelchair, ambulance)
- Person who accompanied the client
- Where client is going (eg, home, nursing home)
- Any active health problems

Documentation Methods

Institutional policies and procedures determine the format for documenting progress notes. This section discusses seven documentation methods: narrative, "SOAP," Focus® Charting, "PIE," "PART," charting by exception, and integrated plans of care (IPOCs).

Narrative, Chronological Charting

Narrative notes (eg, Figure 8–3), written in paragraph form, are the traditional charting format. Nurses write interventions, client responses, and events in chronological order. To make it easier to find data about a specific problem, specific flowsheets (eg, 24-hour intake and output record) are often used along with the progress notes. Narrative notes may be combined with flowsheets, as in Figure 8–5 on page 365.

SOAP Charting

The SOAP method (see Table 8–3) began with the problem-oriented records system, in which caregivers from all disciplines write on the same progress notes. However, it is now used in other systems as well. The chart contains a master problem list identified by the whole healthcare team. Each SOAP note refers to a specific problem; multiple problems require multiple notes. SOAP is an acronym for the following (notice that the definitions for "O" and "A" are different from the traditional nursing process definitions):

S – **Subjective data**. This is what the patient tells you. It describes the patient's perspectives, perceptions, and experience of the problem. When possible, quote the patient's words; otherwise, summarize his statement. Include subjective data only when they are important and relevant to the problem.

O – **Objective data**. This is information that can be measured or observed by use of the senses (eg, vital signs, bowel sounds, x-ray results). You will also use this section to record care that has been given (eg, "Taught procedure for drawing up insulin").

A – **Assessment**. In this method, "assessment" is an interpretation or explanation of the "S" and "O" data. During the initial assessment, the "A" entry contains statements of the patient's problems (eg, a nursing diagnosis). In subsequent SOAP notes, the "A" represents evaluation. It describes the patient's condition and level of progress toward goals, and is not merely a restatement of the diagnosis.

P – **Plan**. This is the plan of care designed to resolve the stated problem. The person who enters the problem on the record writes the initial plan (eg, for a medical problem, the physician writes orders for tests and treatments). The plan is continued, updated, or discontinued in subsequent SOAP notes.

SOAPIE and SOAPIER are variations of the SOAP format, in which the interventions (*I*) are written separately from the objective data (*O*), and an evaluation section (*E*) is added. The SOAPIER format adds a section for revisions of the plan (*R*). APIE is a similar format (Groah and Reed 1983, p. 1184). In this format, the assessment (*A*) includes both subjective and objective data and the nursing diagnosis; the plan (*P*) includes predicted outcomes with the nursing orders; and implementation (*I*) and evaluation (*E*)

DATE	TIME	NOTES	SIGNATURE
9-6-01	0800	Refused breakfast. States, "I feel too sick." abd. firm but not distended. No bowel sounds heard ⫽ auscultating for 5 min. in ® quadrant. Using PCA (morphine) frequently for incision pain (see med. Record).	S. Fried, RN
	0900	200 cc. clear, yellow emesis ————	S. Fried, RN
	0930	100 cc. clear, yellow emesis. c/o severe nausea. Compazine 5 mg. given I M in LVG area. Closed door + advised to lie still ⱷ decrease sensation of nausea.	S. Fried, RN
	1030	States still nauseated, but less severe. No further emesis. T.E.D. hose removed for 15 min + reapplied. No edema or redness on legs. Dangled ® bedside for 5 min. Moves c̄ much reluctance. States, "Hurts too much." ————	S. Fried, RN

Shawnee Mission Medical Center
PATIENT PROGRESS RECORD

Figure 8–3
Patient Progress Record. *Source*: Courtesy of St. Lukes-Shawnee Mission Medical Center, Merriam, KS.

Table 8–3   Comparison of the SOAP, SOAPIER, and APIE Formats

SOAP Format	SOAPIER Format	APIE Format
9/6/01 #5. Nausea 1030	9/6/01 #5. Nausea 1030	9/6/01 #5. Nausea 1030
S–Refused breakfast."I feel too sick." c/o severe nausea during AM. Stated less severe after IM Compazine. **O**–Abd. firm but not distended. No bowel sounds heard after auscultating for 5 min. @ quadrant. Vomited × 2: total 300 mL clear, yellow emesis. Closed door; advised to lie still to decrease sensations of nausea. Compazine 5 mg given IM in LVG area at 0930. **A**–Post-op nausea r/t decreased peristalsis; Compazine somewhat effective. Possible ileus. **P**–Continue to observe for N&V. If nausea unrelieved by Compazine, notify MD. Continue I&O. Assess hydration q shift. Offer fluids 40 mL/hr if no further emesis.	**S**–Refused breakfast."I feel too sick." c/o severe nausea during AM. **O**–Abd. firm but not distended. No bowel sounds heard after auscultating for 5 min. @ quadrant. Vomited × 2: total 300 mL clear, yellow emesis. **A**–Post-op nausea r/t decreased peristalsis; Compazine somewhat effective. **P**–Instruct to lie still to decrease sensations of nausea. Medicate with Compazine. Continue I&O. Continue to assess for N&V. Assess hydration q shift. **I**–Instructed to lie still to decrease sensations of nausea. Compazine 5 mg given IM in LVG area at 0930. **E**–States still nauseated but somewhat relieved after Compazine. Lying still most of AM. No emesis after Compazine. **R**–Offer fluids 40 mL/hr if no further emesis. If nausea unrelieved by Compazine, notify MD.	**A**–Post-op nausea & vomiting. Refused breakfast."I feel too sick." Abd. firm, not distended. No bowel sounds heard after auscultating 5 min. @ quadrant. Vomited × 2; total 300 mL clear, yellow emesis. **P**–Decrease nausea: Instruct to lie still. Compazine per order. Prevent fluid deficit: Continue to assess N&V. Assess hydration q shift. Continue I&O. If nausea and vomiting continue, notify MD. **I**–Instructed to lie still. Compazine 5 mg given IM in LVG area at 0930. **E**–Lying still most of AM. No emesis since Compazine given. States still nauseated, but less severe.

are the same as in the SOAPIE format. See Table 8–3 for a comparison of the SOAP, SOAPIER, and APIE formats. Compare these entries to Figure 8–3 on page 361 and Figure 8–4, on page 363, which contain information about the same incident of nausea.

PIE and PART Charting

PIE charting is similar to SOAP charting. PIE is an acronym for <u>P</u>roblems, <u>I</u>nterventions, and <u>E</u>valuation of patient responses to care. This system supplements the patient progress notes with a flowsheet for assessments and routine care. The nurse keeps a master problem list and rewrites and renumbers it every 24 hours. As in SOAP charting, there may not be a separate care plan.

PART is similar to PIE. However, the problem list is seen as continuous and ongoing, so it is not redone every 24 hours. This method makes use of standards of care, so an individualized plan is not required. However, the nurse records all actual interventions in the chart (Gropper and Dicapo 1995). PART is an acronym for the following:

P – Problem. This is usually a nursing diagnosis.

A – Actions. This section consists of all interventions actually implemented. It *does not* contain the plan of care.

R – Response. This section reflects actual patient outcomes. It consists of subjective and objective data describing the patient's responses to the actions/interventions.

T – Teaching. The nurse records all patient and family teaching in this separate section of the progress notes. This is meant to remind the care providers of the importance of this aspect of care.

Focus® Charting

Like SOAP notes, Focus ® Charting (Lampe 1985) uses key words to label and organize the progress notes, but the subject of the note is not necessarily a problem (see Figure 8–4). A focus can be a condition, strength, nursing diagnosis, behavior, sign or symptom, significant change in the patient's condition, or significant event. Because the focus should be something requiring

Date/Time	Focus	Progress Notes
9/6/01 1430	Post-op nausea	**D**—Refused breakfast. Stated, "I feel too sick." c/o severe nausea throughout A.M. Vomited × 2, total of 300 mL clear, yellow emesis. Abd. firm but not distended. No bowel sounds auscultated after listening for 5 min. @ quadrant.
		A—Closed door. Advised to lie still to decrease sensations of nausea. Compazine 5 mg given IM in LVG at 0930 per order. Continue to assess for N&V. If unrelieved by Compazine, notify MD. Continue I&O. Assess hydration × 1 per shift. Increase p.o. fluids to 40 mL/hr if no further emesis.
		R—Nausea somewhat relieved by Compazine. Stated "less severe." No emesis since Compazine administered. See flow sheet for I&O and VS.————————R. Keeler, RN

Figure 8–4
Example of a Focus® Charting Note

nursing care, it should *not* be a medical diagnosis. It can, however, describe needs and conditions associated with a medical diagnosis. For example, foci for a patient with a fractured femur might include preoperative teaching, Pain, Risk for Constipation, and cast/traction assessment. The progress notes column is organized as follows:

D – Data include observations of patient status and behaviors. This might include data from flowsheets (eg, vital signs). It includes both subjective and objective data, but they are not labeled "S" and "O." This section corresponds to the assessment phase of the nursing process.

A – Action entries include interventions just performed as well as plans for further action—corresponding to the planning and implementation steps of the nursing process.

R – Response entries describe patient responses to nursing and medical interventions. Data in this section consist of measurements and interventions, many of which will be recorded on flowsheets and checklists. This section corresponds to the evaluation phase of the nursing process.

The focus method is useful for health promotion activities because the nurse can organize around positive headings instead of problems.

Charting by Exception

Charting by exception (CBE) is a system in which only significant findings or exceptions to stated norms are recorded. An agency using CBE must develop its own specific, detailed standards that identify (1) the norms for patient assessments and (2) the minimum criteria for patient care (Murphy and Burke 1990). The following are examples of standards of care that an agency might develop for hygiene:

The patient will receive or be offered oral care t.i.d.

The patient will receive or be offered a bath and backrub daily, and a shampoo once a week

Figure 8–5 provides an example of a portion of a form used for CBE. The nurse writes a progress note only when patient data or care deviates from the norms printed in the first column. Completed interventions are recorded in the progress notes or flowsheets. Since the initial development of CBE, commercial vendors and healthcare agencies have developed many variations of this system. It has been shown to significantly reduce documentation time as well as costs associated with paper use. It is a legally sound approach if properly implemented and adhered to (Cummins and Hill 1999).

IPOCs—Charting Integrated Into Plan of Care

As a part of managed care, many agencies have developed critical pathways for common diagnoses and procedures (review "Managed Care," on pp. 344–345;

THE WESTERN PENNSYLVANIA HOSPITAL

PATIENT CARE FLOW SHEET

BASELINE PHYSICAL ASSESSMENT: Date 6/19/01 ___ Time 0800 ___ RN/GN *J.Reed RN*

	NORMALS:	DEVIATIONS:	TIME	PROBLEM/VARIANCE	PROGRESS NOTES
BEHAVIOR/ EMOTIONAL	Behavior and emotions appropriate to situation WNL ☒	☐ Agitated ☐ Depressed ☐ Angry ☐ Anxious ☐ Other ___	08	Neuro	O₂ sat. 70%.
NEUROLOGICAL	Alert & oriented to person, place, time and situation. Speech clear. Follows simple commands. PERL. Sensation intact. WNL ☐	Disoriented to: ☒ Person ☐ Place ☐ Time ☐ Situation ☐ Does not follow commands LOC: ☒ Lethargic ☐ Nonresponsive ☐ Responsive to ___ ☐ Speech deficit ☐ Pupils ☐ R ☐ L ☐ Deficits ___ ☐ Other ___			O₂ admin. per nasal cannula @
					3L/min *J.Reed RN*
			0815	Neuro	O₂ sat. 94% *J.Reed RN*
			0830	Neuro	WNL. *J.Reed RN*
CARDIO-VASCULAR	Apical regular and HR WNL. Heart tones audible. Peripheral pulses +3. No edema. Capillary refill time <3 secs. WNL ☒	☐ Heart rhythm abnormal ___ ☐ Rate abnormal ___ ☐ Abnormal pulses ___ ☐ Calf tenderness ☐ R ☐ L ☐ Edema (loc/severity) ___ ☐ Other ___			

Figure 8–5

Example of a Portion of a Form Used for Charting by Exception. *Source:* Hill, Labik, and Vanderbilt (1997). Managing skin care with the CareMap system. *Journal of Wound, Ostomy, and Continence Nursing,* 24(1):29. Used with permission.

"Using Nursing Diagnoses with Critical Pathways," on pp. 161–162; and "Multidisciplinary Care Plans," on pp. 260–261, as needed). Most critical pathways are "integrated plans of care" (IPOCs) that serve both as a care plan and a form for documenting progress notes (eg, Figure 8–6). This charting model uses graphics and flowsheets along with the IPOC. Progress notes typically use some type of charting by exception. For example, nurses using Figure 8–6 circle "met" or "not met" for each of the stated goals. If a goal is met, no further charting is required. Goals that are not met are called **variances**. They are deviations to what is planned on the critical pathway—unexpected occurrences that affect the planned nursing activities or the patient's responses to them. When a goal is not met, the nurse writes a note describing the unexpected event, the cause, and actions taken to correct the situation or justify the actions taken (see the "Pain Mgmt." and "Discharge Plan/Education" sections of Figure 8–6). Some agencies provide separate forms on which to record variances.

Computerized Documentation

Use of computerized nursing care plans is widespread. In addition, the use of computers for charting is one of the strongest trends in nursing documentation throughout Canada and the United States (Iyer and Camp 1995, p. 237). Some agencies have a terminal at each bedside, enabling the nurse to document care immediately after it is given.

Computers make documentation relatively easy. To record nursing actions and client responses, the nurse either chooses from standardized lists of terms or types of narrative information into the computer (refer to Figure 8–7 for an example of a computerized progress note). Automated speech recognition technology now allows some nurses to do voice-activated documentation.

Because information can be easily retrieved in a variety of forms, multiple flowsheets are not needed in computerized systems. For example, a nurse could obtain the results of a client's blood test, a schedule of all clients on the unit who are to have surgery during the day, a suggested list of interventions for a nursing diagnosis, a graphic chart of a client's vital signs, or a printout of all the progress notes for a client. Selected pros and cons of computer documentation are shown in Box 8–7.

Documenting With Standardized Language

Chapters 5–7 discussed the use of standardized terminology for nursing care plans. Those concepts apply to documenting patient progress as well. For computerized documentation systems, standardized terminology is essential. It is also useful in pen-and-paper systems. Among benefits described in previous chapters, standardized language allows the nurse to concentrate on the clinical judgment aspects of the nursing process, rather than spending time searching for the "right words" to describe interventions and patient responses.

	OUTCOME INTERVENTION	T	I		EXCEPTIONS/*	OUTCOME STATUS: I S
Pain Management	Patient will verbalize/indicate comfort or tolerance of pain. *Location & pain rating (0-10 pain scale) q 4 hrs w/a. PCA/CEA/IM analgesics. Comfort measures _Back rub_ .		1700 _LJ_	1600 1800	c/o pain of "10" in R knee c̄ CEA at 6 cc/hr. ↑ to 8 cc/hr. c̄ no relief. Notified Dr. Green. Percocet tabs ÷ given p.o. (see MAR). Still c/o pain at "8" on scale.	1800 _LJ_ M (N) 0600 ____ M/N
Endocrine	Patient will have no s/s of hypo/ hyperglycemia.					1800 _LJ_ (M) N 0600 ____ M/N
Psychological/ Emotional	Patient/s.o. will indicate ability to cope c̄ prescribed treatments. Use encouragement, praise & listening skills. Encourage verbalization of concerns by patient/s.o.	0800 ____ ____	_LJ_ ____	1800	Pt. has not felt like talking today — Slept in a.m. and was too uncomfortable (see "Pain Mgmt.")	1800 ____ (M) N 0600 ____ M/N
Discharge Plan/ Education	Patient(s.o.) will verbalize & demonstrate understanding of total knee precautions. Discuss pain management plan c̄ patient (s.o.) Encourage BSC for BM's. Patient/s.o. will demonstrate understanding and mutually agree with plan of care. Patient/s.o. will demonstrate understanding and mutually agree with daily procedures. *Special procedures _none_ Indicate readiness to learn: Responsive _s.o._ If unready *document e.g., denies need, uninterested, confused, physical barrier, etc. Circle response to education: _s.o. only_ (Verbalizes understanding, interacts freely, attentive, asks appropriate questions, returns demonstration, *needs reinforcement.)	1400 ____ 1400	_LJ_ _LJ_	1400	Wife receptive. Pt. in too much pain today. Goals met with regard to s.o., but not pt.	1800 _LJ_ (M) N 0600 _LJ_ M/N 1800 _LJ_ (M) N 0600 _LJ_ M/N 1800 _LJ_ M (N) 0600 _LJ_ M/N
Other	*Dr. notification:			1600	Dr. Green. See "Pain Mgmt." _LJ_	

Signature	Initials	Signature	Initials	Signature	Initials
Laura Jimenez	LJ				

Date @ 0700: _2/1/01_   To Date @ 0700: _2/2/01_

Total Knee Replacement - Chart/Documentation
Integrated Plan of Care - Post-op Day 2

Figure 8–6
Portion of a Critical Pathway/Documentation Form. *Source:* Courtesy of Shawnee Mission Medical Center, 9100 W. 74th St., Shawnee Mission, KS 66204-4019

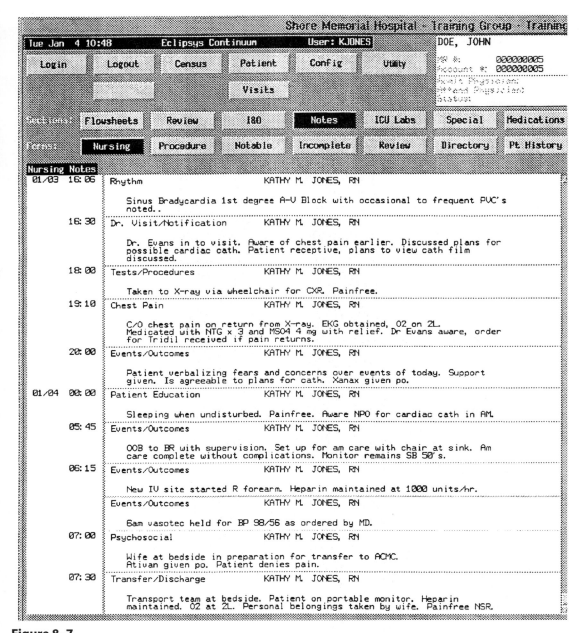

Figure 8–7

Computer Screen Showing Nurse's Notes. *Source:* Courtesy of Shore Memorial Hospital, Somers Point, NJ. Used with permission.

BOX 8–7

Some Pros and Cons of Computer Documentation

Pros

Improves productivity; reduces documentation time.

Improves accuracy and reliability of documentation.

Increases nurse satisfaction and professional practice.

Information can be retrieved easily in a variety of forms; multiple forms not needed.

Client information, requests, and results are sent and received quickly.

Terminals can record data directly from monitoring equipment.

Bedside terminals eliminate need to take notes on a worksheet before recording.

Information is current.

Information is legible.

Standardized terminology improves communication.

The system incorporates and reinforces standards of care.

Allows for creation and sharing of huge data files to be used for research and quality improvement.

Cons

Additional security measures needed to assure patients' privacy.

Breakdowns make information temporarily unavailable.

Initial purchase of hardware and software is very expensive.

Extended training periods may be required.

Sources: Catanzano 1994; Kozier et al 2000; Town 1993

Guidelines for Charting

Requirements for record keeping vary among agencies. Agency policies may describe which personnel are responsible for recording on certain forms, the frequency with which entries are to be made, which abbreviations are acceptable, and the preferred way to handle an error in recording. In addition to legal and policy requirements, you should also observe the following general guidelines (when, what, and how).

When to Chart

1. *Date and time each entry*. Timing guidelines are critical for legal and safety reasons.
2. For each entry, *indicate both the time the entry was made and the time the observation or intervention occurred*, if different. For example, in a chart entry timed 1445, you might write, "Drank 150 mL water at 1245, vomited 200 mL clear fluid at 1310."
3. *Record the nursing action or client response as soon as possible after it occurs*. This helps ensure that the client will not be medicated or treated a second time by a different nurse. It is usually acceptable to record routine repetitive nursing actions at the end of the shift (eg, hourly position changes, mouth care), but keep notes on a worksheet. Don't rely on memory.
4. *Never leave the unit for an extended break unless all important information has been charted*. Rationale is similar to that for Guideline 3.
5. *Do not document interventions before carrying them out*. The client might refuse the treatment or you might encounter an emergency situation that prevents you from carrying out the intervention. Another staff member, seeing it charted, might conclude the action has been done and not wish to repeat it. The result would be that the client does not get the care he needs.
6. *Document in chronological order*. If you forget to chart something, record it as soon as possible, marking it "Late Entry." If there is a lengthy delay in charting, explain why (eg, "9/24, 1215–Late entry-Chart not available 9/24 at 1030. Patient c/o shortness of breath. Notified physician").

What to Chart

1. *As a rule, do not chart actions performed by someone else*. In some situations, it is permissible to do so but your note should identify the person who actually gave the care (eg, Assisted to car by nursing assistant. L. Woods, RN").
2. *Progress notes must be accurate and correct*. If you are not absolutely sure of an assessment, ask someone else to check before you chart.
3. *Go beyond flowsheet data—chart judgments about the data* to indicate whether the patient is doing better or worse. Compare current patient status with previous data (eg, "Incision becoming redder and beginning to ooze serous fluid").
4. *Progress notes should be factual*. Chart what you see, hear, smell, or observe. To improve the precision of your charting, think, "Exactly what happened, and how, when, and where did it happen?" For example, you would chart, "Talking constantly, pacing the floor; pulse 120," rather than "Patient is anxious."

KEY POINT
Report the facts. DO NOT chart:

- Words suggesting errors (eg, "accidentally," "unintentionally," by mistake").
- That an incident report has been filed.
- Staff conflicts, critical comments about the behaviors or care given by other team members.
- Staffing problems or staff shortages (use a confidential memo or incident report instead).

5. *Progress notes should be clear and specific.* Do not use vague generalities, such as *good, normal,* or *sufficient.* It is better to say "a 2 × 2 cm area of blood" than "a small amount of blood."

6. *Do not use negative, prejudicial terms* (eg, *uncooperative, noncompliant, unpleasant*). Instead, describe what the client did that was uncooperative (eg, "Yelled, 'Go away!' and threw his tray on the floor").

7. *To organize a narrative entry, include D—I—E.* Don't actually label the entry with these letters or words; use them as a memory device.

Data	What did you observe about the patient (*S-O*)?
Intervention	What actions did you take? What did you do?
Evaluation	What was the patient's response to the actions? What did he say or do? How did his condition change?

8. *Chart entries should be appropriate and relevant.* You do not need to record everything you know about the client. Recording irrelevant data is a waste of time, and it is sometimes an invasion of privacy (eg, do not chart "slept well" unless this is unusual).

9. *Progress notes should be complete.* This is essential for communication among caregivers, as well as for legal purposes. For example, if there is no record of turning and skin care, nurses may be found negligent if the client develops a dermal ulcer.

10. *Be brief.* Omit unnecessary words, such as *patient.* It is assumed the entry refers to the patient. Progress notes are usually written in incomplete sentences, but be sure to end each thought with a period. For example, write "300 mL clear emesis," rather than "The patient vomited 300 mL of clear fluid."

11. *Balance concisenessness with completeness.* When deciding on the right amount of detail to record:

   ■ Ask "What would someone else need to know to understand what is going on with the patient?"
   ■ Include enough detail to justify any conclusions or judgments you have made (see Item 3).
   ■ Remember that busy caregivers will not read a long, wordy note carefully. They will skim over it to save time. (Rubenfeld and Scheffer 1999, p. 245)

Refer to Box 8–8 for essential information to include in nursing progress notes.

How to Chart

1. *Use dark ink.* Most agencies specify black ink. Erasable ink is not acceptable.
2. *Write legibly, or print.* Narcan and Marcaine are different drugs, but they may look very much alike if handwriting is illegible or messy.
3. *Use correct grammar, spelling, and punctuation.*

BOX 8-8

Essential Information to Chart

1. **A physical symptom** that:
   Is severe (eg, extreme shortness of breath)
   Recurs or persists (eg, vomiting after every meal)
   Is not normal (eg, elevated temperature)
   Becomes worse (eg, fever increases from 102° to 104° F)
   Is not relieved by prescribed actions (eg, patient unable to sleep after taking sleeping pill)
   Is a symptom of a complication (eg, inability to void after surgery)
   Is a known danger signal (eg, a lump in the breast)
2. **Changes in physical function**, such as loss of balance or difficulty seeing or swallowing.
3. **Behavior changes**, such as:
   Strong expressions of emotion (eg, crying, yelling, expressing fear)
   Marked changes in mood
   Change in level of consciousness or orientation
   Changes in relationships with family or friends
4. **Nursing interventions**, especially those performed in response to symptoms and changes in patient status. For example:
   Medications administered
   Treatments/therapies (both dependent and independent)
   Patient teaching
5. **Patient responses to nursing interventions; evaluation of outcomes/goal achievement.**
6. **Inability to carry out prescribed treatments, or patient's refusal of treatments/interventions.** Include your teaching about the need for treatment and the possible consequences of refusal.
7. **Patient's ability to manage care after discharge.**
8. **All medical visits and consultations.** Note time, date, what was discussed, directions given by the physician, and actions you took.
9. **Discussions with the physician about concerns with medical orders.** Note time; date; what directions the physician gave about confirming, canceling, or modifying the orders; and the actions you took.

4. *Use standard symbols, terminology, and abbreviations.* Many agencies have a list of abbreviations and terminology they accept. If not, use only those that are standard and used universally. If you are in doubt about an abbreviation, write the term out fully.
5. *Sign each entry with your name and title* (eg, "Kay Wittman, RN" or "K. Wittman, RN").

6. *The nurse who makes the entry should sign it.* You should not sign some-one else's notes. Remember that the person signing the entry is account-able for the entry.

7. *Chart entries on consecutive lines. Never skip a line or leave a line blank.* Draw a line through any blank spaces before or after your signature. For example, "Lungs clear to auscultation. Skin warm and dry.————————————K. Wittman, RN."

8. *Correct errors by drawing a single line through the mistaken entry* and writ-ing the word *error* above it. Initial the error, and then rewrite the entry correctly (or follow agency policy). Never try to erase or obliterate the entry; the incorrect entry should still be visible. Do not insert words above the line or between words.

9. *Be sure the client's name and identification number are on every page.*

Home Health Care Documentation

Home health care is different from institutional care in that fewer caregivers are present to provide and witness the care. The home care record is usually the only evidence of how patient care decisions were made, the only basis for insurance coverage, the only legal record, and the main source of communi-cation among health team members, who do not see each other as frequently as those in a hospital. Home health documentation is often in the form of a **progress summary**—a brief narrative report of a client's health status and needs, nursing interventions performed, and client outcomes and responses. In home health care, progress summaries are used in two ways:

1. They provide the information the physician needs to determine whether to continue medical treatments, to monitor client progress, and to be aware of any new health or treatment problems that develop.

2. They are sent to third-party payers to establish the continuing need for home health care. Medicare regulations, for example, require that progress summaries be written every 60 days to be sure the client meets Medicare requirements. Therefore, the nurse must be sure to address the following in the summary (Eggland and Heinemann 1994, pp. 171–172):

   - The client is homebound and still needs skilled nursing care.
   - The potential for rehabilitation is good; or the client is dying.
   - Client status is not stabilized.
   - The client is making progress in expected outcomes of care.

The nurse should be certain that the checklists, progress summaries, and other forms also reflect how and why the skills of a professional home care nurse are needed (Marelli and Hilliard 1996, p. 199)—that is:

- Why home care was initiated
- What the skilled interventions are and why they are needed

- The plan of care (patient outcomes or goals of care)
- Discharge plans (including rehabilitation potential)

A unique problem in home care documentation is that the nurse may need some parts of the client's record in the home while, at the same time, those records are needed in the office. For this reason, some home health agencies provide nurses with laptop computers. In this way, records are available in multiple locations, and nurses can upload new client information to agency records without even traveling to the office.

Long-Term Care Documentation

The principles of documentation in long-term care are the same as those explained in this chapter. However, federal and state regulations usually require nurses to document less frequently in long-term care than in acute-care settings. Some long-term care facilities require weekly client progress summaries; others require summaries only every 90 days. Charting should reflect the client's current status (eg, vital signs, skin condition, status of admitting diagnoses), daily functioning (eg, mobility, self-care abilities, sleep patterns), and progress toward expected outcomes, with focus on preventive measures and restorative care.

■ ORAL REPORTS

In addition to written records, nurses use oral reports to communicate nursing interventions and client status. When the client's condition is changing rapidly, physicians and other caregivers must be constantly informed. Oral reports are also given when a client is transferred from one unit to another (eg, from the emergency department to a medical floor), at change of shift, and when family members request reports of the client's condition. A report is given to communicate specific information about what has been observed, done, or considered. It should be concise, but still contain all pertinent information.

A **change-of-shift report** is given to the on-coming nurse by the nurse who has been responsible for the patient. Reports may be given in a meeting, on walking rounds, or on audiotape. Tape-recorded reports are less time-consuming, but do not allow for questions and clarification. A typical change-of-shift report includes the following:

1. *Basic identifying information for each client.* Name, room number, age, medical diagnosis or reason for admission, admission date, and physicians. This will vary depending on the setting (eg, in a long-term care facility, you might omit the admission date).
2. *A description of the client's present condition.* Include only significant measurements. It is not necessary to report that the vital signs are normal, unless this is a change for the client (eg, "After medication, her temperature returned to 98.6°").

3. *Significant changes in the client's condition.* Report both deterioration and improvement in condition (eg, "At 1400 her blood pressure was 150/94; baseline was under 130/80 until that time"). When reporting changes, organize your report as follows: State what you observed, its meaning (if appropriate), what action was taken, the client's response, and the continuing plan for the on-coming nurse.

EXAMPLE: "Her respirations are slow and shallow, and she has weak cough effort. I helped her turn and cough hourly. Her lungs are clear, but she still does not deep breathe well. You should continue to have her cough and deep breathe hourly unless you see improvement."

4. *Progress in goal achievement for identified nursing diagnoses* (eg, "Mrs. Martin has risk for impaired skin integrity. We are presently meeting our goal of intact skin").
5. *Results of diagnostic tests or other therapies performed in the last 24 hours* (eg, "Blood cultures were negative").
6. *Significant emotional responses* (eg, "She has been crying since she was told she won't be able to go home").
7. *Description of invasive lines, pumps, and other apparatus* (eg, Foley catheter).
8. *Description of important activities* that occurred on your shift. This should not be a detailed catalog of the patient's day. Report only significant activities (eg, there is no need to report that all clients showered and ambulated in the hall).
9. *Description of care the on-coming nurse needs to do.* This does not include routine care, such as the daily linen change or routine vital signs, unless it is something you were unable to accomplish (eg, "Her bed still needs to be changed"). Include laboratory and diagnostic tests and preps that the on-coming nurse should do or special observations that she should make (eg, "She is scheduled for surgery in the morning, and should be NPO after midnight").
10. *Patient-centered information*, not a report of the nurse's activities over the shift. Using a shift report sheet such as Figure 8–8 will help to keep your shift reports patient centered.

■ ETHICAL ISSUES IN IMPLEMENTATION

As client advocates, nurses are obligated to protect clients' humanity. During implementation of care opportunities exist for humanization or depersonalization of care. Issues of confidentiality and dignity arise frequently in implementation. In addition, Item 6 of the ANA Code for Nurses (1985) indicates that delegation of care has ethical implications (see Appendix A).

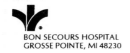

SHIFT:_____

DATE:_____

CHANGE OF SHIFT REPORT

Room No.	Name/Age		Hx / Dx	Problem #1	Problem #2	Problem #3	Special Procedures/ Diet/Abnormal Labs or Diagnostics	Meds	Teaching D/C Prep	Comments
328	Marks	81	CVA	Skin – Turn q 2 h.			CT-09	9,1,5,11 (HS) Pre-op		Speech eval.
329	Smith	60	Lap. Chole.	Pain: 3 pain	Resp: Lungs clear			9, 1, 5, 11 HS Pre-op	Enc. amb.	probable discharge
329	Warren	69	Heart Failure	Cardiac Output	Resp: O2@2L		24 hr. urine	9, 1, 5, 11 HS Pre-op	S.S. to see	
								9, 1, 5, 11		

Figure 8–8

Sample Change of Shift Report. *Source:* Courtesy of Bon Secours Hospital, Grosse Point, MI. Used with permission.

Respect for Dignity

Item 1 of the ANA Code of Ethics emphasizes *respect for human dignity*. Many of the procedures performed during implementation are invasive or require the client to be exposed or assume awkward positions. Nurses are obliged to show respect by providing adequate draping and privacy for such interventions as enemas, catheterizations, and bed baths. These may seem like routine procedures to a busy nurse, but they can be very depersonalizing for the patient. The more skilled you become in technical procedures, the more you will be able to adopt and respect the patient's perspective on what is occurring.

The manner in which you address the patient can also preserve or diminish his dignity. It is easy to fall into the habit of addressing everyone as *dear* or *honey*. Some nurses do this in an effort to express caring; others do it because it is hard to remember the patient's names. However, patients lose their individuality when they all have the same name—even if it is a "nice" name. This is a particularly disrespectful practice when the patient is older than the nurse. You should not call a patient by his first name unless you know that he prefers it, or you are on a reciprocal first-name basis with him.

Privacy and Confidentiality

Privacy and confidentiality are related to the issue of client dignity. Item 2 of the ANA Code treats these subjects: "The nurse safeguards the client's right to privacy by judiciously protecting information of a confidential nature." When you provide good nursing care, patients feel comfortable with you. They may trust you enough to disclose important and personal information (eg, "This baby does not belong to my husband, but he doesn't know"). Do not chart such information unless it is important to the care plan, and do not share it with other staff members. Nurses are free to share only information that is pertinent to the client's health.

The law restricts access to the client's written record. Even if it did not, nurses have a moral obligation to protect the confidentiality of the record. This means that insurance companies and other agencies have no right to the information in the record without the client's permission; nor does the client's family. Legally, the client must sign an authorization for review, copying, or release of information from the chart. When charts are used for educational or research purposes, the student or researcher is obligated to avoid using the client's name or identifying her in any way.

Widespread use of computer-based record systems increases the risk that the client's privacy will be accidentally or intentionally violated. Be aware of the potential for abuse of computer data systems. Angry employees may break through system security to destroy, change, or distribute data, or computer hackers may break into the system simply for the challenge. Refer to Box 8–9 for ways to assure the confidentiality of computer records.

■ LEGAL CONSIDERATIONS

For legal protection, you should adhere to professional standards of nursing care and follow agency policy and procedures for interventions, delegation, and documentation, especially in high-risk situations. An even more important measure for preventing lawsuits is to develop an attentive, caring rela-

---

BOX 8–9

Keeping Computer Records Confidential

1. Follow agency policies and procedures regarding computer documentation.
2. A personal password is needed to enter and sign off computer files. Do not share this password with anyone, including other health team members.
3. After logging on, never leave a computer terminal unattended.
4. Do not leave client information displayed on the monitor where others may see it.
5. Know and follow agency procedures for documenting sensitive material, such as a diagnosis of AIDS.

tionship with patients. Patients are less likely to sue if they feel you are respectful and attentive to their needs.

The *legal* purposes of documentation are to show that care was provided and that there was continuity of care. The preceding "Guidelines for Charting" will help you to chart in a legally prudent manner. In addition, the following discussion focuses on some of the more common legal pitfalls for nurses. In some situations, the healthcare agency may require you to fill our an incident report. If so, document the facts of the incident in the progress notes, but do not chart that an incident report has been completed (Springhouse 1996, p. 130).

Falls

Hospitals and long-term care agencies have a duty to take reasonable measures to ensure patient safety. Most have policies and routines for identifying patients who are likely to fall and taking the necessary precautions. Documentation should include data about level of consciousness, balance, and mobility; precautions taken to prevent falls (eg, helping with ambulation); and any comments by the family that they have accepted some responsibility for helping to prevent falls.

Restraints

Use restraints only according to your agency's policies and procedures (refer to a basic nursing text for information about restraints). Document the reasons the patient is restrained, the method of restraint used, the time and duration of application, frequency of observation, patient responses, safety outcomes, and assessment of the continued need for restraint.

Questioning Medical Orders

When a physician prescribes an order that you do not understand or that you believe to be incorrect, you must be diligent in getting your questions answered before implementing the order. Ask your nurse manager or supervisor for help, and call the attending physician if necessary. Be sure to document the fact that you questioned the order and were assured that it was correct, by whom, and under what circumstances (Tammelleo 1997).

Patient Behaviors That May Contribute to an Injury

Risk managers use the phrase, "**potentially contributing patient acts**" to refer to patient behaviors that may contribute to injury. Documenting such acts may help the nurse defend against a malpractice suit, as in the following situations:

Refusal or Inability to Provide Information　When the client refuses to or cannot give accurate, complete information (eg, about health status, history, or medications), you should try to obtain information from other sources. Document any difficulties in communicating with the client, and reflect his understanding of the importance of the information.

> EXAMPLE OF CHARTING: When asked how she received the bruises on her face and head, client replied, "I don't have to answer that. It's none of your business." Discussed with her the possibility that her dizziness and blurred vision may be caused by her injuries and that the source of injury may be an important piece of information. She turned her face to the wall and did not reply.————RJones, RN

Noncompliance With Medical and Nursing Interventions   (eg, failure to follow medical orders for medications, diet, or staying in bed). When this occurs, chart instructions given to the patient, what the patient did that specifically contradicts instructions, and actions taken to try to encourage compliance.

> EXAMPLE OF CHARTING:
>
> 0700 – Ate all of prescribed diabetic diet.————RJones, RN
> 0830 – Friends visited. Client found eating sweet rolls and chocolate milk. Reviewed with him the possible effects of not following diet. He stated, "I get tired of the stuff they bring me here." He continued eating. RJones, RN

Possession or Use of Unauthorized Personal Items   (eg, heating pad, hair dryer, alcoholic beverages, street drugs, tobacco). Progress notes should describe what was found, what was done with it, and any persons notified.

> EXAMPLE OF CHARTING:
>
> 0900 – Client found using hair dryer from home. Sent dryer to biomedical department to be checked before further use.——RJones, RN

Tampering With Medical Equipment   (eg, changing the IV flow rate, removing traction, adjusting monitoring equipment). Document any observations that might indicate that the patient or family is manipulating equipment. Describe what was done about the problem (eg, instructing the patient, notifying the physician).

> EXAMPLE OF CHARTING:
>
> 0900 – IV infusing at 100 mL/hr with 500 ml. in bag.————RJones, RN
> 0930 – IV found barely dripping, 475 mL in bag. Site not inflamed or infiltrated; tubing patent. Rate increased to 100 mL/hr. Pt. and wife deny touching IV tubing; however, their 2 small children have been in the room this AM. Roller clamp repositioned high on IV pole; cautioned wife to watch children closely around medical equipment.————RJones, RN

■ CULTURAL AND SPIRITUAL CONSIDERATIONS

By now, it should be clear that providing holistic, individualized care means including culture and spirituality in every phase of the nursing process. Certainly it is important to assess, diagnose, and plan for cultural and spiritual needs; but it is during implementation that you have the best opportunity to interact with patients and to demonstrate cultural and spiritual competence.

Cultural Care

To provide meaningful nursing care, you must reflect on and understand your own values, beliefs, and behaviors. This includes your own culture. Box 8–10 offers suggestions for providing culturally competent nursing care.

BOX 8–10

Providing Culturally Competent Care

- Convey respect for the individual and respect for the individual's values, beliefs, and cultural and ethnic practices.
- Learn about the major ethnic or cultural groups with whom you are likely to have contact.
- Increase your knowledge about different beliefs and values and learn not to be threatened when they differ from your own.
- Analyze your own communication (eg, facial expression and body language) and how it may be interpreted.
- Recognize differences in ways clients communicate, and do not assume the meaning of a specific behavior (eg, lack of eye contact) without considering the client's ethnic and cultural background.
- Understand your own biases, prejudices, and stereotypes.
- Recognize that cultural symbols and practices can often bring a client comfort.
- Support the client's practices and incorporate them into nursing practice whenever possible, and not contraindicated for health reasons; for example, provide hot tea to a client who drinks hot tea and never drinks cold water.
- Don't impose a cultural practice on a client without knowing whether it is acceptable; for example, Vietnamese clients may prefer not to be touched on the head.
- Review your own attitudes and beliefs about health and objectively examine the logic of those attitudes and beliefs and their origins.
- Remember that during illness clients may return to preferred cultural practices; for example, the client who has learned English as a second language may revert to the primary language.

Spiritual Care

When orienting patients to the nursing unit, you can provide information about hospital services and arrange for them to participate in these as they are able. Many hospitals have full-time chaplains to assist with spiritual needs and many nursing units have a list of clergy in the community who are on call for spiritual care.

To intervene effectively for patients with Spiritual Distress, you should have already examined and clarified your own spiritual beliefs and values. If you feel uncomfortable with spiritual interventions (eg, praying with a patient who requests it), you should verbalize your discomfort and offer to get someone else to help. It is important to respect and support the patient's beliefs, but it is equally important to not feel guilty about your own discomfort.

When there is true conflict between the client's spiritual (or cultural) beliefs and medical therapy, you should encourage the client and physician to discuss the conflict and consider alternative therapies. As a nurse, you should always support the client's right to make an informed decision.

■ SUMMARY

Implementation

- is action-focused.
- occurs in the environments created by healthcare systems such as managed care and case management.
- requires nurses to perform or delegate dependent, independent, and collaborative actions.
- may use a variety of models of allocating nursing tasks and authority (eg, functional, team, and primary nursing, and differentiated practice).
- should preserve confidentiality and client dignity.
- relies on client readiness and the nurse's cognitive, technical, and interpersonal skills.
- includes teaching strategies to enhance learning and promote compliance with therapies.
- includes delegating the right activities to the right person, as well as supervising the activities.
- requires reflection and critical thinking to assure safe, effective, and efficient care.
- is completed when the nursing actions have been carried out and recorded, along with the client's reactions to them. (The client record or chart is a permanent, legal document of the client's health care and status.)
- is documented in flowsheets and progress notes and reported orally at change of shift and when a client is transferred.

- is documented on forms and in the format (eg, narrative, SOAP) determined by individual institutions.
- must be documented according to accepted guidelines and agency policies and procedures.
- provides the opportunity for culturally and spiritually competent nursing care.
- carries some legal risks that can be minimized by prudent documentation.

IMPLEMENTATION—THINKING QUICK-CHECK

- ❏ Did I consider the patient's readiness before implementing?
- ❏ Did I communicate effectively with the patient?
- ❏ Did I make periodic observations of the patient's condition during the intervention?

NURSING PROCESS PRACTICE

CASE STUDY: Read the following case study. Several of the exercises will refer to it.

Nancy Atwell is a 32-year-old teacher who lives alone. She has had rheumatoid arthritis for approximately 4 years. This has made her knees painful and has limited the motion and weight-bearing ability of her knee joints. Medical treatment has not been successful in relieving her joint pain. She has a recent diagnosis of endometrial cancer. At 7AM, she enters the hospital to have an abdominal hysterectomy. Her surgery is scheduled for 2 PM.

On a previous admission, she was quiet, withdrawn, and extremely concerned for her privacy. Now she seems more outgoing and less overtly concerned about privacy. When questioned, Ms. Atwell states she has had no previous surgical experience, but denies feeling nervous about the operation. She says she is having "quite a bit" of abdominal cramping now. Her preoperative orders include the following:

1. S.S. enema on admission
2. NPO
3. Shower this AM
4. Pre-op med: Demerol 75 mg at 1330
5. Ibuprofen 500 mg p.o. every 3–4 hr prn for abdominal or joint pain
6. IV: 1,000 cc D_5LR at 125 mL/hr

1. Which of the preoperative orders could you delegate to your nursing assistant?

2. What activities may be a threat to Ms. Atwell's privacy and dignity?

3. A discharge planning nurse diagnosis for Ms. Atwell is "Risk for Impaired Home Maintenance Management: Inability to manage own care on dismissal r/t single state (no one to help out), pain in knees, and post-op pain and weakness."

   a. What collaborative (interdependent) nursing action might be performed for this nursing diagnosis?

   b. What independent nursing action might be performed?

4. Ms. Atwell's nursing assistant is preparing to implement the order for a shower. What should the nurse tell her about the rationale for the shower?

5. If you were Ms. Atwell's nurse, what would you do to prepare her before you implement the following new medical order: Nembutal 100 mg p.o. at H.S.?

6. What is an example of therapeutic communication that might be needed by Ms. Atwell either preoperatively or postoperatively? (One example is given for you.)

EXAMPLE: Talking to her to assess for feelings of grief related to her inability to bear children after the hysterectomy.

7. State the guideline for implementing nursing strategies that is demonstrated by the following situations (refer to Box 8–5 on page 355).

a. It is important for Ms. Bates to be turned frequently, but it causes her a great deal of pain. It is 15 minutes past time to turn her, but she has a visitor—the first one she has had in several weeks. In order to meet Ms. Bates's emotional needs, the nurse decides to wait until the visitor leaves to do the turning.

Guideline:

b. The physician has ordered Bromocriptine 2.5 mg p.o. The nurse does not know the side effects of this drug, so he looks it up in the hospital formulary.

Guideline:

c. The nurse pulls the curtain around the bed and drapes the client's legs and perineum before inserting an indwelling catheter.

Guideline:

d. The nurse asks a colleague to double-check her insulin dosage.

Guideline:

e. The nurse uses sterile technique to insert the urinary catheter.

Guideline:

f. The nurse takes the client's blood pressure before administering an antihypertensive medication.

Guideline:

8. a. Chart the following information in DAR format (Focus® Charting): Mr. Jarrett says his head hurts. He has his eyes shut tightly; he says the light makes them hurt. The nurse places a cool cloth on his head and closes the door to his room. She gives him Tylenol #3, tabs 1, p.o., at 6 PM, as ordered. When she reassesses Mr. Jarrett in 1 hour, he says it still hurts. She plans to disturb him as little as possible and keep the room dark. She wants the evening nurse to call Dr. King if Mr. Jarrett's headache is unrelieved after the second dose of medication. The nurse charted the information at 8 PM on August 6, 2001.

    b. Chart the same information, but this time chart at 6 PM and again at 7 PM.

9. Chart in SOAP format all the data that are pertinent for the problem, Risk for Noncompliance with pre- and post-op instructions r/t lack of knowledge. Your plan for this problem will be to (1) remind her not to drink anything, (2) place an "NPO" sign in her room, and (3) remind any visitors that she cannot eat or drink.

    Data
    Ms. Atwell seems outgoing and not overtly concerned about privacy. When questioned, she denies feelings nervous about the operation. She gets up to go to the bathroom and walks about in the room several times during the morning. She walks erect and with a steady gait.

At 9 AM, you give her a soapsuds enema; she has a large, unformed stool. You tell her that she cannot have anything to eat or drink today, explaining the rationale for this restriction. She says she understands this. You take this opportunity to do the rest of her preoperative teaching. She states, "I understand."

Your assessment reveals that her oxygenation function is normal. She has +1 edema of her left ankle, which she says is normal for her. Her pedal pulses are strong and equal bilaterally; she has no numbness or tingling in her extremities. Her skin is warm and dry.

She is alert and oriented. She says she is havng "quite a bit" of abdominal cramping now. You give her the ibuprofen at 10 AM as ordered, and record it in the medication record (MAR). At 11 AM she says, "I feel better now."

10. As the RN, you are working with a nursing assistant to care for seven patients, all of whom require intense help with hygiene and other self-care. Mrs. Appleby has had a stroke, but her condition is stable now. She is very thin and almost completely immobile. The nurse on the previous shift tells you that Mrs. Appleby has developed a red area over her sacrum, but that the skin is intact.

A. Underline any of the following activities (for Mrs. Appleby) that you could delegate to the nursing assistant.

- vital signs q4hrs
- bedbath and linen change
- p.o. medication (stool softener)
- turn and reposition q2hrs
- feeding her lunch to her
- skin assessment

B. If you decided to delegate the bedbath to the nursing assistant, what instructions should you give him/her?

C. Which of the activities in "A" could you perform yourself and combine with the skin assessment? _____

D. How would you evaluate whether the delegated activities were performed satisfactorily? Write the details of your plan.

E. Suppose that Mrs. Appleby's condition changes, and you diagnose Risk for Aspiration r/t Impaired Swallowing. How would this new diagnosis change the activities you delegate? Why?

F. Suppose, even though Mrs. Appleby has Risk for Aspiration, you still must delegate the feeding to the nursing assistant (eg, because of other patient emergencies that develop). What would you do to assure Mrs. Appleby's safety?

CRITICAL THINKING PRACTICE: REASONING

Review "Reasoning," in Chapter 2, pages 56–60. When reasoning about problems and solutions, nurses must use critical thinking to (1) evaluate sources of information and (2) explore the implications, consequences, advantages, and disadvantages of the interventions they are considering. The following exercises provide practice with those skills.

I. EVALUATING SOURCES OF INFORMATION

When identifying problems and choosing interventions, you must base your decisions on good information. One way to do this is to evaluate the *source* of the information. For example, as a beginning student, you may have asked a nursing assistant questions about a patient's breathing, when it would have been better to get that information from a nurse. As another example, when you weigh a baby, the scale is the source of information; so you must be sure that the scale is correctly calibrated. In addition to the questions in Box 2–8, page 59, ask:

- Does the source have a good track record for accuracy, honesty, and so forth?
- Are there conflicting sources? (eg, two textbooks may give different ranges of normal for pulse rate.)
- Are there confirming sources? (eg, even when information is provided by another professional, you may need to look it up in a textbook.)

A. Evaluate the credibility of the source of information in each of the followng situations. Ask the preceding questions and those in Box 2–8. Answer the questions and mark each person's "credibility rating" on the line shown. If you need more information in order to evaluate someone's credibility, state what it is and how you would get it.

1. When giving report, the night nurse says, "Mrs. Alexander has been asking for more pain medication—at least an hour before it is due. Her pain doesn't seem that severe to me though. I think she just wants attention." (Who is/are the information sources to evaluate in this case? Are there conflicting sources? Focus on the credibility of the source(s) rather than on the data about pain, but do not ignore the data given.)

|_____|_____|

Not at all credible   Completely credible

2. Mrs. Domingo says her post-thoracotomy pain is unbearable. Her sister says that although Mrs. Domingo loves needlepoint, she is having too much pain to continue with this hobby. (Does the sister's information conflict with or confirm Mrs. Domingo's? Did the sister observe directly, or did she have to make inferences about Mrs. D's pain? What is the sister's purpose for providing the information?)

|_____|_____|

Not at all credible   Completely credible

3. Mrs. Laurent says, "I have tried all kinds of pain medications, but I have a kidney disease, and they make me so dizzy and nauseated that I can't stand taking them." (You are evaluating Mrs. Laurent's credibility, but with regard to *what*?

|_____|_____|

Not at all credible   Completely credible

4. Mrs. Laurent says, "I have tried all kinds of pain medications, but I have a kidney disease, and they make me so dizzy and nauseated that I can't stand taking them." The clinical

nurse specialist says, "Yes, she does have kidney disease; but the analgesic she is taking now is metabolized mainly in the liver." (CNS is the source.)

Not at all credible		Completely credible

5. You have received a brochure from a pharmaceutical company providing information about the advantages of their new medication for migraine headaches.

Not at all credible		Completely credible

B. You have read in a journal that beta-endorphins increase with exercise. Assuming that you have unlimited time and resources, how could you confirm this? What other sources could you consult?

II. EXPLORING IMPLICATIONS, CONSEQUENCES, ADVANTAGES, AND DISADVANTAGES

Some questions to ask when choosing interventions are: If I perform this activity, (1) what are the implications, (2) what are the possible consequences (effects), and (3) what are the advantages and disadvantages? Be sure you understand the difference between implications and consequences (refer to Chapter 2). To *imply* something is to express it indirectly, suggesting it without stating it. A *consequence* is the *effect* or *result* that is caused by something. To help identify implications, ask "What is the *meaning* of this action?" To help identify consequences, ask "What will *happen* if I do this?"

EXAMPLE: The physician has ordered either p.o. acetaminophen with codeine or IM morphine for Ms. Amot's pain, as needed. The nurse chooses to give the p.o. medication.

This *implies* (for one thing) that the nurse believes Ms. Amot's pain is not severe enough to merit use of morphine. The *expected consequence* is that the p.o. med will adequately relieve the pain.

A. Fill in the blanks. Does the statement represent an implication or a consequence?

(1) _____ Mr. Hill does not eat very much, so he must really be serious about losing weight this time.

(2) _____ If I exercise more and eat less, I will lose weight.

(3) _____ If we turn Mrs. Abbott frequently, we may be able to prevent skin breakdown.

(4) _____ I am going to explain the treatment more fully to the patient because I do not believe anyone else will do it, and I think he needs to know.

B. Mr. X has hepatitis, a liver disease. When you make a home visit, he tells you that he has a headache and wonders if he can take some acetaminophen, which you know to be metabolized in the liver. You are considering a cold cloth to the forehead and some relaxation and visualization exercises as alternative interventions.

1. What are two possible consequences of his taking the acetaminophen? (What is the possible therapeutic effect? An undesirable side effect?)

2. What consequences do you expect if you proceed with the alternative interventions?

3. Instead of using the cold cloth and relaxation, you decide to call Mr. X's physician to ask for a different analgesic. What does this imply (ie, what is your reasoning)?

C. Mrs. B has a nursing diagnosis of Chronic Confusion. You are considering the following nursing activities:

- Teaching her husband ways to deal with delusional thinking.
- Reassuring Mrs. B. frequently with touch and therapeutic communication.
- Orienting Mrs. B. (eg, to staff, to the room) as needed.

1. What are the implications of the teaching activity?

2. Given those implications, what do you need to find out before deciding whether to use the teaching intervention?

3. Refer to Box 2–9, page 60. What questions should you ask about the "reassuring" intervention before deciding to use it?

4. Which of the three interventions can you probably choose even without knowing the etiology or symptoms of Mrs. B.'s chronic confusion?

Case Study: Applying Nursing Process and Critical Thinking

Brad Williams is a 72-year-old man who had a cerebrovascular accident (stroke) due to right cerebral thrombosis 1 week ago. He has been taking antihypertensive medications for 2 years, but his wife says that he often forgets to take it. Mr. Williams is drowsy but responds to verbal stimuli, although he cannot talk. He nods his head to indicate "yes" or "no" when asked questions, and becomes agitated and tearful when he cannot understand or be understood. He cannot move his left arm and leg; flaccid paralysis is present in both (he is left-handed). He does not respond to touch in those extremities. Although he voids when offered a urinal, he is occasionally incontinent of urine. He is receiving heparin sodium by continuous intravenous drip; the dose is adjusted according to the results of a partial thromboplastin time (PTT), which is performed every 4 hours. The nurse has identified the following nursing diagnoses for Mr. Williams:

- *Impaired Physical Mobility* related to left hemiplegia secondary to neurologic deficits
- *Risk for Impaired Skin Integrity* related to inability to change position secondary to left-sided paralysis
- *Feeding Self-Care Deficit* related to paralysis of left hand and arm
- *Impaired Verbal Communication* related to cerebral tissue injury

1. Based just on the information given, what other actual or potential nursing diagnoses should the nurse write?

2. The NANDA definition of *Self-Esteem Disturbance* is: Negative self-evaluation/feelings about self or self-capabilities, which may be directly or indirectly expressed. Does Mr. Williams have this diagnosis (yes/no)? What risk factors exist that may cause Mr. Williams to develop *Self-Esteem Disturbance*?

3. In addition to "inability to change position," what other etiological factor should be added to the diagnosis, *Risk for Impaired Skin Integrity*? Why?

4. For the nursing diagnosis of *Risk for Impaired Skin Integrity* related to inability to change position secondary to left-sided paralysis, the nurse wrote the following expected outcome: "Maintains skin integrity." What assessments should the nurse make to evaluate whether this goal is being met? Be specific.

5. For the diagnosis of *Risk for Impaired Skin Integrity* related to inability to change position secondary to left-sided paralysis, the nurse has included in the care plan the NIC intervention, "Pressure Ulcer Prevention." NIC lists the following nursing activities for Pressure Ulcer Prevention (2000, p. 535).

   - Remove excess moisture on the skin resulting from perspiration, wound drainage, and fecal or urinary incontinence
   - Turn every 1 to 2 hours, as appropriate
   - Inspect skin over bony prominences and other pressure points when repositioning at least daily
   - Provide trapeze to assist patient in shifting weight frequently
   - Use specialty beds and mattresses, as appropriate

6. Refer to Box 2–9, page 60. What questions should you ask about the "reassuring" intervention before deciding to use it?

7. Which of the three interventions can you probably choose even without knowing the etiology or symptoms?

   (a) Underline the activities that are appropriate for Mr. Williams. If some are only partially appropriate, draw lines through the words that do not apply to Mr. Williams.

   (b) Which activity needs to have details added to make it more specific? What is needed?

8. What collaborative problem is associated with heparin administration?

9. When delegating bathing and oral care for Mr. Williams, what safety precautions should the nurse give to the aide, keeping in mind that Mr. Williams is receiving heparin?

10. Keeping in mind Mr. Williams' nursing diagnoses, what specific instructions should the nurse give to the aide regarding the linen change?

11. Write a reasonable long-term goal for Mr. Williams' diagnosis of *Feeding Self-Care Deficit*.

12. There are some safety issues associated with Mr. William's *Impaired Verbal Communication*.

   (a) What do you think they might be?

   (b) What nursing actions could you take to address these risks?

13. For the nursing diagnoses she identified, what referrals might the nurse need to make? Why?

14. Write a nursing order to address Mr. Williams' *Impaired Physical Mobility*.

■ SELECTED REFERENCES

American Nurses Association (1985). *Code for Nurses with Interpretive Statements*. Kansas City, MO: ANA.

American Nurses Association (1996). *Registered Professional Nurses and Unlicensed Assistive Personnel*. 2nd ed. Washington, DC: ANA.

American Nurses Association (1998). *Standards of Clinical Nursing Practice*. 2nd ed. Washington, DC: American Nurses Publishing.

Barter, M. (1999). Delegation and supervision outside the hospital. *AJN* 99(2):24EEE–24FFF, 24HHH.

Canadian Nurses Association (1987). *Standards for Nursing Practice*. Ottawa, Ontario: CNA.

Carson, K., J. E. Burke, and S. Nick (1997). Changing roles in case management: some reflections. *Continuum* 17(4):1, 3–9.

Catanzano, F. (1994). Nursing information/documentation system increases quality care, shortens stay at Desert Samaritan Medical Center. *Computers in Nursing* 12(4):184–185.

Chapman, G. F. (1999). Charting tips. Documenting an adverse incident. *Nursing 99* 29(2):17.

Chase, S. K. (1997). Charting critical thinking: nursing judgments and patient outcomes. *Dimen Crit Care Nurs* 16(2):102–111.

Charting made incredibly easy. (1998). Springhouse, PA: Springhouse.

Cummins, K. M. and M. T. Hill (1999). Charting by exception: a timely format for you? *AJN* 99(3):24G.

Eggland, E. T. and D. S. Heinemann (1994). *Nursing documentation. Charting, recording, and reporting*. Philadelphia: J. B. Lippincott.

Eskreis, T. R. (1998). Seven common legal pitfalls in nursing. *AJN* 98(4):34–40.

Groah, L. and E. Reed (1983). Your responsibility in documenting care. *Ass Oper Room Nurses J* 37(May):1174–85.

Gropper, E. I., and Dicapo, R. (1995). The P.A.R.T. system. *Nurs Manage* 26(4):46, 48.

Guzzetta, C. (1987). Nursing diagnoses in nursing education: effect on the profession. 1. *Heart Lung* 16(November):629–635.

Hill, M., M. Labik, and D. Vanderbilt (1997). Managing skin care with the CareMap system. *J Wound Ostomy Continence Nurs* 24(1):26–37.

Iyer, P. W. and N. H. Camp (1995). *Nursing documentation: A nursing process approach.* 2nd ed. St. Louis: Mosby.

Kayser-Jones, J. and E. Schell (1997). The effect of staffing on the quality of care at mealtime. *Nursing Outlook* 45(2):64–72.

Kennedy, J. (1999). An evaluation of non-verbal handover. *Prof Nurse* 14(6):391–394.

Kozier B., G. Erb, A. Berman (2000). *Fundamentals of nursing: Concepts, process, and practice* (6th ed.). Upper Saddle River, NJ: Prentice-Hall.

Krul, R. (1997). Nurses as case managers: an evolution of the nursing process. *Nurs Spectrum* (Illinois ed.) 10(4):11.

Lampe, S. (1985). Focus charting: streamlining documentation. *Nurs Manage* 16(7):43–46.

London, F. (1998). Improving compliance. What you can do. *RN* 61(1):43–46.

Marelli, T. M. and L. S. Hilliard (1996). Documentation and effective patient care planning. *Home Care Provider* 1(4):198–201.

McKenna, L. G. (1997). Improving the nursing handover report. *Prof Nurse* 12(9):637–639.

Mosher, C. and R. Bontomasi (1996). How to improve your shift report. *AJN* 96(8):32–34.

Murphy, J., and L. J. Burke (1990). Charting by exception: A more efficient way to document. *Nursing 90* 20:65–69.

National Council of State Boards of Nursing (1995). *Delegation: Concepts and decision-making process.* Chicago: Author.

National Council of State Boards of Nursing, Inc. (1997). *Delegation decision-making grid* (based on a concept developed by the American Association of Critical Care Nurses). Available at: http://www.ncsbn.org/files/uap/delegationgrid.pdf. Accessed 12/20/99.

National Council of State Boards of Nursing, Inc. (1997). *Delegation decision-making tree.* Available at: http://www.ncsbn.org/files/uap/delegationtree.pdf. Accessed 12/20/99.

National Council of State Boards of Nursing, Inc. (1997). *The five rights of delegation.* Available at: http://www.ncsbn.org/files/uap/fiverights.pdf. Accessed 12/20/99.

Parkman, C. A. (1996). Delegation. Are you doing it right? *AJN* 96(9):43–47.

Philipsen, N. and P. McMullen (1993). Charting basics 101. *Nursing Connections* 6(3):62–64.

Phillips, E. (1998). Directing UAPs—safely. *RN* 61(6):53–56.

Quigley, P., A. Mathis, and V. Nodhturft (1994). Improving clinical documentation quality. *J Nurs Care Quality* 8(4):66–73.

Rubenfeld, M. G. and B. K. Scheffer (1999). *Critical thinking in nursing.* Philadelphia: Lippincott.

Springhouse. (1996). *Nurse's legal handbook.* 3rd ed. Springhouse, PA: Author.

Sticklin, L. A. (1994). Putting the nursing process back into charting. *MEDSURG Nurs* 3(3): 232–233.

Tammelleo, A. D. (1997). Legal case briefs for nurses. Did physician prescribe excess dosage?: Did nurse err in administering meds? *The Regan report on nursing law* 38(7):3.

Town, J. (1993). Changing to computerized documentation—PLUS. *Nurs Manage* 24(7): 44–46, 48.

Walton, J. C. and M. Waszkiewicz (1997). Managing unlicensed assistive personnel: tips for improving quality outcomes. *MEDSURG Nurs* 6(1):24–28.

Zimmerman, P. G. (1997). Delegating to unlicensed assistive personnel. *Nursing 97* 27(5):71.

9
Evaluation

Learning Outcomes

On completing this chapter, you should be able to do the following:

- Define evaluation as it relates to (1) the nursing process and (2) quality assurance.
- State the importance and purpose of evaluation in (1) the nursing process and (2) quality assurance.
- Explain how nurses use critical thinking when evaluating.
- Describe the process of evaluating client progress toward outcome achievement.
- Given predicted outcomes and client data, write two-part evaluative statements.
- Describe a process for modifying the nursing care plan.
- Explain the relevance of culture and spirituality to evaluation in the nursing process.
- Describe a process for nursing quality assurance.
- Differentiate between criteria and standards.
- Explain how quality-assurance evaluation supports the moral principles of beneficence and nonmaleficence.

■ INTRODUCTION

Nurses make frequent and varied evaluations. Because the client is the nurse's primary concern, the most important evaluations involve the following:

1. The client's progress toward health goals
2. The value of the nursing care plan in helping the client to achieve desired outcomes
3. The overall quality of care given to defined groups of clients

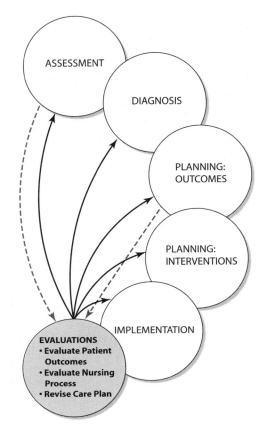

Figure 9–1
The Evaluation Phase of the Nursing Process.

This chapter examines the universal characteristics of evaluation, discusses evaluation as a step of the nursing process (see Figure 9–1), and explains the process of quality assurance.

◼ GENERAL CHARACTERISTICS OF EVALUATION

Before examining evaluation as it is used in the nursing process, it may be helpful to analyze a more general definition of the term. In general, **formal evaluation** is a deliberate, systematic process in which a judgment is made about the *quality, value, or worth* of something by comparing it to *previously identified criteria or standards*. Almost anything can be the subject of evaluation (eg, a painting, a highway system, a teaching method, or a person's character). Furthermore, various aspects or properties of a thing can be evaluated. If you are evaluating a painting, for instance, you can assess the artist's use of color or the extent to which the painting elicits emotion. If you were evaluating teaching methods, you might measure the teacher's ability to hold student interest or minimize student stress. The important thing to remember is that you must decide *in advance* what properties you are going to consider and how you will measure those properties.

Standards and Criteria

Although *standards* and *criteria* are sometimes used interchangeably, most texts differentiate between these terms. A **standard** is established by authority, custom, or consensus as a model of what should be done. In nursing, standards describe quality nursing care and are used for comparison when evaluating job performance. Some standards, like those written for routines of care on a nursing unit, are specific enough to serve as criteria. Others are broad and abstract, as in the ANA's *Standards of Care* (1998). When standards or criteria are broad, as in Box 9–1, more specific criteria must be developed to guide the collection of data for evaluation. **Criteria** are measurable or observable qualities that describe specific skills, knowledge, behaviors, attitudes, and so on. In Box 9–1, the criteria for ANA Standard VI are labeled. For CNA Standard II, in the lower half of the box, the first statement (5) is the standard. Statements 5.1 through 5.7 are the criteria used for evaluating whether the standard is met.

Concrete, specific criteria serve as guides for collecting evaluation data, as well as for making judgments about such data. The patient outcomes you learned to write in Chapter 6 are examples of criteria.

Criteria should be both valid and reliable. A criterion is **valid** if it actually measures what it is intended to measure. For example, the white blood cell count is often used to "measure" the presence of infection. However, it would not be valid if used alone, because the white cell count is not elevated in all infections; in addition, the white cell count is sometimes elevated when there is no infection. More valid indicators might be a blood culture or a bacterial count of a body fluid. A **reliable** criterion yields the same results every time it is used, no matter who uses it (eg, determining a patient's age by asking his friends is less reliable than asking the patient or checking his birth certificate). Box 9–2 presents a comparison of standards and criteria.

■ EVALUATION IN NURSING PROCESS

In the nursing process, **evaluation** is a planned, ongoing, deliberate activity in which the client, family, nurse, and other healthcare professionals determine (1) the client's progress toward outcome achievement and (2) the effectiveness of the nursing care plan. The nurse and client determine the *quality* of the client's health by using as *predetermined criteria* the predicted responses (outcomes) identified in the planning step. They determine the *value* of the nursing care plan by using as *standards* the excellent application of each step of the nursing process.

KEY POINT
Evaluation is a planned, ongoing, deliberate activity in which the nurse, client, significant others, and other healthcare professionals determine:

1. the extent of client outcome achievement, and
2. the effectiveness of the nursing care plan.

BOX 9–1

Nursing Standards of Care

ANA Standard VI: Evaluation

The nurse evaluates the patient's progress toward attainment of outcomes.

Measurement Criteria

1. Evaluation is systematic, ongoing, and criterion-based.
2. The patient, family, and other healthcare providers are involved in the evaluation process, as appropriate.
3. Ongoing assessment data are used to revise diagnoses, outcomes, and the plan of care, as needed.
4. Revisions in diagnoses, outcomes, and the plan of care are documented.
5. The effectiveness of interventions is evaluated in relation to outcomes.
6. The patient's responses to interventions are documented.

Source: Reprinted with permission from American Nurses Association, *Standards of Clinical Nursing Practice* (2nd ed.) © 1998 American Nurses Publishing, American Nurses Foundation/American Nurses Association, 600 Maryland Avenue, SW, Suite 100W, Washington, DC 20024–2571, pp. 9–10.

CNA Standard II (Nursing Process)

Evaluation

5. Nurses are required to evaluate all steps of the nursing process in accordance with their conceptual model for nursing. The nurse in any practice setting:
    5.1 observes the results of nursing actions
    5.2 compares the results of nursing actions with those stated in the short- and long-term objectives
    5.3 judges, within the context of client participation, the degree to which the objectives have been met in accordance with the conception of the expected results
    5.4 communicates with appropriate others regarding evaluation
    5.5 revises with the client and relevant others the objectives, priorities and nursing actions as indicated
    5.6 implements the modified plan of action
    5.7 continues in cyclical fashion the entire nursing process until the client–nurse relationship is terminated

Source: Canadian Nurses Association (1987). *Standards for Nursing Parctice.* Ottawa: Ontario, p. 5.

BOX 9–2

Comparison of Nursing Standards and Criteria

	Standards	Criteria
Similarities	Describe what is acceptable or desired	Describe what is acceptable or desired
	Serve as basis for comparison	Serve as basis for comparison
Differences	Describe nursing care	Describe expected nurse or client behaviors
	May be broad or specific	Are specific, observable, measurable
Example	ANA standards	Patient outcomes on a care plan

General Definition of Evaluation

Determination of quality or value

Use of predetermined criteria or standards

Nursing Process Definition

1. of the client's health.
2. of the nursing care plan.

1. Use of the outcomes identified in the planning phase.
2. Use of the nursing process according to guidelines such as those in Table 6–9 on p. 280.

Evaluation begins with the initial baseline assessment and continues during each contact with the client. Frequency of evaluation depends on frequency of contact, which is determined by the client's status or the condition being evaluated. When a patient has just returned from surgery, the nurse may evaluate for signs of change in status every 15 minutes. The following day, the nurse may evaluate the client only every 4 hours. As the client's condition improves and she approaches discharge, evaluation gradually becomes less frequent.

Relationship to Other Phases

Effective evaluation depends on the effectiveness of the steps that precede it. Assessment data must be accurate and complete so that the outcomes written in the planning step will be appropriate for the client. The desired outcomes (planning) must be stated in concrete, behavioral terms if they are to be useful for evaluating actual client outcomes. Finally, without the implementation step, there would be nothing to evaluate.

Evaluation overlaps with assessment. During evaluation, the nurse collects data (assessment), but for the purpose of evaluating (evaluation), rather than diagnosing. The *act* of data collection is the same; the differences are in (1) when it is collected and (2) how it is used. In the assessment step the nurse uses data to make nursing diagnoses; in the evaluation step, data are used to assess the effect of nursing care on the diagnoses.

	Assessment Data	Evaluation Data
When Collected	In assessment phase	In evaluation phase
	Before interventions	After interventions
Purpose/Use	Make nursing diagnosis	Evaluate goal achievement
	Determine present health status	Compare "new" health status to desired health status

Although it is the final step in the nursing process, evaluation does not end the process; the information it provides is used to begin another cycle. After implementing the care plan, the nurse compares client responses to predicted outcomes and then uses this information to review the care plan and each step of the nursing process.

Evaluating Patient Progress

In the context of the nursing process, outcome evaluation focuses primarily on the client's progress toward achieving health goals. After giving care, the nurse compares the clients' health status (responses) to the predicted outcomes identified during the planning phase and makes a judgment about whether or not they have been achieved.

Evaluation of client outcomes may be ongoing or intermittent. **Ongoing evaluation** is done while (or immediately after) implementing an intervention, enabling you to make on-the-spot modifications. **Intermittent evaluation**, performed at specified times, shows the amount of progress toward outcome achievement; it enables you to correct any inadequacies in the client's care and modify the care plan as needed. Evaluation continues until the client's health goals are achieved or until he is discharged from nursing care.

Terminal evaluation indicates the client's condition at the time of discharge. It includes understanding of follow-up care and status of outcome achievement, especially with regard to self-care abilities. Most agencies have a special Discharge Record for the terminal evaluation, as well as for instructions regarding medications, treatments, and follow-up care. As you work with the client throughout her stay, you should prepare her for eventual discharge by gradually promoting more self-care and talking about the time when she will be leaving.

Professional Standards of Practice

Professional standards of practice (see Box 9–1 on page 398) identify evaluation as a mutual nurse-client activity. Family and other team members provide data and participate, but the nurse is responsible for initiating and recording the evaluation.

By performing organized, systematic evaluation of client outcomes, nurses demonstrate caring and responsibility. Examining outcomes shows that nurses care not only about planning and delivering care, but also about its effect on those whose lives they touch. Without evaluation, nurses would not know whether the care they give actually meets the client's needs.

Evaluation enables the nurse to improve care. It promotes efficiency by eliminating unsuccessful interventions and allowing the nurse to focus on actions that are more effective. Only by evaluating the client's progress in relation to the plan of care can the nurse know whether to continue, change, or terminate the plan.

Finally, by linking nursing interventions to improvements in client status, evaluation can demonstrate to employers and consumers that nurses play an important role in achieving client health.

Process for Evaluating Client Progress

The professional nurse responsible for the care plan is also responsible for evaluating the client's responses to care. The following discussion provides a six-step guide for evaluating client progress:

1. *Review the desired outcomes (indicators).* Outcomes and indicators identified in the planning phase are the criteria used to evaluate the patient's responses to nursing care. Desired outcomes (indicators/goals) have two purposes: (1) they establish the kind of data that need to be collected, and (2) they provide standards against which the data are judged. For example, given the following desired outcomes, any nurse caring for the patient would know what data to collect.

- Urine output will be at least 50 mL/hour
- Oral fluid intake will be at least 2,000 mL per 24 hours

2. *Collect evaluation data.* Collect data about the client's responses to the nursing interventions. Use the nursing diagnosis and its list of outcomes from the care plan to guide your ongoing focus assessment. Evaluation data are collected by observing the client's behavior and responses, examining client records, and talking to the client, family, friends, and other health team members. In the example in Table 9–1, in order to get the data under "Actual Outcomes" during interactions with Sam Rizzo, the nurse focused on his facial expression and muscle tension and listened for statements reflecting his level of anxiety and his knowledge of routines and treatments.

Table 9–1   Evaluation Example: Sam Rizzo

Nursing Diagnosis: Moderate Anxiety r/t unfamiliar environment and dyspnea		
Compare Desired Outcomes . . .	**to Actual Outcomes (Data) . . .**	**Conclusion**
Broad goal: Will experience reduced anxiety, as evidenced by outcomes:		
1. verbalization of feeling less anxious	When dyspneic, states "What should I do? Can you help me?"	Outcome not achieved.
2. relaxed facial muscles	Face relaxed except during episodes of dyspnea.	Outcome partially achieved.
3. absence of skeletal muscle tension	No skeletal muscle tension except during episodes of dyspnea.	Outcome partially achieved.
4. verbalization of understanding of hospital routines and treatments	States, "I feel better since you explained about the fire drill. I thought there was a real fire."	Outcome achieved.
	States, "I understand about the hospital routines and the breathing treatments. Those things really aren't causing any anxiety."	

The nature of the outcome determines the type of information you will collect. Outcomes can be classified as cognitive, psychomotor, or affective, or as pertaining to body appearance and functioning. For cognitive outcomes, you might ask the client to repeat information or apply new knowledge (eg, choose low-fat foods from a menu). For psychomotor outcomes, you could ask the client to demonstrate a skill, such as drawing up insulin. For affective outcomes, you might talk to the client and observe her behavior for cues to changes in values, attitudes, or beliefs. You can obtain data about body appearance and functioning by interviewing, observing, and examining the client, as well as from secondary sources, such as laboratory results. Some examples of data-collection methods for the different types of outcomes appear in Table 9–2.

3. *Compare patient status with desired outcomes, and draw a conclusion.* If the nursing process has been effective up to this point, it is relatively simple to determine if a goal has been met. Is the client's response (actual outcome) what you wanted it to be (desired outcome)? Is it at least the best you can expect given the time and circumstances? Include the client in decisions about the level of outcome achievement. Go over the desired outcomes with the client, and ask him if he believes they have been achieved. You can draw three possible conclusions about outcome achievement.

Outcome achieved   The desired client response occurred; that is, the actual response is the same as the desired outcome.

Table 9–2 Evaluation Data-Collection Methods

Type of Outcome	Outcome Statement	Example of Data Collection Activity
Cognitive	By the end of the week, names foods to avoid on a low-fat diet.	Using a chart of the Food Guide Pyramid, ask the client to tell you which foods to avoid.
Psychomotor	Within 24 hours after delivery, positions baby correctly at breast.	Observe the mother breastfeeding the infant.
Affective	After orientation to routines and procedures, states he is feeling less anxiety.	Listen for spontaneous statements about anxiety, or ask, "How are you feeling?"
Body function and appearance	Heart rate < 100 at all times.	Auscultate apical heart rate.

Outcome partially achieved	Some, but not all, desired behaviors were observed, or the predicted outcome is achieved only part of the time.
Outcome not achieved	The desired client response did not occur by the target time, or the actual outcome does not match the desired outcome.

Table 9–1 shows how actual outcomes would be compared to predicted outcomes in order to draw conclusions about Sam Rizzo's goal achievement.

4. *Write the evaluative statement.* An evaluative statement consists of two parts: (a) the judgment about whether the outcome was achieved ("Conclusion" in Table 9–1) and (b) data to support the judgment ("Actual Outcomes" in Table 9–1). Following are the evaluative statements that would be written for Sam Rizzo, using the data and conclusions in Table 9–1.

Desired Outcome	Evaluative Statement
Verbalization of feeling less anxious	2/14. Outcome not achieved. When dyspneic, states, "What should I do? Can you help me?" No statements of feeling less anxious.
Relaxed facial muscles	2/14. Outcome partially achieved. Face relaxed except during episodes of dyspnea.
Absence of skeletal muscle tension	2/14. Outcome partially achieved. No skeletal muscle tension except during episodes of dyspnea.

| Verbalization of understanding of hospital routines and treatments | 2/14. Outcome achieved. States, "I feel better since you explained about the fire drill. I thought there was a real fire." Also states, "I understand about the hospital routines and the breathing treatments. Those things really aren't causing any anxiety." |

When using NOC or other standardized outcomes and indicators, evaluative statements may take a different form. Recall from "The Nursing Outcomes Classification (NOC)" on pp. 273–274, and Table 6–4 on p. 273, that goals may be written by writing the label, the indicator, and the scale number of the desired outcome. Goals and evaluation statements are written in exactly the same manner. For example, for a patient with Impaired Transfer Mobility, the goal might be to transfer independently; after interventions, reassessment shows that the patient can transfer using crutches. The goal and evaluative statements would read as follows:

Goal: Transfer performance: 5
Evaluation Statement: Transfer performance: 4

Figure 9–2 is an example of NOC outcomes used in computerized care planning. It is a screen that provides the definition and indicators for an NOC outcome. Figure 9–3 shows, in the same automated system, the patient's status on admission (Initial Scale), the patient goal (Expected Scale), and the evaluation statement (Outcome Scale).

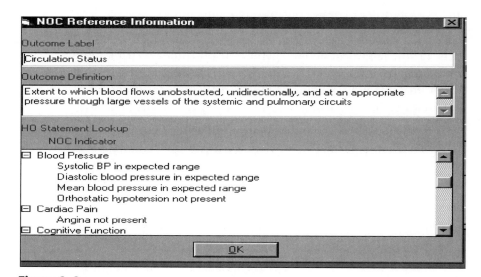

Figure 9–2
Computer Screen: NOC Outcome Reference. *Source*: Copyright © Courtesy of Ergo Partners, L.C.: Boulder, CO. All rights reserved.

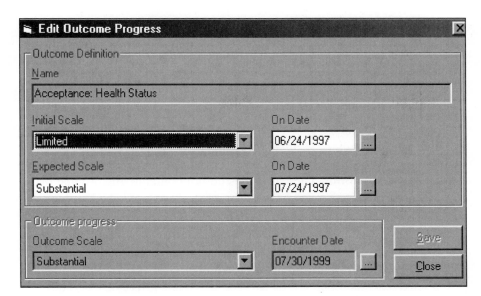

Figure 9–3
Computer Screen: NOC Outcome Progress. *Source*: Copyright © Courtesy of Ergo Partners, L.C.: Boulder, CO. All rights reserved.

Some care plans have a special column for the evaluative statement; in other systems you may record the evaluative statement in the progress notes. In still other systems you may record the evaluation data but not the conclusion about goal achievement.

5. *Relate nursing interventions to outcomes.* It is important to establish whether or not the patient outcomes were actually caused by the nursing actions. You should not assume that a nursing intervention was the reason a goal was or was not met. A number of variables can affect outcome achievement, for example:

Actions and treatments performed by other healthcare professionals

Influence of family members and significant others

Client's attitudes, desire, and motivation

Client's failure to give accurate or sufficient information during data collection

Client's prior experiences and knowledge

Nurses cannot control all the variables that might influence the outcome of care; therefore, in determining the effect of a nursing action, you should try to identify other factors that might have promoted or interfered with its effectiveness.

Evaluating/Revising the Care Plan

After finishing the outcome evaluation, examine the nursing care plan to see if it needs to be changed. You will probably modify the care plan if the client's condition changes or if the health goals were not met. In evaluating a care plan, you need to (1) draw conclusions about the status of client problems and (2) review each step of the nursing process and the manner in which it was performed.

Some agencies use a pink or yellow highlighter to mark through discontinued sections of the care plan. Others have a status column in which to write the date of any revisions. These methods do not obliterate the original plans; thus they can be photocopied or used for reference as needed. Computerized care plans are easily changed on-screen, and a copy of the revised plan can be printed out.

???

THINKING POINT

> Mrs. Adams needed to lose 60 lb (28 kg). With her input, the nurse included in the care plan a goal to "Lose 6 lb (2.8 kg) by 5/2/01." A nursing order in the care plan was to "Explain how to plan and prepare a 1,000-calorie diet." When Mrs. Adams weighed herself on May 2, she had lost 10 lb. The goal had been met.
>
> - Does this mean that the nursing order was effective?
> - What do you need to know in order to decide if that nursing action led to the weight loss?
> - What other factors might have caused Mrs. Adams to lose weight?
> - If Mrs. Adams says, "I forgot what you said about the diet, so I just ate out a lot," what conclusion would you draw about the nursing strategy?

Draw Conclusions About Problem/Health Status

You will use judgments about goal achievement to determine whether the care plan was effective in resolving, reducing, or preventing patient problems. This is important in deciding whether to continue or modify the care plan.

When Goals Have Been Met You can draw one of the following conclusions about the status of the patient's nursing diagnoses:

- *The actual problem has been resolved.* If all the outcomes for the nursing diagnosis have been achieved, you can conclude that the problem has been resolved. This means that nursing care is no longer needed for that nursing diagnosis. Document that the goals were met and discontinue the nursing diagnosis. In Mr. Rizzo's case (Table 9–1), the Anxiety problem can be considered resolved when Outcomes 1, 2, and 3 have been achieved.
- *The actual problem or wellness need still exists.* Even if a goal has been achieved, the problem may still exist, particularly if the goal was only one

of several written for the problem. The Anxiety diagnosis in Table 9–1 illustrates this point. Mr. Rizzo did verbalize understanding of hospital routines and treatments. However, other goals were not met, so the nursing diagnosis of anxiety should remain on the plan. Nursing orders related to explaining routines and treatments could be discontinued, but other interventions for Anxiety should be continued or changed to make them more effective.

■ *The potential problem has been prevented.* If the risk factors have been removed, the nursing diagnosis can be removed from the care plan. However, risk factors may still be present even though the problem still has not occurred. This means that nursing care is still required, so you would not remove the diagnosis from the care plan.

EXAMPLE: Tamara Jordan's nursing diagnosis is Risk for Puerperal Infection r/t membranes having ruptured several days before delivery of her baby. The goal is that she will not develop puerperal infection. When the home health nurse evaluates her progress on postpartum day 3, Tamara's temperature is normal and she has no other signs of infection. However, she could still develop an infection, so the nurse keeps the nursing diagnosis in the care plan and will continue to assess for it.

■ *A possible problem has been ruled out.* In this case, discontinue the problem, goals/outcomes, and nursing orders.
■ *All problems have been resolved; there are no new problems.* When this is the case, the patient is discharged from nursing care. In an acute-care setting this is not likely to occur before dismissal from the institution.

When Goals Have Been Partially Met   You may have some, but not enough, evidence that the outcome has been achieved; or perhaps it is being demonstrated at one time and not another. Mr. Rizzo, for instance, demonstrates absence of muscle tension at times, but not when he is dyspneic. In such instances, you can draw the following conclusions about the nursing diagnosis:

■ *The problem has been reduced and the care plan needs revisions.* As in Mr. Rizzo's case, nursing interventions are still needed. Because the goal is not being fully met, the care plan may need to be modified to make it more effective.
■ *The problem has been reduced; continue with the same plan but allow more time for goal achievement.* Perhaps the interventions are effective, but the client needs more time to achieve the outcome. To decide, you must assess why the outcome has not been fully demonstrated.

When Goals Have Not Been Met   This means that the problem still exists. Even so, you cannot assume that the care plan needs revision. Recall that patient, family, and other variables also influence outcome achievement. Therefore, you must reexamine the entire care plan and each step of the nursing process and decide whether to continue with the same plan or revise the plan.

Evaluating Collaborative Problems   The evaluation process is slightly different for collaborative problems and nursing diagnoses. For both, the nurse collects and evaluates data about changes in the patient's condition. However, in the nursing process, the nurse compares patient responses to the desired outcomes (goals) on the care plan and concludes, "goal met" or "goal not met." For collaborative problems, the nurse compares data to established norms (eg, normal blood glucose) and concludes that the data are or are not within an acceptable range. If the collaborative problem is becoming worse, the nurse notifies the physician.

Critically Review All Steps of the Nursing Process

As you can see, whether or not outcomes have been achieved, there are several decisions to make about continuing, modifying, or terminating nursing care for each problem. Before making specific changes, you must first determine why the plan was not effective. This requires that you review the entire care plan and the nursing process steps involved in its development. This section provides a checklist of questions and actions for use in your review of each step of the nursing process. Table 9–3, on pp. 409–412, provides questions to help you review each step of the nursing process and make decisions about revising the care plan. For in-depth evaluation of each step, refer to the guidelines and critical thinking standards in Chapters 3, 4, 6, 7, and 8.

Assessment Review   Examine the initial and ongoing assessment data in the client's chart (eg, database, progress notes). Errors or omissions in data influence subsequent steps of the nursing process and may require changes in every section of the care plan. You may find that new data have become available since the client's initial assessment, or perhaps the client's condition has changed.

> EXAMPLE: Wasumita Singh answers the nurses in brief phrases; she does not initiate conversation. Her nurses initially believed her communication problem was caused by her difficulty with English. When evaluating her progress, the nurse concludes that her impaired verbal communication problem still exists. However, on reviewing Ms. Singh's chart, she finds new data: a psychiatric consultation note indicating that Ms. Singh is deeply depressed. The nurse realizes now that Ms. Singh's communication problem is more than simply a language barrier.

Diagnosis Review   If your examination of the assessment step results in a revision of the database, you may need to revise or add new nursing diagnoses. Even if data were complete and accurate, you must still analyze the diagnostic process and each of the diagnostic statements. The nursing diagnosis could be incorrect because of errors in the diagnostic process, or the diagnostic statement may have been poorly written. Perhaps the nurse who wrote the statement had a clear idea of the client's problem, but was unable to commu-

Table 9–3   Evaluation Checklist

Instructions: Check the appropriate box and follow the associated instructions.

Assessment Review

1. Were the assessment data complete and accurate?

❑ Yes. No action.   ❑ No. Reassess client. Record the new data. Change care plan as indicated.

2. Have all data been validated, as needed?

❑ Yes. No action.   ❑ No. Validate with client (by interview and physical examination), significant others, or other professionals. Record validation (or failure to validate). Change care plan as indicated.

3. Have new data become available that require changes in the plan (eg., a different problem etiology, new goals/outcomes, new medical orders)?

❑ No. No action.   ❑ Yes. Record the new data in the progress notes; redefine problem, goals, nursing orders, as needed.

4. Has the patient's condition changed?

❑ No. No action.   ❑ Yes. Record data about present health status. Change care plan as indicated.

Move to a review of the diagnosis step.

Diagnosis Review

1. Is the diagnosis relevant and related to the data?

❑ Yes. No action.   ❑ No. Revise the diagnosis.

2. Is the diagnosis well supported by the data?

❑ Yes. No action.   ❑ No. Collect more data. Support or revise diagnosis.

3. Has the problem status changed (actual, potential, possible)?

❑ No. No action.   ❑ Yes. Relabel the problem.

4. Is the diagnosis stated clearly?

❑ Yes. No action.   No. Revise the diagnostic statement.

5. Does the etiology correctly reflect the factors contributing to the problem?

❑ Yes. No action.   ❑ No. Revise the etiology.

(continues)

Table 9–3   Evaluation Checklist *(continued)*

Instructions: Check the appropriate box and follow the associated instructions.

6. Is the problem one that can be treated primarily by nursing actions?

❑ Yes. No action. ❑ No. Label as collaborative and consult appropriate health professional.

7. Is the diagnosis specific and individualized to the patient?

❑ Yes. No action. ❑ No. Revise diagnosis. Revise outcomes and nursing orders as suggested by the new nursing diagnosis.

8. Does the problem (diagnosis) still exist?

❑ Yes. No action. ❑ No. Delete diagnosis and related outcomes and nursing orders.

Proceed to a review of client goals.

Planning Review: Outcomes

1. Have nursing diagnoses been added or revised?

❑ No. No action. ❑ Yes. Write new outcomes.

2. Are the outcomes realistic in terms of patient abilities and agency resources?

❑ Yes. No action. ❑ No. Revise outcomes.

3. Was sufficient time allowed for outcome achievement?

❑ Yes. No action. ❑ No. Revise time frame.

4. Do the outcomes address all aspects of the client's problem?

❑ Yes. No action. ❑ No. Write additional outcomes.

5. Do the expected outcomes, as written, demonstrate resolution of the problem specified in the nursing diagnosis?

❑ Yes. No action. ❑ No. Revise outcomes.

6. Have client priorities changed, or has the focus of care changed?

❑ No. No action. ❑ Yes. Revise outcomes.

7. Is the client in agreement with the goals?

❑ Yes. No action. ❑ No. Get client input. Write outcomes valued by the client.

Proceed to review of nursing orders

Table 9–3 Evaluation Checklist *(continued)*

Instructions: Check the appropriate box and follow the associated instructions.

Planning Review: Nursing Orders

1. Have nursing diagnoses or outcomes been added or revised in previous review steps?
   - ❏ No. No action.
   - ❏ Yes. Write new nursing orders.

2. Are the nursing orders clearly related to the stated patient outcomes?
   - ❏ Yes. No action.
   - No. Revise or develop new nursing orders.

3. Is the rationale sufficient to justify the use of the nursing order?
   - ❏ Yes. No action.
   - ❏ No. Revise or develop new nursing orders.

4. Are the nursing orders unclear or vague, so that other staff may have had questions about how to implement them?
   - ❏ No. No action.
   - ❏ Yes. Revise nursing orders. Add details to make more specific or individualized to the patient.

5. Do the nursing orders include instructions for timing of the activities?
   - ❏ Yes. No action.
   - ❏ No. Revise nursing orders—add times, schedules.

6. Was an order clearly and obviously ineffective?
   - ❏ No. No action.
   - ❏ Yes. Delete it.

7. Are the orders realistic in terms of staff and other resources?
   - ❏ Yes. No action.
   - ❏ No. Revise orders or obtain resources.

8. Have new resources become available that might enable you to change the goals or nursing orders?
   - ❏ No. No action.
   - ❏ Yes. Write new goals or nursing orders reflecting the new capabilities.

9. Do the nursing orders address all aspects of the client's health goals?
   - ❏ Yes. No action.
   - ❏ No. Add new nursing orders.

Proceed to review of implementation step.

Implementation: Review

1. Did the nurse get client input at each step in developing and implementing the plan?
   - ❏ Yes. No action.
   - ❏ No. Obtain client input, revise plan and implementation as needed.

2. Were the nursing interventions acceptable to the patient?
   - ❏ Yes. No action.
   - ❏ No. Consult patient; change nursing orders or implementation approach.

(continues)

Table 9–3 Evaluation Checklist *(continued)*

Instructions: Check the appropriate box and follow the associated instructions.

3. Did the nurse prepare the patient for implementation of the nursing order (eg, explain what the patient should expect or do)?

   ❏ Yes. No action. ❏ No. Continue same plan, but prepare patient before implementing. Reevaluate.

4. Did the nurse have adequate knowledge and skills to perform techniques and procedures correctly?

   ❏ Yes. No action. ❏ No. Continue same plan. Have someone else implement or help the nurse to acquire the needed knowledge or skills. If neither of these is possible, delete nursing order.

5. Did client or family comply with the therapeutic regimen? Were self-care activities performed correctly?

   ❏ Yes. No action. ❏ No. Reassess motivation, knowledge, and resources. Add outcomes and nursing orders aimed at teaching, motivating, and supporting patient in carrying out the regimen. Set time for reevaluation.

6. Did other staff members follow the nursing orders?

   ❏ Yes. No action. ❏ No. Implement the omitted nursing orders or ensure that others will do so. Set time for reevaluation. Find out why order was not carried out.

7. Was the plan of care implemented in a manner that communicated caring?

   ❏ Yes. No action. ❏ No. This is a problem that must be addressed by personal and staff development.

After making the necessary revisions to the care plan, implement the new plan and begin the nursing process cycle again.

nicate the idea when writing the diagnostic statement. Other nurses might therefore have focused their interventions inappropriately.

Planning Review: Outcomes If you have made additions to the data or changed the nursing diagnosis, you will need to revise the outcomes. If the data and the diagnostic statement are satisfactory as initially written, the reason for lack of outcome achievement may lie in the outcomes themselves. Perhaps they were unrealistic, or perhaps the target time was too soon.

Planning Review: Nursing Orders If you have revised the nursing diagnoses or desired outcomes, you will need to change the nursing orders as well. You may wish to revise them anyway for clarification or to add more effective strategies.

Implementation Review   If all sections of the nursing care plan appear to be satisfactory, perhaps the lack of outcome achievement is due to the manner in which the plan was implemented. To find out what went wrong in the implementation step, consult the progress notes, the client, significant others, and other caregivers.

■ REFLECTING CRITICALLY ABOUT EVALUATION

After you have reviewed each step of the nursing process (eg, using Table 9–3), you should also reflect on the thinking you used in evaluating the plan and the patient's health status. The following questions will guide your reflection (critical thinking standards are shown in parentheses):

1. (**Clarity**) Is my evaluation statement clear: Goal met + supporting data?
2. (**Accuracy**) Have I compared reassessment data to the goals on the care plan? Is the patient being honest about goal achievement, or is he trying to please?
3. (**Precision**) Is my evaluation statement precise, using patient statements and behaviors, rather than such statements as "Tolerated well"?
4. (**Relevance**) Did I collect reassessment data that relates to the stated goals?
5. (**Depth**) Am I missing anything? Have we covered all the bases? If interventions did not produce desired outcomes, do I need consultation?
6. (**Breadth**) How does the patient describe the outcomes/goal achievement?
7. (**Logic**) In what way did the interventions contribute to goal achievement? Could we have done better?
8. (**Significance**) Is there still a need for nursing care? Do we need to make a plan to prevent further problems?

Evaluation Errors

Probably the most common evaluation error is failure to perform systematic evaluation of patient outcomes. Many nurses are more action-oriented than analytic and reflective. It is relatively easy in the press of a busy day to make a plan and act; however, you may have to make determined efforts to find time to observe and record the client's responses to the actions. Remember that quality care is not guaranteed by simply implementing the nursing orders. Only when you evaluate client outcomes can you be assured that the care has met the client's needs.

Usually nurses do, in fact, observe the client's response, but they may not document it or consciously use it in an evaluation process that would enable them to modify interventions. You must be sure to document the evaluative statements so that other nurses will be able to judge the effectiveness of your interventions. Otherwise, they might continue with approaches that you have already discovered to be ineffective.

Another error occurs when a nurse uses irrelevant data to judge the level of goal achievement. Consider only data that are clearly related to the predicted outcome. Box 9–3 provides examples of both relevant and irrelevant data related to Mr. Rizzo's anxiety problem from Table 9–1 (on page 402).

Errors are also possible in judging the congruence between actual and predicted client outcomes; actual outcomes may be measured inaccurately, or data may be incomplete. In the example of Table 9–1, if the nurse observed Sam Rizzo only during periods when he was not dyspneic, she might erroneously conclude that his anxiety was relieved.

Ethical Considerations

The moral principle of **beneficence** holds that we ought to do good things for other people, that is, benefit them. A nurse who holds the hand of a dying patient honors this principle. The principle of **nonmaleficence** holds that we should not harm others. For example, a nurse upholds this principle when she withholds morphine from a client whose respirations are already depressed. You can think of these principles as being on a continuum, with the duty to do no harm taking precedence over the other duties. It is easy to see how the first situation is a stronger duty than the last one.

Quality assurance evaluation (to be discussed on pp. 417–420) and evaluation of client progress fulfill the obligation of beneficence by enabling nurses to improve the quality of care they deliver. Quality assurance can also produce changes in the total healthcare system and improve communication and collaboration between healthcare disciplines. The ANA code of ethics (1985) in Appendix A includes at least four items that imply that evaluating care is a nursing responsibility:

BOX 9–3

Relevant and Irrelevant Data: Sam Rizzo

Relevant data   When dyspneic, states "What should I do? Can you help me?"

Face relaxed; no skeletal muscle tension except during episodes of dyspnea.

States, "I feel better since you explained about the fire drill. I thought there was a real fire."

States, "I understand about the hospital routines and the breathing treatments. Those things really aren't causing any anxiety."

Irrelevant data   Temperature 98.6° F.

Watching television except when wife is here.

Item 4. The nurse assumes responsibility and accountability for individual nursing judgments and actions.

Item 8. The nurse participates in the profession's efforts to establish, implement, and improve standards of nursing.

Item 9. The nurse participates in the profession's efforts to establish and maintain conditions of employment conducive to high-quality nursing care.

Item 11. The nurse collaborates with members of the health professions and other citizens in promoting community and national efforts to meet the health needs of the public.

Cultural and Spiritual Considerations

When desired outcomes have not been achieved, review the client's cultural values, beliefs, and practices to determine what effect they may have had. You must consider these factors in addition to other physiologic, psychologic, social, and developmental factors when you review the nursing process and revise the treatment plan. Complete evaluation includes evaluating your own ability to provide culturally competent care and to determine whether you need to improve your ability to work with clients from culturally diverse backgrounds.

When evaluating whether clients have accomplished spiritual goals, you will need skill in observation, helping relationships, and communication. You will need to observe the client when he is alone and when he is interacting with others, and listen to what the client says and does not say. The following are characteristics that indicate spiritual well-being and achievement of spiritual goals: a sense of inner peace, compassion for others, reverence for life, gratitude, appreciation of unity and diversity, humor, wisdom, generosity, ability to transcend the self, and the capacity for unconditional love (Carson 1989).

Some indicators for the NOC (2000, p. 407) outcome of Spiritual Well-Being are as follows:

- Expressions of faith, hope, meaning and purpose in life, serenity, love, or forgiveness
- Mystical experiences
- Prayer, worship, or participation in spiritual rites and passages
- Interaction with spiritual leaders
- Meditation or spiritual reading
- Connectedness with others to share thoughts, feelings, and beliefs

■ QUALITY ASSURANCE/IMPROVEMENT

In addition to evaluating goal achievement for individual patients, nurses are involved in evaluating and improving the overall quality of care for groups of patients (eg, in a hospital). Government programs (eg, Medicare), regulatory agencies (eg, The Joint Commission for Accreditation of Healthcare Organizations), and state boards of nursing require institutions to provide documentation that nursing care is being given according to nursing standards. Various programs exist for this purpose, including quality assurance (QA), quality improvement (QI), continuous quality improvement (CQI), total quality management (TQI), and persistent quality improvement (PQI). While focuses and approaches may vary, all such programs involve the evaluation of care provided in the agency. Table 9–4 compares quality assurance and nursing process evaluation.

Quality assurance programs make use of **peer review**, which means that members of the profession delivering the care develop and implement the process for evaluating that care. This usually involves a **nursing audit**, in which patient records are reviewed for data about nursing competence. A committee establishes standards of care (eg, for safety measures, documentation, preoperative teaching), and charts are randomly selected and reviewed to compare nursing activities against these standards.

Computerized Records and Standardized Nursing Languages

In agencies with computerized patient records, the laborious task of manual chart audits can be avoided; information is simply retrieved in the form of reports. When records systems make use of standardized nursing languages (ie, NANDA, NIC, NOC), specific data about nursing care can be retrieved from the database. This means that data about individual patients can be combined to create data about groups of patients (eg, all the patients on a unit). Such data can be used to support unit, organizational, and

Table 9–4   Comparison of Quality Assurance and Nursing Process Evaluation

	Nursing Quality Assurance	The Nursing Process
Scope of evaluation	Groups of clients	Individual clients
Subject of evaluation	Overall quality of care	1. Progress toward achieving client outcomes. 2. Review of nursing care plan.
Type of evaluation	Structure, process, outcome	1. Outcome evaluation of patient progress 2. Process evaluation of nursing care plan
Responsibility for evaluation	Chief nurse in the institution	Nurse caring for client

national policy decisions and to compare the care given in different institutions.

Types of QA Evaluation

Quality assurance requires evaluation of three components of care: structure, process, and outcome (see Table 9–5). Each type of evaluation requires different criteria and methods, and each has a different focus. All three must be considered because they work together to effect care.

Structure evaluation focuses on the setting in which care is given. It asks the question, What effect do environmental and organizational characteristics have on the quality of care? To answer that question, it uses information about policies, procedures, fiscal resources, facilities, equipment, and the number and qualifications of personnel. Examples of criteria that might be written for structure evaluation include:

- Call light is within reach
- Narcotics are kept in double-locked cabinet
- Policies for medication errors are written and easily accessible

Table 9–5 Comparison of Structure, Process, and Outcome Evaluation

Aspect of Care	Focus	Criterion Examples
Structure	Setting	Exit signs are clearly visible. A resuscitation cart will be housed on each unit. There is a family waiting room on each floor.
Process	Caregiver activities	Initial interview is completed within 8 hours after admission of client. Client responses to medications are charted. Patients will receive oral hygiene on each shift. Nurse introduces self to client before giving care.
Outcome	Patient responses	B/P < 140/90 at all times. Walks to bathroom unsupported by third day. Abdomen will be soft and nontender by day 5.
	Grouped patient responses	Temperature < 100° F 24 h after surgery (*Expected compliance = 90%*) Patient will not fall during hospital stay (*Expected compliance = 95%*)

Although adequate staff and resources do not guarantee high-quality care, they are certainly important factors. Without them, it is difficult to meet process and outcome criteria.

Process evaluation focuses on how the care was given—on the activities of the nurses. It answers questions such as: Is the care relevant to the patient's needs? Is the care appropriate, complete, and timely? The ANA *Standards of Clinical Nursing Practice* (1998) are examples of process standards. Other examples include:

- Checks client's identification band before giving medication
- Explains procedures (eg, catheterization) before implementing
- Medications are administered on time

Of course, even perfect processes do not guarantee good outcomes. For example, a patient's health or the agency infection rate may become worse no matter how expertly nurses perform. But overall, good nursing care should improve patient and agency outcomes.

Outcome evaluation focuses on demonstrable changes in client's health status as a result of care. Currently, outcomes evaluation is extremely important, as accreditation and certification agencies and managed care companies are demanding outcomes data. For example, the Health Care Financing Adminstration (HCFA) requires home health agencies to use their "OASIS" tool to measure and report changes in patient status at various times (Raffa 1997). In an effort to standardize patient outcomes that are sensitive to nursing care, the ANA developed a nursing care "report card" for use by healthcare organizations. It includes the following outcome measures: mortality rate, length of stay, adverse incidents, complications, and patient satisfaction with nursing care (ANA 1995).

For agency evaluation, criteria are written in terms of client responses or health states, just as they are for evaluation of individual client progress. In addition, for QA evaluation the criterion states the percent of clients expected to have the outcome when nursing care is satisfactory.

EXAMPLE: Skin over bony prominences is intact and free from redness. *Expected compliance: 100%*

Taken alone, this means that you would expect that with good care, no clients in the institution will develop redness over a bony prominence. However, that fails to consider the effect of variables other than nursing care—some clients' nutritional and mobility status may be so compromised that no amount of care could prevent redness. For example, a process evaluation for a client might show that a plan to turn the client hourly was written and implemented; this would indicate that nursing care was adequate even though the outcome was poor. A structure evaluation might also show that the nursing unit was chronically understaffed, which would validate a process evaluation that reveals that the client often went for more than 2 hours without being repositioned. That would explain the reason for the poor outcome and processes.

It is not always easy to demonstrate the relationship between nursing care and client outcomes. Medical, or disease-related, outcomes are easy to observe. For instance, a temperature of 98.6° F and a white blood cell count of 8,000 provide good evidence that there is no infection, and it is easy to attribute these results to the effects of the antibiotic that was prescribed. The nursing perspective is more holistic, so it is sometimes difficult even to define the outcomes desired. Emotional, social, or spiritual responses, for instance, are hard to write in measurable terms. It is also difficult to measure the degree to which the outcome was caused by the nursing care, because many variables contribute to improvement (or deterioration) in the client's health (eg, the nature of the client's illness, medical interventions, quality of nursing care, availability of resources, client motivation, and family participation).

However, the ANA (1997) has reported a study demonstrating nursing's impact on selected patient outcomes. It included the following findings:

- Higher nurse staffing was associated with shorter patient lengths of stay.
- A high ratio of RNs to non-RNs was related to patients' having fewer preventable conditions (eg, pressure ulcers, pneumonia, postoperative infections, and urinary tract infections).

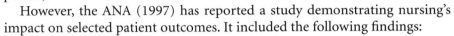

THINKING POINT

In the past 3 months, several medication errors have been made on your nursing unit. The unit has instituted some policies and procedures to improve the safety of this task. Develop criteria to use to evaluate whether this practice problem has been solved. Include criteria to measure structure, process, and outcomes. To begin, answer these questions:

- What is the purpose of the evaluation?
- What is being evaluated; what is the function of the "thing" being evaluated?
- What different points of view may exist?

A Procedure for Quality-Assurance Evaluation

The quality-assurance process is similar to the nursing process; it involves data collection, comparison of data to criteria, identification of problems, generation and implementation of solutions, and reevaluation. It is different in that it focuses on nurses and institutions rather than patients and is concerned with groups of clients, rather than individuals. The following steps are included in the quality-assurance models of most organizations:

1. *Decide the topic to be evaluated.* The topic might be the care for a group of clients with a particular medical diagnosis, care for all clients in a hospital, or record keeping on a nursing unit.

2. *Identify standards of care.* Determine whether structure, process, or outcome standards are appropriate. Recall that standards are broad guidelines and are not measurable or useful in data collection. Therefore, this step is sometimes omitted and only the criteria are actually written.

3. *Establish criteria* for measuring the standards of care. Process and outcome criteria are specific, observable characteristics that describe the desired behaviors of the nurse or client.

4. *Determine expected compliance or performance levels.* A performance level is the percentage of times you would expect the criterion to be met. This may vary from 0% to 100%, depending on how the criterion is stated. For example, you might expect that 95% of the time, an admission database would be completed within 4 hours after the client was admitted.

5. *Collect data related to the criteria.* Data may be obtained from client interviews, chart audits, direct observation of nursing activities, questionnaires, or special evaluation tools, depending on the criterion being evaluated.

6. *Analyze the data.* Identify discrepancies between the data and the criteria. Determine reasons for the discrepancies, using information about structures, processes, and outcomes. Identify problems. In the example in Item 4, if fewer than 95% of the admission databases were completed in the specified time, it would be important to find out why this is happening.

7. *Generate solutions for correcting discrepancies and solving problems.* For instance, more in-service education may be needed for nurses, or perhaps the staffing pattern should be changed, or a new data collection form used.

8. *Implement the solutions.* The purpose of evaluation is to maintain the quality of care being delivered. Once problems have been identified, action must be taken to see that they do not recur.

9. *Reevaluate* to determine if the solutions were effective.

QA enables nursing to demonstrate accountability to society for the quality of its services. Consumers, administrators, and bureaucrats do not always clearly see the relationship between good nursing care and improved patient outcomes. Professional survival requires that nurses demonstrate this link. Additionally, the present payment systems encourage agencies to keep patients for as short a time as possible, raising both professional and consumer concerns about quality. Providing adequate care is difficult under these circumstances, and nurses are challenged to monitor and promote good care.

■ SUMMARY

Evaluation

- is a deliberate, systematic process in which the quality, value, or worth of something is determined by comparing it to previously identified criteria or standards.
- considers *structure* (focusing on the setting in which care is given), *process* (focusing on nursing activities), and *outcomes* (focusing on the changes in client health status that result from nursing care).
- in nursing process, is a planned, ongoing, deliberate activity in which the nurse, client, significant others, and other healthcare professionals determine the client's progress toward goal achievement and the effectiveness of the nursing care plan.
- does not end the nursing process, because the information it provides is used to begin another cycle.
- involves five steps: (1) *review* of the stated client goals or predicted outcomes, (2) *collection* of data about the client's responses to nursing interventions, (3) *comparison* of actual client outcomes to the predicted outcomes and drawing a conclusion about whether the goals have been met, (4) *recording* of evaluative statements, and (5) *relating* the nursing interventions to the client outcomes.
- requires the nurse to consider all variables, including cultural and spiritual, that may have influenced goal achievement and to modify the care plan as needed.

Quality-assurance evaluation

- is an ongoing, systematic process designed to evaluate and promote excellence in healthcare.
- is usually concerned with the care given to groups of clients.
- frequently refers to evaluation of the level of care provided in an agency; it may be as limited in scope as an evaluation of the performance of one nurse or as broad as the evaluation of the overall quality of care in an entire country.
- commonly uses the methods of retrospective chart audit and peer review.
- reflects the moral principles of beneficence and nonmaleficence.

EVALUATION—THINKING QUICK-CHECK

- ❏ Do the data indicate goal achievement?
- ❏ Which nursing interventions did or did not contribute to goal achievement?
- ❏ Have I reexamined each step of the nursing process?
- ❏ Did I get patient input during evaluation?

Nursing Process Practice

1. Place a check mark (✓) beside the criteria that are specific, measurable, or observable.

   a. _____ The nurse gives safe care.

   b. _____ Medications are recorded at the time they are given.

   c. _____ Every patient will have an arm band with name and hospital number.

   d. _____ Temperature will be less than 100.1° F during entire stay.

   e. _____ Each unit will have an adequate number of wheelchairs.

   f. _____ Data collection is systematic.

2. Match the data source to the letter of the type of evaluation for which it would be used.

   a. Structure

   b. Process

   c. Outcome

   1. _____ Charts (patient records)

   2. _____ Procedure manuals

   3. _____ Verbal data from the client

   4. _____ Observation of the client (eg, VS)

   5. _____ Observation of nursing activities

   6. _____ Staff orientation plans

   7. _____ Most performance evaluation forms

   8. _____ System for measuring client acuity

3. Match the criterion (or question) to the letter of the type of evaluation for which it would be used.

   a. Structure

   b. Process

   c. Outcome

   1. _____ Client will state he is free from pain.

   2. _____ The nurse washes her hands before drawing up the medication.

   3. _____ How many wheelchairs are kept on the unit?

   4. _____ Client's B/P will be < 130/90 mm Hg.

   5. _____ All direct caregivers are registered nurses.

   6. _____ Bed is in low position with wheels locked.

   7. _____ Are all monitors in working order?

4. Your client has a nursing diagnosis of Altered Oral Mucous Membrane r/t prolonged NPO and mouth breathing. Some of the nursing orders follow:

1. Instruct client to rinse mouth as needed with a solution of 25% acetic acid and water.

2. Reinforce importance of oral hygiene after meals and as needed.

3. Remind client to breathe through nose as much as possible.

4. Lubricate lips with mineral oil.

    a. Write at least two outcome criteria you could use to determine whether this problem has been resolved.

    b. State how you would obtain the data needed to determine if each criterion has been met (eg, interview the patient, etc.)

CASE STUDY: Refer to the following case study for Exercises 5 and 6.

Ms. Nancy Atwell is a 32-year-old unmarried teacher who was diagnosed with rheumatoid arthritis 4 years ago. This change has made her knees painful and has limited the motion and weight-bearing ability of the knee joints themselves. She has recently been diagnosed with uterine cancer, and now enters the hospital to undergo a hysterectomy. On her previous admission for treatment of her arthritis, she had been quiet, withdrawn, and extremely concerned for her privacy. Now she seems more outgoing and less overtly concerned about privacy. When questioned, Ms. Atwell states that she has had no previous surgical experience, but denies feeling nervous about the operation. Her preoperative orders follow:

1. S. S. enema at 0900
2. Nembutal 100 mg p.o. at HS
3. NPO
4. Pre-op med: Demerol 75 mg IM at 1 PM.

---

5. The nurse identified for Ms. Atwell a diagnosis of "Risk for Anxiety r/t lack of knowledge of effects and procedure of hysterectomy." Her goal is to find out whether Ms. Atwell is anxious and if she is, to relieve her anxiety. (The first answer is provided for you.)

   a. Give an example of a verbal cue that would indicate achievement of this objective.

      Ms. Atwell states, "I'm confident everything will go all right. I certainly don't have any experience with this kind of thing, but I know you will tell me what I need to know. I feel pretty relaxed, actually."

   b. Give an example of a nonverbal cue that would indicate achievement of this objective.

   c. Give an example of a verbal cue that would indicate the objective has not been achieved.

   d. Give an example of a nonverbal cue that would indicate the objective has not been achieved.

6. The following nursing diagnoses and outcomes appear on Ms. Atwell's care plan. Using the new data charted by the nurse after implementing care for each diagnosis, write an evaluative statement for each diagnosis.

Nursing Diagnosis	Outcomes	New Data (Progress Notes)
Risk for Anxiety r/t lack of knowledge of effects and procedure of hysterectomy	Will state not anxious about effects of surgery	Pre-op teaching done. States understanding of surgical procedure.
	Will show no physical signs of anxiety.	Says she expects to have some post-op pain, but is sure she can manage with meds. No facial tension, hands folded loosely in lap while talking.
Evaluate statement for care plan:		

Nursing Diagnosis	Outcomes	New Data (Progress Notes)
Risk for Grief r/t loss of childbearing ability 2° hysterectomy	Will express her feelings about sterility/desire for children, before discharge.	During pre-op teaching, ct. was told she would not have periods after her hysterectomy and would not be able to become pregnant. She stated "Periods are a nuisance anyway," but did not comment further.
Evaluative statement for care plan:		

Nursing Diagnosis	Outcomes	New Data (Progress Notes)
Risk for Noncompliance with NPO order r/t lack of understanding of importance	Will state reasons for remaining NPO for OR after pre-op teaching. Will remain NPO after midnight.	9 PM—Pre-op teaching done. States relationship of NPO to anesthesia, aspiration, etc. this evening. 11:50 PM—Water pitcher removed; NPO sign up. 2:30 AM—Ct. up to bathroom, drinking water from cupped hands. Stated she forgot about drinking restriction and would not drink any more.
Evaluative statement for care plan:		

7. For the three nursing diagnoses in Exercise 6, draw a line through parts of the care plan that could be discontinued after evaluation.

8. The nursing diagnosis is "Risk for Impaired Skin Integrity: Dermal Ulcer r/t inability to move about in bed and poor nutritional status." The desired outcome is, "Skin integrity will be maintained." The nurse notes that the client's skin is intact, with no redness over bony prominences, and concludes that the goal has been met. Circle the letter of the correct action. The nurse should

   a. decide the problem no longer exists, document that the outcome was achieved, and discontinue the nursing care for that outcome.

   b. decide that the problem still exists even though the outcome was achieved, and continue the same nursing interventions.

Critical Thinking Practice: Judging and Evaluating

Review "Judging and Evaluating," Chapter 2, pages 55–56. Recall that judgments are evaluations of facts/information that reflect some criteria, such as our values. When developing evaluative criteria, you should consider: (a) the purpose of the evaluation, (b) the function of the thing being evaluated, and (c) different points of view that may exist. Evaluation criteria should be: (a) made explicit, (b) stated clearly, and (c) applied consistently.

Evaluation statements include goal status (met/not met) and the data (evidence) to support that conclusion. Critical thinkers realize that not everything offered as evidence should be accepted. Data can be complete or incomplete, relevant or irrelevant. Statements of "fact" can be true, questionable, or false. Use the following questions as criteria for evaluating reassessment data and facts.

- What data do I have to show that the goal was met?
- Are the data complete?
- Are there enough data to support my conclusion?
- Where did I get the data; is the source reliable?
- How do I know the data are correct?
- What other data might exist that could change my conclusion?

Learning the Skill

Mary James, age 70 years, lives alone. Today she seems drowsy and is having a little trouble concentrating. She has been type 1 diabetic for many years, and her blood glucose is well controlled, usually between 100 and 200 mg/dL. She wears thick glasses, is frail, and walks with a walker. She has been managing her diabetes on her own, including insulin injections and glucose monitoring, with weekly visits from a home health nurse. Ms. James performs a fingerstick glucose test before meals and at bedtime and keeps a daily record of the results. A goal on her care plan reads: "Maintains blood glucose at 80–200 mg/dL before meals and at bedtime (fingerstick)." You see that all her diary entries for this week are between 60 and 80 mg/dL. These readings are lower than usual for Ms. James. The entries are scribbled and hard to read, but they are all there. Should you conclude that the goal has been met this week?

1. What data do you have to show that the goal was met?

2. Are the data complete?

3. Are there enough data to support your conclusion?

4. Where did you get the data?

5. Is the source reliable (are the data accurate)? Explain your reasoning.

6. What are some things that may have caused her diary entries to be inaccurate?

7. How could you find out if Ms. James' data are accurate?

8. At this point, would you conclude that the goal has been met?

9. What other data might you obtain to help you decide if the data are accurate and the goal has been met?

Now, imagine that you have calibrated the glucose monitor. You find that it is accurate and you can conclude that Ms. James' diary contains accurate information. It is just before lunchtime, and you perform a fingerstick; her blood glucose level is 360 mg/dL.

10. Is the goal being met today? Explain.

11. Does that necessarily mean that Ms. James' diary entries were incorrect? Explain.

12. Now that you have determined that the glucose monitor is working properly, what are some possible explanations for the discrepancy between your readings and those of Ms. James?

13. What must you conclude about the goal status *during the past week*?

14. In light of the preceding possibilities, would you keep this same goal? Why?

15. What goals and nursing orders should you add to her care plan? Consider the following:

   a. Should you increase the frequency of your visits?

   b. What assessments do you need to make in the next several days in order to evaluate her ability to monitor and regulate her blood glucose?

Applying the Skill

Your patient is a 78-year-old woman who had a total hip replacement 48 hours ago. She is receiving morphine via a PCA pump for pain. She has been drowsy and disoriented at times since the surgery. The following collaborative problems and nursing diagnoses appear on her critical pathway, along with their desired outcomes. Use the questions on page 426 to evaluate the associated data and goal achievement.

1. *Potential Complication of Surgery and Immobility: Thrombophlebitis*

   Goal: Will develop thrombophlebitis

   Your Evaluation Data: The patient is wearing antiembolism stockings to improve her peripheral circulation. When you remove and replace them, you note that there is no redness or swelling in her legs; she says they are not tender.

A. Are there enough data to conclude that the goal is being met? If not, explain.

B. If you conclude "goal met," should you remove this collaborative problem from the care plan? Why or why not?

2. *Potential Complication of Foley Catheter: urinary tract infection.*

Goal: No signs/symptoms of UTI (eg, no burning, frequency, or foul urine odor; temperature WNL)

Your Evaluation Data: She had a Foley catheter postoperatively; you remove it at noon. At 3:30 PM, the nursing assistant tells you that the patient has voided 200 cc and that the patient's temperature is 98.9° F.

A. Are there enough data to conclude that the goal is being met? If not, explain.

B. If you conclude "goal met," should you remove this collaborative problem from the care plan? Why or why not?

3. *Risk for Constipation r/t immobility, decreased fluid intake, and morphine.*

Goal 1: Will have bowel sounds in all 4 quadrants by 36 hours postoperatively.

Goal 2: Will pass soft, formed stool by day 3 postoperatively.

Your Evaluation Data: She is taking a full liquid diet with no nausea or vomiting. She has occasional bowel sounds in all 4 quadrants; she states she is not passing flatus. She says, "I had a bowel movement yesterday"; however information in shift report and in the chart indicate "no B.M.," and the nursing assistant tells you that the patient has not had a B.M. today.

A. Are there enough data to conclude that the goal is being met? If not, explain.

B. If you conclude "goal met," should you remove this collaborative problem from the care plan? Why or why not?

CASE STUDY: Applying Nursing Process and Critical Thinking

Carla Jackson, a 55-year-old widow, has come to the clinic for her annual check-up and mammogram. Her history indicates that she has not worked outside the home in over 30 years. She tells the nurse that since the death of her husband a few months ago she has lost interest in her usual physical activities. She no longer attends her swimming and Yoga classes, and does not see the couples she and her husband had as mutual friends. She says she is bored, depressed, and "I hate how I'm beginning to look." She is 5'2" tall and weighs 160 lb. She says, "I've gained 15 lb just in the last 2 months!" She says that her eating habits have changed: "It doesn't seem worth the trouble to cook a meal now. I just snack on whatever is handy—chips, cookies, ice cream. If I crave 'real' food, I buy a fast-food 'burger or something.'" Ms. Jackson's lab results are all normal. She asks the nurse to help her find a way to lose weight. The nurse diagnoses a nutrition problem and together they make the following plan:

Nursing Diagnosis: *Altered Nutrition: More than Body Requirements r/t excess calorie intake and decreased activity expenditure.*

Goals/Desired Outcomes	Nursing Interventions & Activities

Weight Control (NOC #1612).
1. Maintains optimal daily caloric intake
2. Develops an exercise plan that gradually engages her in 30 minutes of daily exercise (by next appointment, in 1 month)
3. Identifies eating habits that contribute to weight gain by day 2.
	1. Weight Reduction Assistance (NIC #1280)
	  a. Determine eating patterns by having pt. keep a diary of what, when, and where she eats.
	  b. Help pt. to develop a daily meal plan with a well-balanced diet, reduced calories, and reduced fat.
	
	2. Nutritional Counseling (NIC #5246)
	  a. Use accepted nutritional standards to assist Ms. Jackson to evaluate the adequency of her dietary intake.
	  b. Discuss food likes and dislikes
	
	3. Behavior Modification (NIC #4360)
	  a. Identify the specific behaviors to be changed.
	  b. Have pt. choose rewards that are meaningful to her, for motivation to follow her plans.

1. Has the nurse omitted any important nursing diagnoses (refer to a nursing diagnosis handbook to check Ms. Jackson's defining characteristics)?

2. What do you think about the nursing diagnosis of Altered Nutrition?

3. How could you make it more descriptive of Ms. Jackson's situation?

4. How could the desired outcomes for Weight Control be improved? When you are deciding the desired amount of weekly weight loss, which of the following principles is *essential* to apply?

   a. Goal setting provides motivation, which is essential for a successful weight-loss program.

   b. A combined plan of calorie reduction and exercise can enhance weight loss, because exercise increases calorie utilization.

   c. Intake must be reduced by 500 calories to obtain a 1 lb/week weight loss.

   d. Overweight people are often nutritionally deprived.

5. Look at Nursing Activity 1b. Which of the preceding principles provides the rationale for this nursing activity?

6. What referrals might be helpful for the nurse to make?

When Ms. Jackson comes to the clinic the following month, she has lost 3 lbs. She brings with her a dietary log. Using nutritional standards to evaluate her diet, she and the nurse determine that she has been planning well-balanced, nutritionally sound, meals. She verbalizes awareness that she feels hungry, and eats, when she is bored and depressed—"but I'm not keeping junk food in the house now, so when I can't resist snacking, at least it is more nutritious food now." She says she has been walking about 20 minutes each day.

7. Discuss the extent to which each of the desired outcomes has been met.

8. Which of the planned nursing activities does the nurse still need to implement at this visit? Why?

9. Ms. Jackson says, "I realize that a lot of my snacking is done while I watch TV. This is one of the behaviors I need to change." Consider this principle: It is easier to increase (or add) a behavior than to decrease (or stop) one.

   a. What specific suggestions can you make, using this principle, to help her change her snacking behavior?

   b. What has Ms. Jackson already done that utilizes this principle?

10. Ms. Jackson's specific plans are to (a) decrease her calorie intake by 500 calories per day, (b) engage in 30 minutes of exercise a day, (c) keep a food diary, and (d) stop snacking in front of the TV. Try to imagine you are Ms. Jackson.

a. How would you reward yourself for modifying these behaviors? Indicate which behaviors you would reward, how often you would reward yourself, and with what (eg, Would you reward yourself every day you decreased your intake by 500 calories, or only after you do it every day for a week?)

b. Explain why each of these rewards would be meaningful to you.

■ SELECTED REFERENCES

American Nurses Association (1985). *Code for Nurses with Interpretive Statements.* Kansas City, MO: ANA.

American Nurses Association (1995). *Nursing report card for acute care.* Washington, DC: ANA.

American Nurses Association (1997). *Implementing nursing's report card. A study of RN staffing, length of stay and patient outcomes.* Washington, DC: Author.

American Nurses Association (1998). *Standards of Clinical Nursing Practice.* 2nd ed. Washington, DC: Author.

Carson, V. B. (1989). *Spiritual dimensions of nursing practice.* Philadelphia: W. B. Saunders.

Dianis, N. L. and C. Cummings (1998). An interdisciplinary approach to process performance improvement. *Nurs Care Quality* 12(4):49–59.

Gordon, M., C. P. Murphy, D. Candee, et al (1994). Clinical judgment: an integrated model. *Advan Nurs Sci* 16(4):55–70.

Irvine, D., S. Sidani, L. M. Hall (1998). Linking outcomes to nurses' roles in health care. *Nurs Econ* 16(2):58–64, 87.

Johnson, M., M. Maas, S. Moorhead (2000). *Nursing Outcomes Classification.* 2nd ed. St. Louis: Mosby.

Keys, P. (1998). The betrayal of the Total Quality Movement in Western management: managed health care and provider stress. *Fam Commun Health* 21(2):1–19.

London, M. R. and C. D. Klug (1998). A framework for improving quality: using project study teams, Providence Health System tackles problem areas. *Health Progress* 79(2): 56–60.

Maas, M. L., C. Delaney, D. Huber (1999). Contextual variables and assessment of the outcome effects of nursing interventions. *Outcomes Manage Nurs Prac* 3(1):4–6.

McCormick, K. A. (1998). New tools—new models to integrate outcomes into quality measurement. *Semin Nurse Managers* 6(3):119–125.

McGourthy, R. J. (1999). Omaha and OASIS: a comparative study of outcomes in patients with chronic obstructive pulmonary disease. *Home Care Provider* 4(1):21–25.

Parlocha, P. K. and S. B. Henry (1998). The usefulness of the Georgetown Home Health Care Classification System for coding patient problems and nursing interventions in psychiatric home care. *Computers in Nursing* 16(1):45–52.

Raffa, C. J. (1997). Proposed conditions of participation shift from process to patient. *Home Healthcare Today* 3(3):10–11.

Saba, B. K. (1997). Why the Home Health Care Classification is a recognized nursing nomenclature. *Computers in Nursing* 15(2):569–576.

Stonestreet, J. S. and S. S. Prevost (1997). A focused strategic plan for outcomes evaluation. *Nurs Clin North Amer* 32(3):615–631.

Strickland, O. L. (1997). Outcomes measurement and management: challenges in measuring patient outcomes. *Nurs Clin North Amer* 32(3):495–512.

Yancey, R., B. A. Given, N. J. White, et al (1998). Computerized documentation for a rural nursing intervention project. *Computers in Nursing* 16(5):275–284.

10

Creating a Care Plan

Learning Outcomes

On completing this chapter, you should be able to do the following:

- Describe the content of a comprehensive patient care plan.
- Compare and contrast standardized and individually written care plans.
- Explain how critical pathways, model care plans, standards of care, protocols, and policies are used in creating a patient care plan.
- Compare and contrast individualized nursing care plans with multidisciplinary care plans or critical pathways.
- List guidelines for writing patient care plans.
- Explain how a well-written care plan supports two conventional ethical principles of nursing.
- Describe the steps necessary in using the nursing process to develop a comprehensive patient care plan.

■ INTRODUCTION

Chapters 3 through 9 presented the six phases of the nursing process and illustrated how each step is applied, using nursing models as frameworks for collecting, organizing, and analyzing data. The nursing process phases are summarized for you in Figure 10–2.

This chapter describes each component of a comprehensive care plan. The Luisa Sanchez case, begun in Chapter 3, is used to demonstrate how to create a comprehensive care plan by combining standardized (preprinted) and individually written care plans. And finally, a step-by-step Care Planning Guide summarizes how the nursing process is used to create care plans.

Most healthcare organizations (eg, hospitals) and regulating bodies (eg, the Joint Commission for Accrediting Healthcare Organizations) require evidence of care planning. However, the care plan may not be found in one place. For example, the nursing assessment may be in one place, a critical pathway with outcomes and interventions in another, medical orders in another, and an individualized nursing diagnosis care plan in another. Sometimes an individualized plan can be found only in the progress notes.

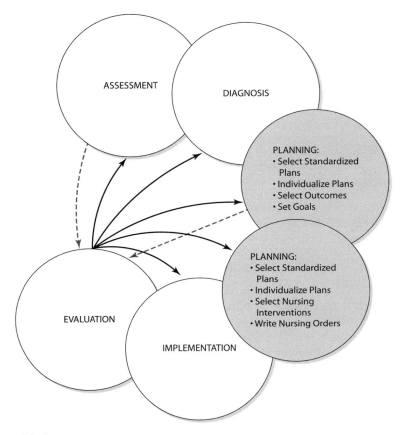

Figure 10–1
Planning: Creating a Care Plan.

■ COMPREHENSIVE CARE PLANS

Nurses use the term *care plan* in two ways: (1) when referring to the outcomes and nursing orders for a single problem or nursing diagnosis, and (2) when referring to the total plan of care for a patient. To avoid confusion, this text uses **nursing diagnosis care plan** for the first meaning and **comprehensive care plan** for the second. A **comprehensive care plan** is made up of several different documents that cover all aspects of the care needed by the patient. Any nurse, even one who does not know the patient, should be able to find in the plan the instructions needed to provide competent care. The plan may consist of a combination of preprinted and hand-written documents, including (1) a brief patient profile, (2) instructions for meeting basic care needs, (3) nursing responsibilities for the medical plan, and (4) the care plan for the patient's identified nursing diagnoses and collaborative problems. Many care plans also include special sections for discharge and teaching plans. Figure 10–3 illustrates the components of a comprehensive care plan.

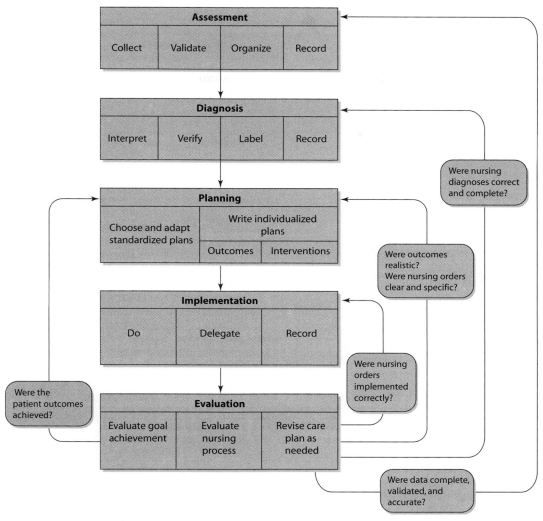

Figure 10–2
The Interdependent Steps of the Nursing Process

Client Profile

The client profile includes the client's name, age, admitting diagnosis, support people, and other pertinent personal or demographic data. This should be a brief summary, available at a glance, to give a quick overview of the client. On a computer care plan (see Figure 10–12 on page 449), some profile data appears at the top of each page. The Kardex (Figure 10–4) shows Luisa Sanchez's profile data, taken from Figure 3–2 in Chapter 3. This profile data is grouped in a section at the bottom of the Kardex. Notice that even if the nurse is not acquainted with Mrs. Sanchez, she can quickly find out how to

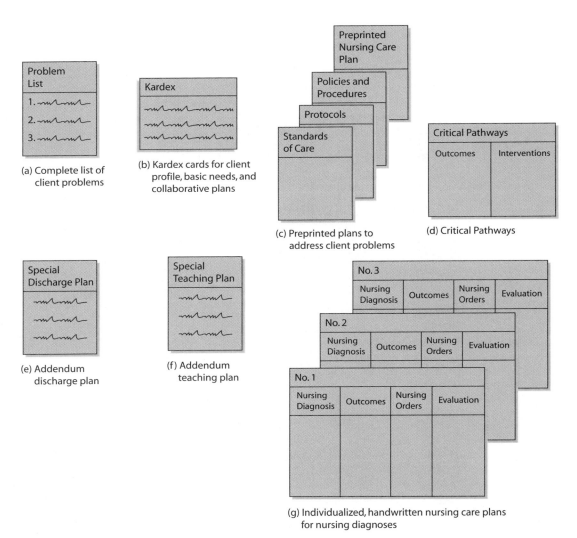

Figure 10–3
Components of a Comprehensive Care Plan

reach Mr. Sanchez in case of an emergency. She can also see the date and type of surgery, as well as the physician to call if she needs medical orders.

Instructions for Meeting Basic Needs

Regardless of the client's nursing diagnoses, the nurse must know what routine assistance is needed for hygiene, nutrition, elimination, and other basic needs. Most comprehensive care plans have a separate section for these instructions, often on a Kardex or basic care flowsheet, where they can be found quickly and conveniently. From Figure 10–4, the nurse can quickly

SHAWNEE MISSION MEDICAL CENTER

Date ord.	Radiology	Date Sch	DONE	Date ord.	Laboratory	Date Sch	DONE	Date ord.	Special Procedures	Date Sch	DONE
4/16/96	Chest X ray PA + lateral	4/16	✔	4/16	Blood Culture	4/16	✔	4/16	C+S Sputum		✔
				4/16	urine specific gravity	4/16	✔	4/16	24-hr urine		
				4/16	Blood gases	4/16	✔				
				4/16	serum Electrolytes	4/16	✔				
				4/16	CBC with diff.	4/16	✔				

Ancillary Consults

Daily Tests

Daily Weight

Diet: Clear liquid, then as tol.

Food Allergies: none

Hold:

Feeding/Fluids

☒ Self
☐ Assist
☐ Feeder
☒ Force 3,000 ml/day
☐ Restrict c̄ IV

	meal	Ext	IV
7-3			
3-11			
11-7			

☒ I&O
☒ IV O₃ LR, 100/hr
☐ Other_____

Safety Measures

☐ Siderails
☐ Restraints
☐ Other_____

Activities

☐ Bedrest
☒ BRP
☐ Dangle
☒ Chair
☐ Commode
☐ Up ad Lib
☐ Turn
☐ Ambulate

Transportation
per _____

Hygiene

☐ Bedbath
☒ Assist
☐ Self Bath
☒ Shower
☐ Tub
☐ Vanity
☐ Oral Care

Bowel/Bladder

☐ Foley   IN _____
            OUT _____
☐ Cath care Bid
☐ Incontinent
☐ Colostomy
☐ Ileostomy
☐ Urostomy

Communication

Fowlers or semi-fowlers position

V.S. q̄ 4h

Physical Therapy	Date	Treatments

Cardio-Pulmonary

4/16 Postural drainage 0900 daily
4/16 Incentive spirometer q̄ 3hrs
4/16 O₂ per cannula at 5L
4/16 Nebulizer q4h

Drug Allergies: Penicillin

Isolation: _____ In _____ Out _____

Emergency Instructions: Out of town until 4/17.
Relatives: Michael Sanchez
Phone: 641-1212

Clergy: none
Religion: Catholic

Religious Rites: Last Rites only

Code Blue
Yes

Diagnosis: Pneumonia

Surgery & Dates:

Consults & Dates:

Room	Name	Adm Date	Age	Physician
416	Luisa Sanchez	4-16-01	28	R. Katz

Figure 10–4
Kardex: Client Profile, Basic Needs, Medical Plan. *Source*: Courtesy of Shawnee Mission Health System, St. Luke's-Shawnee Mission, KS

determine that Mrs. Sanchez can feed herself, can have clear liquids and then solid foods as she can tolerate them, can get out of bed to go to the bathroom, has an IV, and should have 3,000 mL of fluids per day. Because instructions for meeting basic needs change rapidly as the client's condition changes, this section of the care plan is usually marked with pencil so it can be easily altered.

You may need to write individualized nursing diagnosis plans for clients who have special basic needs requirements, for example, those with Bathing/Hygiene Self-Care Deficit, urinary incontinence, or altered nutrition. These would be written in the nursing diagnosis care plan section (see Figure 10–3).

Aspects of the Medical Plan to Be Implemented by the Nurse

A comprehensive care plan includes nursing activities necessary for carrying out medical orders, for example, dressing changes and IV therapy. It also includes a section for scheduling prescribed diagnostic tests and treatments to be carried out by other departments (eg, physical therapy). In Figure 10–13, on page 462, this type of information is listed under "Active Doctor's Orders" and "Active Ancillary Orders." In Figure 10–4 it appears mainly in the top section of the form.

It is better to have a separate section for these activities, but you may also see them included as a part of the nursing care plan for a nursing diagnosis or collaborative problem; for example, in the section for "Laboratory" in Figure 10–4, on page 437, a physician-ordered "blood culture." However, if you were creating a student care plan, you might not have a Kardex form to work with. So, for Mrs. Sanchez, you might write a collaborative problem: Potential Complication of Pneumonia: Sepsis. The medical order for a blood culture would then be incorporated into the nursing interventions for that problem.

EXAMPLE:

Medical order (in bold print) included in student care plan.

Problem	Nursing Orders
Potential Complication of Pneumonia: Sepsis	1. **Blood cultures today, per order.** Explain reason for blood cultures 2. Temperature q4hr. Hourly if > 101° F

Nursing Diagnoses and Collaborative Problems

The **nursing diagnosis care plan** is the section of the comprehensive care plan that prescribes the outcomes and nursing interventions for the patient's nursing diagnoses and collaborative problems. A comprehensive care plan usually contains several single-problem care plans. This part of the care plan reflects the independent component of nursing practice and is the part that best demonstrates the nurse's clinical expertise. Figure 10–5 is an example of a care plan for a single nursing diagnosis. Note too, that Luisa Sanchez's care plan (see Figure 10–13, on pages 462–464) also contains nursing diagnosis care plans.

Addendum Care Plans

In many institutions the comprehensive care plan includes separate sections (addendum plans) for discharge planning and special teaching needs. Figure 6–2, on page 255, is an example of a discharge plan.

Teaching needs may be addressed in standards of care, in critical pathways (as in Figures 10–7 and 10–8), or by individually written nursing diagnoses. It is usually better to include teaching interventions as a part of the nursing orders for every nursing diagnosis rather than to use a Knowledge Deficit problem to address all the patient's various learning needs. However, when a patient has complex learning needs (eg, a new mother without a support system), you may wish to develop a special teaching plan to ensure efficient use of nursing time and maximize the patient's learning. Figure 10–6 is an example of a section of an individualized teaching plan.

Standardized Approaches to Care Planning

Obviously it would be inefficient to handwrite every bit of nursing care needed for all patients for whom a nurse provides care. For predictable or routine problems, the outcomes and nursing orders are often available in standardized, preprinted instructions in critical pathways, standards of care, standardized nursing dignosis care plans, protocols, and agency policies and procedures. Regardless of the system used, it is up to the nurse to modify standardized plans or handwrite an individualized plan for unique patient needs. The problem list you develop for the patient (Chapters 4 and 5) will help you to individualize care because each patient, regardless of medical diagnosis, will have a different set of problems and etiologies.

Critical Pathways

As discussed in Chapters 4 and 6, a **critical pathway** is a standardized form of the multidisciplinary plan that outlines the care required for patients with common, predictable conditions (eg, a patient undergoing a renal transplant). It is organized with a column (or sometimes page) for each day of hospitalization. There are as many columns (or pages) on the plan as the preset number of days allowed for the client's diagnostic-related group (DRG). For example, if the expected length of stay for a renal transplant patient is 6 days, the renal transplant critical pathway would have six columns (or six pages). See Figure 10–7 for a portion of a critical pathway. Patients often receive a modified form of their critical pathway so they will know what to expect (see Figure 10–8 for an example).

```
Note Type: PPOC - Gas Exchange, Impairment
Note Time: N/A
Last Stored: 1257 11 April 2000
Stored by: CLARKE, MARY F, RN
```

Genesis Medical Center   **PATIENT PLAN OF CARE**
Davenport, IA

**GAS EXCHANGE IMPAIRMENT: Excess or deficit in oxygenation and/or carbon
dioxide elimination at the alveolar-capillary membrane.**

INITIATED   Date 4/6/2000   Time 1256
Resolved   Date   Time

SIGNS & SYMPTOMS: (observed or reported) (select at least 2)

X Abnormal arterial blood gases	*X* Dyspnea
X Restlessness	*X* Headache upon awakening
Confusion	Somnolence
Irritability	Cyanosis (Neonates)
Vision disturbances	*X* Hypoxemia
X Nasal flaring	Hypercapnea

RELATED FACTORS:
　 Alveolar-capillary membrane changes
X Ventilation/perfusion alterations

OUTCOMES

Scale: 1=0% 2=25% 3=50% 4=75% 5=100%	Admission Date/Time 04/16/2000 1256	Date Time 04/17/2000 1600	D/C Date/Time 04/18/2000
X Respiratory Status: Gas Exchange	2	4	4
－ Neurological status IER			
－ Ease of breathing			
－ Restlessness not present			
－ O$_2$ Saturation WNL			
－ PaO$_2$ WNL			
－ PaCO$_2$ WNL			
－ CXR findings IER			
X Respiratory Status: Ventilation	2	3	4
－Respiratory rate, rhythm IER			
－Dyspenea @ rest not present			
－Adventitious breath sounds not present			
IER: In Expected Range			

Definition of Scoring Scales	1=0%	2=25%	3=50%	4=75%	5=100%
Respiratory Status: Gas Exchange - Alveolar exchange of CO$_2$ or O$_2$ to maintain arterial blood gas concentration.	Extremely Compromised	Substantially Compromised	Moderately Compromised	Mildly Compromised	Not Compromised
Respiratory Status: Ventilation - Movement of air in and out of the lungs.	Extremely Compromised	Substantially Compromised	Moderately Compromised	Mildly Compromised	Not Compromised

---

INTERVENTIONS

	YES	D/C
Acid-Base Management		
Acid-Base Monitoring	X	
Airway Management	X	
Airway Suctioning		
Artificial Airway Management		
Aspiration Precautions	X	
Cough Enhancement	X	
Embolus Care: Pulmonary		
Mechanical Vantilation		
Mechanical Ventilatory Weaning		
Oxygen Therapy		
Respiratory Monitoring		
Resuscitation: Neonate		
Ventilation Assistance		

```
Acct:
MRN:
LUISA SANCHEZ   Age:28
Admit Date: 4/16/00
Admit Phys:      Reed
          Physician
┌──────────────────┐
│  G.M.C.          │
└──────────────────┘
```

Figure 10–5

Computer Printout. Standardized Care Plan for a Single Nursing Diagnosis, Using NANDA, NIC and NOC.
Source: Courtesy of Genesis Health System (Genesis Medical Center and Illini Hospital), Davenport, IA.

Nursing Diagnosis:
Risk for Altered Health Maintenance r/t lack of knowledge of insulin therapy

Met	Learning Objective	Content	Teaching Strategy	Learning Strategy
	1st Session Client will describe the basic pathophysiology of diabetes mellitus (cognitive).	Location and function of pancreas How cells use glucose Function of insulin Effects of insulin deficiency (elevated blood sugar, mobilization of fats and proteins, ketones, etc.)	Explain. Transparency of the pancreas.	Read pamphlet, "Your Pancreas."
	2nd Session Ct. will demonstrate ability to draw up correct amount of insulin (psychomotor).	Syringe markings Sterile technique Preparation	Point out on enlarged drawing; then actual syringe. Demonstrate and discuss. Demonstrate and discuss: How to mix insulin. Read label carefully, be sure syringe and label concentrations match. Clean top of bottle with alcohol. Withdraw correct amount.	Practice with syringe and vial of sterile water.

Figure 10–6
Sample Teaching Plan (Partial): Diabetes Mellitus

Critical pathways can result in cost savings and increased patient satisfaction (Gage 1994), and the communication that occurs in creating them tends to enhance collaborative practice. Nevertheless, they are time-consuming to develop, and there is concern that individualized care may be lost in this system. The focus of such plans is usually more medical than holistic; and the need to achieve outcomes within rigidly specified time frames creates the danger of focusing on efficiency more than quality of care.

Unit Standards of Care

Unit standards of care are standardized, preprinted directions for care, developed by nurses for groups of clients, rather than for individuals. They are

HOSPITAL OF THE UNIVERSITY OF PENNSYLVANIA

RENAL TRANSPLANT RECIPIENT - CLINICAL PATHWAY OVERVIEW:
Immediate Graft Function

Eligibility Criteria: All renal transplant recipients (living related and cadaver). Individualize pathway if kidney develops delayed graft functionor rejection.

Expected LOS: 6 Days Cadaver, 7 Days Living Related Recipient

ADDRESSOGRAPH

Clinical pathway is a collaborative plan meant to guide the care of routine patients and should be modified on the basis of clinical indications.

TIMEFRAME	POSTOP - DAY OF SURGERY	POSTOP DAY 1
LOCATION	PACU/Rhoads 4	RHOADS 4
OUTCOMES		•Pain ≤ midpoint on pain scale

ASSESSMENTS	•Notify MD if
	    -temp > 100.4 po
	    -SBP > 180
	    -DBP > 100
	    -Decrease in hourly u/o by 50% or >
	•Assess operative dressing
	•VS q 15 min till stable, q 30 x 4 hrs, q 1 hr, then q 4 hr
	•Breath sounds
	•I&O; hourly urine output x24hrs
	•Assess pain q4h and document
	•Fistula/shunt precautions
		•Individualize pathway if kidney has delayed graft function
		•Review antihypertensive regimen with nephrology
		•Daily wt
		•Breath sounds
		•Assess bowel function
		•Assess operative dressing q shift
		•VS q 4 hr
		•I&O
		•Assess pain q4h and document

CONSULTS		•Consult Diabetologist for patients with DM
TESTS	•K⁺, Hgb stat 2hrs after surgery •Fingerstick glucose	•CBC •Electrolytes: BUN, Cr, Glu, Ca⁺, Phos •Renal scan - if oliguric or Creat. has not lowered by 2mg/dl
TREATMENTS	•Foley •Cough & deep breathe & splint q 2hr while awake •Incentive spirometry q 1 hr while awake •Pneumatic stockings	•Foley •Cough & deep breathe q 2hr while awake •Dialysis: if hyperkalemic, volume overloaded, or uremic •Incentive spirometry q 1 hr while awake •Pneumatic stockings while in bed
MEDICATIONS/IVS	•Urine output cc/cc replacement .45 NSS alternate with .45 NSS with 1 amp NaHCO₃/L •Analgesia - morphine PCA 1mg basal/1mg intermittent •Ancef 500mg IV q 12 hr x 2 doses •Lasix 200-300mg IV prn oliguria as long as u/o adequate	•Continue IVF •Analgesia - MSO₄ PCA 1mg basal/1 mg intermittent •MVI 1 po QD •Alutabs 2 tabs qid (d/c if phos < 4.0) •Clotrimazole troche 5 times/day •Colace 100mg po bid •Zantac 150 mg po bid •Bactrim ss 1 po qd •Acyclovir 800mg po qid if creat < 3. Adjust dose according to renal function. •Acyclovir 200mg po BID if donor and recipient are CMV negative •Neoral 4mg/kg q12h •Cellcept 1 gm po q12h •Prednisone 1.5mg/kg/day-taper by 10mg/day until 30 mg/day
ACTIVITY/FUNC-TIONAL LEVEL	•Bedrest	•OOB to chair
NUTRITION/ELIMINATION	•NPO except ice chips	•Clear liquids - advance as tol
PATIENT/FAMILY EDUCATION	•Reinforce postop teaching •Pain scale •Incentive spirometer •PCA pump	•Review patient pathway •Review medications, activity, diet •Provide kidney transplant discharge booklet
DISCHARGE PLANNING		•Transplant Coordinator to assess need for prescriptions •CRC to assess need for home care, home infusion •Social Work to assess each patient for financial and psychosocial issues including insurance coverage of meds.

Figure 10–7

Portion of a Renal Transplant Critical Pathway. *Source:* Courtesy of Hospital of the University of Pennsylvania, Philadelphia, PA.

Patient's Overview for Total Knee Replacement

NOTE: This is a guide ONLY. Your Plan of Care may vary depending on doctor orders, your individualized needs, and/or your response to treatment.

Category	Operative Day	Post-Op Day 1–2	Post-Op Day 3–Discharge
Exercise/Rest	–You will be on bedrest. –You may be started on gentle knee movement using continuous passive motion machine (CPM) –You will be assisted to turn from side to side approximately every 2 hours after surgery, unless you have a CPM machine.	–Out of bed activity progresses from sitting on side of bed to sitting in chair. –Physical Therapy starts with exercises and progresses to walking with walker/crutches. The amount of weight you can put on your operative leg may be limited according to your doctor. –If you have a CPM, the degree of bend will be increased daily.	–Your activity will continue to progress from sitting in a chair to walking in halls. –You will continue to walk with walker/crutches. The amount of weight you can put on your operative leg may remain limited. –Your goal is 90° bend by discharge with Physical Therapy and/or CPM. –Your CPM will continue to be increased daily.
Nutrition/Fluids	–You will have an IV. –Liquids are allowed upon arrival to the nursing unit following surgery. –Solid foods may be permitted for the evening meal if you are not nauseated.	–IV continued.	–IV stopped on third day. –Diet as tolerated.

Figure 10–8

Portion of a Critical Pathway Given to Patients. *Source:* Courtesy of St. Luke's-Shawnee Mission Health System, Shawnee Mission, KS. Used with permission.

detailed guidelines for the care to be given in defined situations, for example:

- A medical diagnosis (eg, abdominal hysterectomy)
- A treatment or diagnostic test (eg, colonoscopy)
- A nursing diagnosis (eg, anticipatory grieving)
- A situation such as relinquishment of a newborn

Standards of care describe achievable rather than ideal nursing care, taking into account the circumstances and client population of the institution. They do not contain medical orders. They are different from critical pathways in that they are not time-sequenced and they define only interventions for which nurses are held accountable. Standards of care are usually not placed in the client's medical record, but are reference documents, stored as permanent hospital records. They are either filed on the unit or in the computer for easy reference. When they are not a part of the care plan, the problem list (see Table 10–1 on page 457) should indicate which standards of care apply to the patient. Standards of care may or may not be organized according to nursing diagnoses. Figure 10–9 is an example of standards of care that list only the nursing interventions, without identifying the problems to which they apply. Clearly, though, it focuses on the collaborative problem of Potential Complication of Thrombophlebitis: Pulmonary Embolus.

Model (Standardized) Care Plans

Do not confuse **standardized care plans** with *standards of care*. To avoid confusion, some nurses prefer to call them **model care plans**. Although they have some similarities, there are important differences between standards of care and model care plans:

1. Model care plans are kept with the client's active care plan (in the Kardex or computer). When no longer active, they become a part of her permanent medical record. This is not usually true of standards of care.
2. Model care plans provide more detailed instructions than standards of care. They contain deviations (either additions or deletions) from the standards for the agency.
3. Unlike standards of care, model care plans take the usual nursing process format:

Problem → Outcomes → Nursing orders → Evaluation

4. Model care plans allow you to add addendum care plans. They usually include checklists, blank lines, or empty spaces to allow you to individualize goals and nursing orders. This is not usually true for standards of care.

Model care plans are similar to standards of care in that they are preprinted guides for nursing interventions for a specific nursing diagnosis or for all the nursing diagnoses associated with a particular situation or medical condition. They are developed by nurses, and while they are not standards of care, following them ensures that acceptable standards of care are provided. Refer to Figure 10–10 for a portion of a preprinted model care plan. Figure 10–5, on page 440, is a computerized model care plan for a single nursing diagnosis. Both of these examples use NANDA, NIC, and NOC.

Many commercial books of model care plans are available. They can be used as guides when developing your care plans, but remember that they do not address the client's individualized needs, and they can cause you to focus on predictable problems and miss cues to important special problems the

STANDARDS OF CARE: Patient with Thrombophlebitis

Goal:
1. To monitor for early signs and symptoms of compromised respiratory status.
2. To report any abnormal signs and/or symptoms promptly to the medical staff.
3. To initiate appropriate nursing actions when signs and/or symptoms of compromised respiratory status occur.
4. To institute protocol for emergency intervention should the client develop cardiopulmonary dysfunction.

SUPPORTIVE DATA: The purpose of these standards of care is to prevent, monitor, report, and record the client's response to a diagnosis of thrombophlebitis. Thrombophlebitis places the client at risk for pulmonary embolism. The hemodynamic consequences of embolic obstruction to pulmonary blood flow involve increased pulmonary vascular resistance, increased right ventricular workload, decreased cardiac output, and development of shock and pulmonary arrest.

CLINICAL MANIFESTATIONS: Nursing assessments performed q3–4h should monitor for the following signs/symptoms:

- Dyspnea (generally consistently present)
- Sudden substernal pain
- Rapid/weak pulse
- Syncope
- Anxiety
- Fever
- Cough/hemoptysis
- Accelerated respiratory rate
- Pleuritic type chest pain
- Cyanosis

PREVENTIVE NURSING MEASURES:

- Encourage increased fluid intake to prevent dehydration.
- Maintain anticoagulant intravenous therapy as prescribed (See Protocol for Anticoagulant Administration).
- Maintain prescribed bedrest.
- Prevent venous stasis from improperly fitting elastic stockings; check q3–4h.
- Encourage dorsiflexion exercises of the lower extremities while on bedrest.

INDIVIDUALIZED PLANS/ADDITIONAL NURSING/MEDICAL ORDERS

Do not massage lower extremities.

Intake and output q8h.

Initiated by: _S. Ibarra, RN_   Date: _4-9-01_

Figure 10–9
Example of Non–Problem-Oriented Standards of Care

client is experiencing. If you use a model care plan as a student, do the following:

1. Consult your instructor to be sure you are using a reliable source.
2. Perform a nursing assessment and make your own list of all the client's actual and potential problems. You can then consult the model care plan to be sure your list is complete.

Patient Name: _____

PLAN OF CARE   Medical Record Number: _____

NURSING DIAGNOSIS	INTERVENTION	OUTCOME		
Impaired Physical Mobility Related To:	**Exercise Therapy: Ambulation**	Outcome	Indicators	Scale
☐ Intolerance to activity/ decreased strength and endurance	**ACTIVITIES** Medicate with prescribed analgesic prior to Physical Therapy session to enhance level of mobility.	**Mobility Level** (Ability to move purposefully)	Transfer performance Ambulation: walking	(circle one) Date: _____ Initials: _____ 1 2 3 4 5
☐ Pain/discomfort	Gait training per Physical Therapy.			Date: _____ Initials: _____ 1 2 3 4 5
☐ Perceptual/cognitive impairment	Transfer training per Physical Therapy.			
☐ Neuromuscular impairment	Bed mobility / activity training per Physical Therapy.			Date: _____ Initials: _____ 1 2 3 4 5
☐ Depression/severe anxiety	Monitor patient's use of walking aids/ adaptive devices.			Date: _____ Initials: _____ 1 2 3 4 5
	Instruct patient about safe transfer and ambulation techniques.			
	Place side rails (upper and/or lower) to assist patient with mobility and aid patient in turning and repositioning.			Date: _____ Initials: _____ 1 2 3 4 5
	Ensure post-operative hip precautions are followed, as appropriate.			Date: _____ Initials: _____ 1 2 3 4 5
	Active exercise per Physical Therapy: _____			Date: _____ Initials: _____ 1 2 3 4 5
	Passive exercise per Physical Therapy: _____			Date: _____ Initials: _____ 1 2 3 4 5
	CPM per Physical Therapy: _____			Date: _____ Initials: _____ 1 2 3 4 5
	E Stim per Physical Therapy: _____			Date: _____ Initials: _____ 1 2 3 4 5
	Other: _____			Date: _____ Initials: _____ 1 2 3 4 5
Self-Care Deficit:	**Self-Care Assistance**	**Self-Care: Activities of Daily Living** (Ability to perform the most basic physical tasks and personal care activities)	Dressing	Date: _____ Initials: _____ 1 2 3 4 5
☐ Bathing/Hygiene Self-Care Deficit	**ACTIVITIES** Monitor patient's ability for independent self-care.		Eating	Date: _____ Initials: _____ 1 2 3 4 5
☐ Dressing/Grooming Self-Care Deficit	Monitor patient's need for adaptive devices for personal hygiene, dressing, grooming, toileting and eating.		Toileting	Date: _____ Initials: _____ 1 2 3 4 5
☐ Toileting Self-Care Deficit	Provide assistance until patient is fully able to assume self-care.			Date: _____ Initials: _____ 1 2 3 4 5
Related To:	Assist patient in accepting dependency needs.			Date: _____ Initials: _____ 1 2 3 4 5
☐ Decreased or lack of motivation	Encourage patient to perform normal activities of daily living to level of ability.			Date: _____ Initials: _____ 1 2 3 4 5
☐ Perceptual or cognitive impairment				
☐ Neuromuscular impairment				
☐ Musculoskeletal impairment				Date: _____ Initials: _____ 1 2 3 4 5
☐ Discomfort				

Scale Descriptors: **1** = Dependent, does not participate, **2** = Requires assistive person and device, **3** = Requires assistive person,
4 = Independent with assistive device, **5** = Completely independent

Figure 10–10
Portion of a Model Care Plan (Using Standardized Nursing Lanuage). *Source*: Courtesy of Grant/Riverside Methodist Hospital, Columbus, OH.

3. Using client input, establish specific, individualized goals before consulting the model care plan. Consulting the model first may inhibit your creativity.
4. Be sure the nursing interventions in the model are appropriate for your client and possible to implement in your institution. Delete any that do not apply.

5. Individualize the outcomes and nursing orders to fit your client.

   EXAMPLE:

   Standardized Nursing Order
   Force fluids as ordered or as tolerated by patient.

   Individualized Nursing Order
   Force fluids to 2400 mL per 24 hours:
   7-3: Offer 200 mL water or apple juice hourly.

   3-11: Offer 200 mL water or apple juice hourly while awake.

   11-7: Offer water or juice when awakening patient for VS or meds.

   Pt. prefers ice in his water or juice.

Protocols

Protocols are standardized and preprinted (see Figure 10–11 for an example). Like standards of care and model care plans, they cover the common actions required for a particular medical diagnosis, defined situation, treatment, or diagnostic test. For example, there may be a protocol for admitting a patient to the intensive care unit, or a protocol covering the administration of magnesium sulfate to a preeclampsia patient. Protocols are different, however, because they may include both medical orders and nursing orders. When a protocol is used, it can be added to the nursing care plan and become a part of the patient's permanent record. An alternative is to keep all protocols in the hospital's file of permanent records and write "See protocol" on the care plan, as in Table 10–1 on page 457.

Policies and Procedures

When a situation occurs frequently, an institution is likely to develop a **policy** to govern how it is to be handled. For example, a hospital may have a policy that specifies the number of visitors a patient may have. Policies and procedures may also be similar to protocols and specify, for example, what actions are to be taken in the case of cardiac arrest. As with protocols and standing orders, the nurse must recognize the situation and then use judgment in implementing the policy. Hospital policies must be interpreted to meet patient needs.

   EXAMPLE: While on a business trip, Fred Gonzalez was in an automobile accident. He has been hospitalized in serious condition for several days. It is 8:55 PM, and Mr. Gonzalez's wife has just arrived on the unit for her first visit. Even though hospital policy requires that visitors leave at 9 PM, the nurse decides that implementing the policy would not meet Mr. Gonzalez's needs.

If a policy covers a situation pertinent to the patient care plan, it is usually simply noted on the care plan (eg, "Make Social Service referral per Unit

Expected Outcome: The patient's amniotic fluid level will be increased in attempt to eliminate variable decelerations or to dilute the amount of meconium in the amniotic fluid.

Supportive Data:

Contraindications:
Late decelerations
Fetal tachycardia
Absence of variables
Bleeding
Fetal presentation other than vertex

Possible Complications:
Prolapsed cord
Elevation of intrauterine pressure
Polyhydramnios
Abruption
Infection

Policy:
The physician will place the IUPC.

When the fetus is premature the fluid will be warmed through a blood warmer during administration.

When the fetus is at term the fluid may be at room temperature.

Preparation/Administration:
1. Connect 1000ml normal saline to infusion pump tubing. Flush the tubing.
2. Zero and assist the physician with insertion of the IUPC.
3. Attach infusion tubing to the amnio port on the IUPC.
4. To treat variable decelerations:
   a. Bolus infusion of 250ml-500ml in 10 min before connecting to infusion pump.
   b. Place the tubing on the pump after the bolus and run @ 3ml/min or 180ml/hr.
5. To prevent variable decelerations:
   a. Infuse @ 10ml/min for 1 hr (Set infusion pump @ 600ml/hr).

Intervention:

Assess/Document:

1. FHR per standards of practice
2. Intrauterine pressure q 30 min
3. Character/amount of leakage
4. Amount of NS infused
   Note: Amount of fluid infused must not exceed amount leaked by 500ml/1000ml to maintain amniotic fluid volume at all times.

Maintain lateral recumbent position (right/ left side).

CAUTION! If resting tone is >25mmg or no uterine relaxation—STOP and notify the physician.

Initiated by: _____

Date: _____

Figure 10–11
Protocol for Amnio Infusion. *Source*: Courtesy of St. Luke's-Shawnee Mission Health System, 9100 W. 74th Street, Shawnee Mission, KS 66204.

Policy"). Hospital policies and procedures are institution records, not patient records, so they are not actually placed in the care plan.

■ COMPUTERIZED CARE PLANS AND STANDARDIZED LANGUAGE

Computers are used to create both standardized and individualized care plans. Figure 10–5, on page 440, is a printout of a standardized care plan for Gas Exchange Impairment that is stored in the computer and individualized by checking the signs and symptoms, outcomes, and interventions that

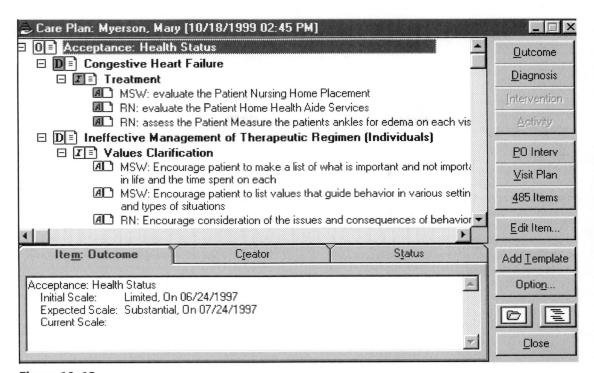

Figure 10–12

Care Plan (Computer Screen) Using NANDA, NIC, NOC and Medical Diagnosis. *Source:* Courtesy of Ergo Partners, L.C. All Rights Reserved.

apply to a particular patient. Figure 10–12 shows how a section of a care plan might look on the computer screen. Both of these examples use standardized nursing language (i.e., NANDA, NIC, and NOC) to label problems, outcomes, and interventions. Figure 10–13 (pages 462–464) is also a computer-generated care plan, but it does not use standardized language for outcomes and interventions. It is an individualized plan, created specifically for Luisa Sanchez, for the two nursing diagnoses of Anxiety and Sleep Pattern Disturbance. Outcomes and interventions were typed in by the nurse, using her own wording.

■ CARE PLANNING GUIDE

Now that you are familiar with the various documents that make up a comprehensive care plan, you should be able to follow the steps of the nursing process and make a care plan for an actual patient. Box 10–1 compresses all the steps of the nursing process into a concise guide to use in planning care. The care plan developed for Luisa Sanchez in this chapter follows this guide.

BOX 10–1

Care-Planning Guide

1. **Collect data.**
   a. Interview, physical examination.
   b. Validate data.
   c. Organize according to framework.
2. **Analyze and synthesize data.**
   a. Group related cues according to framework.
   b. Form new cue clusters as needed.
   c. Identify deviations from normal.
3. **List all problems (working list).**
   a. Human responses that need to be changed.
   b. Medical, nursing, collaborative.
   c. Actual, risk, possible.
4. **Make formal list of labeled problems.**
   a. Label nursing diagnoses (Problem + Etiology)
      (1) Problem: Compare patient data to defining characteristics, definitions, and risk factors.
      (2) Etiology: Related factors (risk, causal, contributing factors).
   b. Label Collaborative Problems (Potential complications of . . .).
5. **Determine which problems can be addressed by**
   a. critical pathways.
   b. standards of care.
   c. model care plans.
   d. protocols.
   e. policies/procedures (eg, note on formal problem list: Risk for Pulmonary Embolus—See Standards of Care).
6. **Individualize model care plans, protocols, and so forth, as needed.**
7. **Transcribe medical, collaborative, activities of daily living, and basic care needs to Kardex.**
8. **Develop individualized care plan for remaining nursing diagnoses and collaborative problems.**
   a. Develop individualized outcomes.
      (1) State desired client responses.
      (2) Opposite of problem response.
      (3) Measurable/realistic.
   b. Write nursing orders.
      (1) Address etiology: reduce/remove related factors.
      (2) Address problem: relieve symptoms.
      (3) Address outcomes: how to bring about desired behaviors.
      (4) Health promotion, prevention, treatment, observation.

(continues)

BOX 10–1

Care-Planning Guide (continued)

(5) Physical care, teaching, counseling, environment management, referrals, emotional support, activities of daily living.

(6) For complex orders, refer to policies and protocol (See "Unit Procedure for IV Therapy").

   c. Include any special or complex teaching or discharge plans.

9. Implement care plan (do or delegate; record in chart).

10. Evaluate results of care.

   a. Compare patient progress to original goals.

   b. Revise care plan as needed.

     (1) Collect more data, if needed.

     (2) Revise, discontinue, or continue problem.

     (3) Change outcomes if unachievable.

     (4) Revise, discontinue, or keep nursing orders.

Each chapter in this book has included a detailed guide for carrying out a particular step of the nursing process. If you need to review any of the steps in the care-planning guide, refer to the appropriate chapter in this book, where the step is expanded for you. In addition to proceeding step-by-step through the care-planning guide, you should refer to Box 10–2 on page 452 when writing care plans.

■ CREATING A COMPREHENSIVE CARE PLAN

Read the following case study, which describes the course of Luisa Sanchez's hospitalization. Then follow the steps of the care-planning guide (Box 10–1) and the guidelines in Box 10–2 to develop a comprehensive plan for Ms. Sanchez.

Case Study: Luisa Sanchez

Framework: Functional Health Patterns, Gordon
Medical Diagnosis: Pneumonia

Luisa Sanchez, a 28-year-old married attorney, was admitted to the hospital with an elevated temperature, a productive cough, and rapid, labored respirations. During the nursing interview, she told Mary Medina, RN, that she has had a "chest cold" for 2 weeks and has been short of breath on exertion. She stated, "Yesterday I started having a fever and pain in my lungs." Mrs. Sanchez's complete assessment data appear in Figure 3–2 in Chapter 3, so they are repeated here only in part. Admission medical orders included:

Guidelines for Writing Care Plans

1. **Include each of these components:**
   a. Client profile
   b. Basic needs
   c. Aspects of medical plan
   d. Nursing diagnoses and collaborative problems
   e. Special or complex teaching or discharge needs
2. **Date and sign the initial plan and any revisions.** The date is important for evaluation; the signature demonstrates nursing accountability.
3. **List or number the nursing diagnoses in order of priority.** Priorities can be changed as the client's needs change.
4. **List the nursing orders for each problem in order of priority** or in the order in which they should be done. For instance, you would assess the client's level of knowledge before you teach him to log-roll.
5. **Write the plan in clear, concise terms.** Use standard medical abbreviations and symbols. Use key words rather than complete sentences. Leave out unnecessary words, like *client* and *the* (eg, write "Turn & reposition q2h" rather than "Turn and reposition the client every 2 hours").
6. **Write legibly, in ink.** When the plan cannot be erased, accountability is emphasized and more importance is placed on what is being written. If a nursing diagnosis is resolved, write "Discontinued" and a date beside it, highlight it, or date a special "Inactive" column. Outcomes and nursing orders can be discontinued similarly.
7. **For detailed treatments and procedures, refer to other sources** (eg, standards of care) instead of writing all the steps on the care plan. You might write, "See unit procedure book for diabetic teaching," or you might attach a standard nursing care plan for a problem (eg, "See standard care plan for ineffective breastfeeding"). This saves time, and focuses the written part of the care plan on the unique needs of the client.
8. **Be sure the plan is holistic.** It should consider the client's physiological, psychological, sociocultural, and spiritual needs.
9. **Be sure the plan is individualized** and addresses the client's unique needs. Include the client's choices about how and when care is given. For example, "Prefers evening shower."
10. **Include the collaborative and coordination aspects of the client's care.** You may write nursing orders to consult a social worker or physical therapist, or you may simply coordinate tests and treatments. The medical plan should be incorporated into the nursing care plan so that the two plans do not conflict.
11. **Include discharge plans** (eg, arrangements for follow-up by a social worker or community health nurse).

CBC with differential
Arterial blood gases
Urine specific gravity
Sputum C & S
Postural drainage daily
Pulse oximeter
IV of D_5 LR, 100 mL/hr
Tylenol 650 mg q4h po for temp
> 101°

PA and lateral chest x-ray
Blood culture (repeat ×2 if temp
over 101°)
24-hour urine
Serum electrolytes
Incentive spirometer q3h
Nebulizer q4h
Vancomycin 0.5 gm IV q6h
O_2 per cannula, 5L

Assessment

Step 1: Collect Data

To begin collecting Mrs. Sanchez's data, you could use a data collection form such as Figure 3–2 in Chapter 3, organized by body systems and specific nursing concerns, rather than one based on a single nursing model. Next you would organize the data according to a nursing model (eg, Gordon's Functional Health Patterns) in order to have a worksheet to use during data analysis. Box 4–4 on pages 164–166 summarizes the admission data collected in each of the patterns.

Diagnosis

Step 2: Analyze and Synthesize Data

Next underline all the cues that seem significant or outside the norm (see Box 4–4, pp. 163–164). For example, in the Role-Relationship pattern, the nurse underlined "husband out of town" and "child with neighbor." Next, think about how the abnormal (significant) cues in one group might be related to cues in another group—inductively forming new cue clusters (refer to Table 4–6 on pp. 169–170). For instance, in the Coping/Stress-Tolerance pattern, Luisa shows signs of Anxiety (eg, tense facial muscles, trembling). You might wonder if the data in the Role-Relationship pattern might be related to that anxiety. Perhaps part of Mrs. Sanchez's anxiety might be caused by worry about her child or by her need for emotional support from her husband, who is away. Because those cues seem related, they are inductively grouped, together with other related cues, into a new cue cluster (Cluster 9 in Table 4–6). Cluster 9 represents a problem that is essentially psychological and fits best in the Self-Perception/Self-Concept pattern.

Notice in Box 4–4 that the cues "urinary frequency and amount decreased ×2 days" and "diaphoretic" cannot be interpreted accurately using only the cues in that pattern. To interpret their meaning, you need to think how those abnormal cues relate to the cues in the Nutritional-Metabolic pattern. Notice, too, that even in the new, inductively formed groupings, a single piece of data may appear in more than one cluster. For example, in Table 4–6, "Can't breathe lying down" appears in Clusters 4 and 6. In Cluster 4, it is one of the causes of sleep pattern disturbance; in Cluster 6, it indirectly causes self-care deficit by causing Mrs. Sanchez to lose sleep and become too tired and weak to perform self-care activities. Examine Box 4–4 and Table 4–6 to see if you can follow the reasoning for each of the cue clusters. If you need to review Functional Health Patterns, refer to Table 3–10 on pages 105–106.

Step 3: Make a Working Problem List

In this step you made a judgment about the most likely explanation for each cue cluster; then decide whether it represents an actual, potential (risk), or possible problem. Also decide whether the problem is medical, collaborative, or a nursing diagnosis. Tentative explanations for Luisa Sanchez are listed in Table 4–6 on pages 169–170.

Cluster 1—no abnormal cues in the Health Perception/Health Management pattern. The pattern represents patient strengths: a healthy lifestyle and understanding of and compliance with treatment regimens (eg, taking her Synthroid as directed).

Cluster 2—problem of inadequate nutrition. A likely explanation is that Mrs. Sanchez's poor appetite is a result of her disease process. Her appetite will probably return on successful medical treatment of the pneumonia. In the meantime, Mrs. Sanchez will need nursing care to assess for and encourage adequate nutrition.

Cluster 3—nursing diagnosis, Fluid Volume Deficit. It is probably caused by excess fluid loss secondary to fever and diaphoresis, as well as inadequate fluid intake because of nausea and poor appetite. Mrs. Sanchez's poor skin turgor, decreased urinary frequency, dry mucous membranes, and hot skin are defining characteristics that help to identify the problem.

Cluster 4—a Sleep/Rest pattern nursing diagnosis. Apparently, when she lies down to sleep, she is unable to breathe. In addition, her cough and pain keep her awake. Undoubtedly her fever, diaphoresis, and chills (in Clusters 3 and 7) also keep her awake. As a result, she feels weak and is short of breath on exertion.

Cluster 5—a medical problem, hypothyroidism, for which Mrs. Sanchez is already receiving medication. Therefore, the problem requires no nursing intervention and would not be included in the care plan. The medication order would appear in the medication record and would be given to Mrs. Sanchez routinely while she was in the hospital.

Cluster 6—nursing diagnosis, either Activity Intolerance or Self Care Deficit. Both are being caused by cues and problems in other clusters. For example, the Sleep-Rest problem in Cluster 4, and the oxygenation problem in Cluster 11 are both contributing to the overall pattern of weakness in Cluster 6.

Cluster 7—problem, Mrs. Sanchez is uncomfortable because she is having chills. The chills are being caused by fever secondary to the pneumonia, and will stop when her illness is treated. The fever will be treated medically (by the order for Ibuprofen); however, there are nursing interventions that can be used to increase Mrs. Sanchez's comfort.

Cluster 8—contains risk factors for a potential nursing diagnosis, Risk for Altered Family Processes. However, there is not enough data to indicate an actual problem. In any event, the problem will resolve itself the next day, as soon as Mr. Sanchez returns home. You might decide to include it in the care plan, to be sure that the necessary follow-up assessments are made.

Cluster 9—nursing diagnosis, Anxiety. Mrs. Sanchez expressed anxiety but she had no other signs of Anxiety, such as trembling and tense facial muscles. She said she was worried about leaving her child with a neighbor, and about getting behind at work. In addition, her Anxiety is obviously caused by periodic difficulty breathing. This is a nursing diagnosis with more than one etiology.

Cluster 10—nursing diagnosis of Chest Pain, which is caused by the pneumonia-induced cough. Until the antibiotic therapy can treat the pneumonia, nursing measures will be needed to promote comfort.

Cluster 11—nursing diagnosis, Ineffective Airway Clearance. Cues are: productive cough, shallow respirations, decreased chest expansion, and inspiratory crackles. The other cues (eg, pale mucous membranes) are signs of pneumonia, the medical problem creating the ineffective airway clearance. You can infer that problems in other patterns are contributing to the oxygenation problem as well: fluid volume deficit creates thick, tenacious mucus, and pain and weakness contribute to shallow respirations and decreased chest expansion.

In addition to the problems identified from the cue clusters, you should identify collaborative problems that exist for Mrs. Sanchez because of her disease process and her IV and medical therapies. Recall that collaborative problems are potential problems for which nursing care focuses on assessment and prevention. The following is a working problem list for Luisa Sanchez, before being put into standard NANDA terminology:

Cue Cluster	Probable Explanation
1	No problem. Strength: Healthy lifestyle; understanding of and compliance with treatment regimens.
2	Actual nursing diagnosis. Altered Nutrition: Less than Body Requirements. Probably caused by nausea and poor appetite; and also by increased metabolism secondary to fever and pneumonia.
3	Actual nursing diagnosis. Fluid Volume Deficit, caused by excess fluid loss (diaphoresis) secondary to fever; and inadequate intake secondary to nausea and loss of appetite.

Cue Cluster	Probable Explanation
4	Actual nursing diagnosis. Difficulty sleeping; probably NANDA label of Sleep Pattern Disturbance, caused by cough, pain, orthopnea, fever, and diaphoresis.
5	No problem as long as patient takes Synthroid. Be sure it is on medical administration record.
6	Actual nursing diagnosis. Probably Self-Care Deficit (perhaps Activity Intolerance). Lack of oxygen and sleep loss are causing weakness and fatigue. As a result, she is unable to perform self-care activities.
7	Actual nursing diagnosis. Chills are causing discomfort.
8	Potential nursing diagnosis. There could be a problem with child care if Mr. Sanchez's return is delayed. Probably Altered Family Processes because both parents are unavailable to care for child; but probably self-limiting (tomorrow).
9	Actual nursing diagnosis. Anxiety. Caused by difficulty breathing, worry about child, and of "getting behind" at work.
10	Actual nursing diagnosis. Chest pain from cough. Medical treatments will help alleviate.
11	Actual nursing diagnosis. Airway clearance problem. Unable to cough up thick sputum, which has been created by infection, fever, weakness, pain, and fluid deficit.

Collaborative Problems

Potential Complication of pneumonia: septic shock
Potential Complication of pneumonia: respiratory insufficiency
Potential Complications of IV therapy: infiltration, phlebitis
Potential Complications of antibiotic therapy: allergic reaction, GI upset

Step 4: Write Problem Statements in Standardized Language

To make the formal list of nursing diagnoses and collaborative problems, refer to the list of NANDA diagnostic labels (see pages i–ii for the list of diagnostic labels organized by Functional Health Patterns). Compare the data in the cue clusters to the defining characteristics in a nursing diagnosis handbook to be sure you have chosen the correct NANDA label for each nursing diagnosis. After verifying the diagnoses with Mrs. Sanchez, you would write them on the care plan in order of priority (see Table 10–1). Note that in addition to listing all the problems identified for Mrs. Sanchez on the day of her admission, Table 10–1 indicates changes that a nurse might make to the list after implementing the care plan and evaluating the outcomes.

Table 10–1 Formal Prioritized Problem List for Luisa Sanchez

Prioritized Problems	Type of Plan Used
1. Ineffective Airway Clearance related to viscous secretions and shallow chest expansion secondary to pain, fluid volume deficit, and fatigue	See "Unit Standards of Care for Pneumonia"
2. ~~Fluid Volume Deficit related to intake insufficient to replace fluid loss secondary to fever, diaphoresis, and nausea~~ Resolved 4/17/01 JW	See Standard Care Plan for Fluid Volume Deficit
3. Anxiety related to difficulty breathing and concerns over work and parenting roles	Individualized nursing diagnosis care plan
4. Sleep Pattern Disturbance related to cough, pain, orthopne·, fever, and diaphoresis	Individualized nursing diagnosis care plan
5. Self-Care Deficit (Level 2) related to Activity Intolerance secondary to Ineffective Airway Clearance and Sleep Pattern Disturbance	See "Unit Standards of Care for Pneumonia"
6. Chest Pain related to cough secondary to pneumonia Risk for 4/17/01 JW	See "Unit Standards of Care for Pneumonia"
7. Altered Comfort: Chills related to fever and diaphoresis	Individualized nursing diagnosis care plan
8. ~~Risk for Altered Family Processes related to mother's illness and temporary unavailability of father to provide child care~~ Resolved 4/17/01 JW	Individualized nursing diagnosis care plan
9. Altered Nutrition: Less than Body requirements related to decreased appetite and nausea and increased metabolism secondary to disease process	See Standardized Care Plan for Altered Nutrition: Less than Body Requirements
10. Potential Complications of Pneumonia: Septic shock and respiratory insufficiency	See "Unit Standards of Care for Pneumonia"
11. Potential Complications of IV Therapy: Infiltration, phlebitis	See Unit Procedures: "IV Insertion and Maintenance"
12. Potential Complications of Vancomycin Therapy: Ototoxicity, Hepatotoxicity, Allergic reaction, GI upset	See "Protocol for Administration of Intravenous Vancomycin"

Planning

Step 5: Determine Which Problems Can Be Addressed by Critical Pathways and Other Standardized Plans

After developing the formal problem list, decide how each of the problems is to be addressed (ie, with preplanned interventions or individualized plans). For each problem, ask the following series of questions.

1. *Is there a **critical pathway** or **standard of care** for this medical diagnosis or situation?* Mrs. Sanchez was admitted to 2-South, a medical unit that has

written standards of care for patients having pneumonia. These standards describe all the care necessary for Problems 1, 5, 6, and 10 (Ineffective Airway Clearance, Self-Care Deficit, Chest Pain, and Potential Complications of Pneumonia). Most patients with pneumonia experience these problems, so it is possible to plan in advance the care these patients are expected to need. Because no special plan is necessary, you would simply list the problems and write beside them, "See Unit Standards of Care for Pneumonia," as shown in Table 10–1.

2. *Is there a **model nursing care plan** for the client's medical diagnosis or condition?* In Mrs. Sanchez's case, because there were standards of care for pneumonia patients, and because her needs did not exceed the standards, you would not look for a model care plan for this medical diagnosis.

3. *For the **collaborative problems** not completely covered by the standards of care, do any of the following exist to direct your interventions?*
   Physician's orders (you may need to call to obtain these)
   Standing orders
   Protocols
   Policies and procedures

Mrs. Sanchez has two collaborative problems not addressed by standards of care: Problems 11 and 12. For Problem 11, the physician's orders specify the type of IV fluid and prescribe the rate of flow. You would note this information on an IV flowsheet or a Kardex form (Figure 10–4 on page 437). The 2-South procedure manual contains a section on IV therapy, which specifies how often IV tubing is to be changed, what focus assessments to make, and so forth. This resource is noted on the formal problem list beside Problem 11 (in Table 10–1).

Because vancomycin is not routinely given to all pneumonia patients, it would not be included in the unit's Standards of Care for Pneumonia. However, because it is often given to patients who are allergic to penicillin, it would not be unusual to give it. Furthermore, the nurses must be aware of assessments and interventions that apply to vancomycin that are over and above those routinely performed when administering penicillin. Therefore, 2-South developed a preprinted multidisciplinary protocol that specifies how the drug is to be administered: for example, that the drug is to be given no faster than 100 mL/hour and that it is never given intramuscularly. It also specifies the important nursing observations to make: for example, monitor for tinnitus, oliguria, hypotensive reaction, rash, chills, and itching. You would simply note on the formal problem list the reference to the protocol (see Table 10–1, item 12).

If there are collaborative problems that are not covered by any of the above documents, they must be written on the care plan, and individualized nursing orders must be developed for them. This is not needed for Mrs. Sanchez.

4. *For the **nursing diagnoses** not covered by the standards of care, determine the following:*

  a. *Which nursing diagnoses really need individualized nursing care plans?* Remember that an individualized plan is needed only if the care is not completely covered by standards of care, protocols, or other routine nursing care. For Luisa Sanchez, Problems 2 through 4 and 7 through 9 need care beyond that specified in the standards of care and unit procedures. You would not expect all pneumonia patients to have these problems (Fluid Volume Deficit, Anxiety, Sleep Pattern Disturbance, Risk for Altered Family Processes, and Altered Nutrition). Therefore, they would not be found on the standardized care plan or on unit standards of care for pneumonia.

  b. *Is there c preprinted model care plan for the nursing diagnosis?* Recall that model care plans may exist for a medical diagnosis or for a single nursing diagnosis. For Problem 2, Fluid Volume Deficit, 2-South has a standardized (model) nursing diagnosis care plan. You would indicate that resource on the formal problem list (Table 10–1).

For beginning student care plans, you might not use the procedure in Step 5 (Planning step); but you will certainly use it when you develop working care plans as a professional nurse. While you are learning to write care plans, your instructors may ask you to make a complete list of the client's nursing diagnoses and collaborative problems, and to write your own outcomes and nursing orders for each problem—even the ones that are routine. You may not have the option of using standards of care, standing orders, protocols, and model care plans.

Step 6: Individualize Standardized Documents as Needed

Besides the handwritten care plans for the three nursing diagnoses, you would use the following documents to direct Mrs. Sanchez's care:

"Unit Standards of Care for Pneumonia"
"Standardized Care Plan for Fluid Volume Deficit"
"Standardized Care Plan for Altered Nutrition: Less than Body
  Requirements"
"Unit Procedures: IV Insertion and Maintenance"
"Protocol for Administration of Intravenous Vancomycin"

Assume that the "Unit Standards of Care for Pneumonia," the "Unit Procedures for IV Insertion and Maintenance," and the "Protocol for Administration of Intravenous Vancomycin" are all in the 2-South files and require no alterations for Mrs. Sanchez. Because they are a part of the permanent agency records and reflect the care given to all patients with those conditions and therapies, you would not add copies of them to Mrs.

Sanchez's comprehensive care plan. However, the standardized care plans for fluid volume deficit and altered nutrition are meant to be individualized to a specific patient. Therefore, you would individualize them and place a copy with Mrs. Sanchez's comprehensive care plan.

Step 7: Transcribe Medical, Collaborative, ADLs, and Basic Care Needs to Special Sections of the Kardex or Computer

Because 2-South uses computerized care plans, you would type the medical orders into the computer. Each day you can obtain a list of orders in effect for that day (see Figure 10–13, "Active Doctor's Orders"). Instructions for Mrs. Sanchez's diet, activity, hygiene needs, IV therapy, and so on, are also found on the care plan; some appear under "Active Ancillary Orders." (Note: page 1 of Mrs. Sanchez's computerized care plan, her Problem List, is not shown in Figure 10–13.)

Step 8: Develop Individualized Care Plan for Remaining Nursing Diagnoses and Collaborative Problems

Examining the formal problem list (Table 10–1 on page 459), you can see that you would need to develop outcomes and nursing orders for Problems 3 (Anxiety), 4 (Sleep Pattern Disturbance), 7 (Altered Comfort: Chills), and 8 (Risk for Altered Family Processes). You would type these into the computer or, in some systems you would be able to choose appropriate outcomes and nursing orders from a list provided by the computer. See Figure 10–13 on pp. 462–464 for an example of what a computerized plan for two of Mrs. Sanchez's nursing diagnoses might look like.

Implementation

Step 9: Implement the Care Plan (Do or Delegate)

On the day of admission, care was instituted immediately for Mrs. Sanchez's two highest-priority problems, Ineffective Airway Clearance and Fluid Volume Deficit. Medical orders for oxygen and intravenous antibiotics were begun, diagnostic tests were performed, and routine nursing care was given according to the Unit Standards of Care for Pneumonia, as well as other documents listed in Table 10–1. Problems 3 and 4 (Anxiety and Sleep Pattern Disturbance) were addressed by nursing orders on the nursing diagnosis care plan, and constant monitoring was done for the collaborative problems (10, 11, and 12). As a part of the Implementation step, all of this care would have been charted and passed on to other caregivers in oral reports.

Evaluation

Step 10: Evaluate Results of Care, Revise Plan as Needed

During evaluation, you will compare patient progress to the predicted outcomes and revise the care plan if necessary. Using a computerized plan, such as Figure 10–13, you would simply key in the changes and print out a new plan. On this form, there is a column for problem "Status" and a "Start/Stop" column in which one can enter the date that a problem is discontinued. Of course, not all agencies have computerized care plans. Table 10–1 on page 457 indicates how changes might be made on a handwritten problem list; Table 10–2 on page 465 shows how changes to Mrs. Sanchez's care plan would look if it were not computerized. For brevity, only Problem 3 is shown in Table 10–2. The following scenario illustrates how the evaluation step might have been done for Mrs. Sanchez on the next morning after her admission.

> The intravenous fluids quickly restored Mrs. Sanchez's fluid balance, and by the next morning, she showed no signs of fluid volume deficit (Problem 2). As you would expect, her ineffective airway clearance, along with Problems 4, 5, 6, and 9, did not improve as rapidly. These problems would resolve more slowly, as the antibiotics gradually controlled the pneumonia and her oxygenation improved. Therefore, Problems 1, 4, 5, 6, and 9 are unchanged in Table 10–1, the problem list.
>
> Improvement was noted in Problem 7. Because the oral ibuprofen was effective in lowering Mrs. Sanchez's temperature, she was no longer experiencing chills. Her husband returned as expected, removing the risk factor for altered family processes (Problem 8). Table 10–1 shows how these problems were redefined to reflect Mrs. Sanchez's changing condition.
>
> The evening and night nurses were able to effectively implement the nursing orders for Problem 3 (anxiety). Resulting changes in the care plan for anxiety are shown in Table 10–2. However, Anxiety remains on the problem list (Table 10–1) because not all the outcomes were achieved.

■ WELLNESS IN THE ACUTE-CARE SETTING

Even in an acute-care setting, nurses do not focus entirely on problems and illness needs. You can increase your wellness focus by being sure to identify client strengths and to use those strengths in working to relieve the client's problems. Mrs. Sanchez's strengths are that she is able to communicate adequately, has a healthy lifestyle, is well educated, and understands and complies with treatment regimens. Realizing this, her nurse could use discussion, pamphlets, and diagrams as nursing interventions. Because Mrs. Sanchez has a stable family situation and finances, a special discharge plan is probably not needed.

```
STORMONT VAIL REGIONAL MED CTR                    04/16/01        17:15
TOPEKA, KS 66604


Patient: SANCHEZ, LUISA
Location: 221A        Sex: F      Age: 28      Birthdate: 1/25/73     Wt.: 125 lbs
Account #: 8-37838-1 MRN: 299333 Vst#: 00279 3      Admitted date: 04/16/01
Discharge Date: / /                                 Admitting Diagnosis: PNEUMONIA
Surgical Procedure: NONE
Drug Allergies: PENICILLIN          Admitting Dr.: KATZ, R
Food Allergies: NONE                Consult Dr. 1:
Other Allergies: NONE               Consult Dr. 2:
Religion: CATHOLIC                  Consult Dr. 3:
Marital Status: MARRIED             Pri Care Phy: KATZ, R
Diabetic? N       Pregnant? N    Smoker? N     Infectious? Y     Fasting? N
Hygiene? Help bath 4/15/96
```

ACTIVE DOCTOR'S ORDERS

	Start	Stop	Entered by
ACTIVITY			
BRP, CHAIR	04/16/01		MLM
INTAKE & OUTPUT	04/16/01		MLM
ROUTINE			
IV THERAPY/FLUIDS			
PERIPHERAL - D$_5$LR @ 100CC/HR	04/16/01		MLM
PULSE OXIMETER	04/16/01		MLM
MEDICATIONS			
VANCOMYCIN 0.5 GM IV q6HR	04/16/01		MLM
TYLENOL 650 MG Q4HR PO FOR TEMP>101°	04/16/01		MLM
OXYGEN PER CANNULA, 5L	04/16/01		MLM

ACTIVE ANCILLARY ORDERS

	Ord#	Freq	Priority	Ord Dt	Status	Entered by
LABORATORY						
CBC WITH DIFF	1	X1	ROUT	04/16/01	ORDERED	MLM
ABG'S	2	X1	STAT	04/16/01	ORDERED	MLM
BLOOD CULTURE	10	X2IF TEMP>101	STAT	04/16/01	ORDERED	MLM
SERUM ELECTROLYTES	12	X1	ROUT	04/16/01	ORDERED	MLM
URINE SPEC GRAVITY	3	X1	ROUT	04/16/01	ORDERED	MLM
24-HOUR URINE	11	X1	ROUT	04/16/01	ORDERED	MLM
SPUTUM C&S	4	X1	ROUT	04/16/01	ORDERED	MLM
DIAGNOSTIC RADIOLOGY						
PA & LATERAL CHEST XRAY	9	X1	STAT	04/16/01	ORDERED	MLM
RESPIRATORY THERAPY						
POSTURAL DRAINAGE	5	DAILY	ROUT	04/16/01	ORDERED	MLM
INCENTIVE SPIROMETER	13	q3HR	ROUT	04/16/01	ORDERED	MLM
NEBULIZER	14	Q4HR	ROUT	04/16/01	ORDERED	MLM

Figure 10–13

Initial Care Plan for Luisa Sanchez. *Source:* Adapted courtesy of Stormont Vail Regional Medical Center, Topeka, KS.

```
         DAILY CARE ACTIVITY SHEET                              PAGE 3

STORMONT VAIL REGIONAL MED CTR                    04/16/01    17:15
TOPEKA, KS 66604
Patient: SANCHEZ, LUISA
Location: 221A      Sex: F      Age: 28      Birthdate: 1/25/73      Wt.: 125 lbs
Account #: 8-37838-1 MRN: 299333 Vst#: 00279 3          Admitted date: 04/16/01
```

NURSING CARE PLAN

```
Prob.
No.                                               Start   Stop  Status
3. Nursing Diagnosis:  ANXIETY (MODERATE)         04/16/01       IN PROGRESS
   Related to:         DIFFICULTY BREATHING AND CONCERNS
                       OVER WORK AND PARENTING ROLES

   Outcomes:           • LISTENS TO AND FOLLOWS INSTRUCTIONS  04/16/01   IN PROGRESS
                         FOR CORRECT BREATHING AND COUGHING
                         TECHNIQUE, EVEN DURING DYSPNEIC
                         PERIODS
                       • VERBALIZES UNDERSTANDING OF          04/16/01   IN PROGRESS
                         CONDITION, TESTS, AND TREATMENTS
                         (BY 04/16/01, 2200).
                       • DECREASED REPORTS OF FEAR AND        04/16/01   IN PROGRESS
                         ANXIETY (NONE WITHIN 12 HOURS).
                       • VOICE STEADY, NOT SHAKY.             04/16/01   IN PROGRESS
                       • RESP. RATE 12-22/MIN.                04/16/01   IN PROGRESS
                       • FREELY EXPRESSES CONCERNS ABOUT      04/16/01   IN PROGRESS
                         WORK AND PARENTING ROLES, BUT
                         PLACES THEM IN PERSPECTIVE IN
                         VIEW OF HER ILLNESS.

   Nursing Orders:     • STAY WITH CLIENT WHEN SHE IS         04/16/01   IN PROGRESS
                         DYSPNEIC. REASSURE HER YOU WILL STAY.
                       • REMAIN CALM; APPEAR CONFIDENT.       04/16/01   IN PROGRESS
                       • ENCOURAGE SLOW, DEEP BREATHING WHEN  04/16/01   IN PROGRESS
                         CLIENT IS DYSPNEIC.
                       • GIVE BRIEF EXPLANATIONS OF
                         TREATMENTS AND PROCEDURES.
                       • WHEN ACUTE EPISODE OVER, GIVE
                         DETAILED INFORMATION ABOUT NATURE
                         OF CONDITION, TESTS, AND TREATMENTS.
                       • AS TOLERATED, ENCOURAGE TO EXPRESS   04/16/01   IN PROGRESS
                         AND EXPAND ON HER CONCERNS ABOUT
                         HER CHILD AND HER WORK. EXPLORE
                         ALTERNATIVES.
                       • NOTE WHETHER HUSBAND RETURNS AS      04/16/01   IN PROGRESS
                         EXPECTED. IF NOT, INSTITUTE CARE
                         PLAN FOR ACTUAL ALTERED FAMILY
                         PROCESSES.
```

Figure 10–13
(continued)

```
DAILY CARE ACTIVITY SHEET                                        PAGE 4
STORMONT VAIL REGIONAL MED CTR                      04/16/01      17:15
TOPEKA, KS 66604


Patient: SANCHEZ, LUISA
Location: 221A      Sex: F      Age: 28      Birthdate: 1/25/73      Wt.: 125 lbs
Account #: 8-37838-1 MRN: 299333 Vst#: 00279 3          Admitted date: 04/16/01



                        NURSING CARE PLAN
Prob.
No.                                                Start   Stop   Status
4. Nursing Diagnosis: SLEEP PATTERN DISTURBANCE    04/16/01       IN PROGRESS
   Related to:        COUGH, PAIN, ORTHOPNEA, FEVER,
                      DIAPHORESIS                  04/16/01       IN PROGRESS

   Outcomes:        • OBSERVED SLEEPING AT NIGHT ROUNDS.   04/16/01   IN PROGRESS
                    • REPORTS FEELING RESTED IN A.M.       04/16/01   IN PROGRESS
                    • DOES NOT EXPERIENCE ORTHOPNEA        04/16/01   IN PROGRESS
                      (BY DAY 2).

   Nursing Orders:  • PROVIDE COMFORT MEASURES, SUCH       04/16/01   IN PROGRESS
                      AS BACK RUB, QUIET ENVIRONMENT,
                      DIM LIGHTS, DRY LINEN WHEN
                      DIAPHORETIC, AND MOUTH CARE.
                    • MONITOR AND INSTITUTE                04/16/01   IN PROGRESS
                      COLLABORATIVE MEASURES TO CONTROL
                      PAIN, FEVER, AND DYSPNEA.
                    • USE FLASHLIGHT WHEN MAKING           04/16/01   IN PROGRESS
                      NIGHT ROUNDS.
                    • USE SEMI-FOWLER'S POSITION IF        04/16/01   IN PROGRESS
                      CLIENT CANNOT FALL ASLEEP IN
                      FOWLER'S.
                    • INQUIRE DAILY IF CLIENT FEELS        04/16/01   IN PROGRESS
                      RESTED
```

Figure 10–13
(concluded)

Clients have health-promotion and illness-prevention needs beyond their admitting medical diagnoses. Sometime before discharge, the nurse might assess whether Mrs. Sanchez's health practices include regular exercise, eating balanced meals, and performing breast self-examinations. Notice, however, that the nurses must first focus on Mrs. Sanchez's more basic and immediate needs—adequate oxygenation, hydration, anxiety, and potential complications of pneumonia. This illustrates the difficulty of addressing wellness needs in an acute-care setting. Still, such an assessment could help Mrs. Sanchez to follow through on her own to improve her health after dismissal.

Table 10–2 Revised Care Plan for Luisa Sanchez (Anxiety Only)

Nursing Diagnosis	Expected Outcomes	Evaluation Statements	Nursing Orders	Rationale
Anxiety r/t difficulty breathing and concerns about work and parenting roles (4/16/01 MM)	Demonstrates decreased anxiety, as evidenced by:		(a) When client is dyspneic, stay with her; reassure her you will stay.	(a) Presence of a competent caregiver reduces fear of being unable to breathe. Control of anxiety will help client to maintain effective breathing pattern.
	1. Listens and follows instructions for correct breathing and coughing technique, even during periods of dyspnea.	1. Outcome met. Performed coughing techniques as instructed during periods of dyspnea.		
			(b) Remain calm, appear confident.	(b) Reassures client the nurse can help her.
	2. Verbalizes understanding of condition, diagnostic tests, and treatments (by end of day 1).	2. Outcome met. See nurses' notes for 3–11 shift. Stated "I know I need to try to breathe deeply even when it hurts." Demonstrated correct use of incentive spirometer and stated understanding of the need to use it. Understands IV is for hydration and antibiotics. (Evaluated 4/17/01 JW).	(c) Encourage slow, deep breathing to feel in control and decrease anxiety.	(c) Focusing on breathing may help client.
			(d) When dyspneic, give brief explanations of treatments and procedures.	(d) Anxiety and pain interfere with learning. Knowing what to expect reduces anxiety.
	3. Reports of fear and anxiety decrease; none within 12 hrs.	3. Outcome met. States, "I know I can get enough air, but it still hurts to breathe."	(e) ~~When acute episode is over, give detailed information about nature of condition, treatments, and tests.~~ *Reassess whether client needs any information about condition, etc. (4/17/01 JW).*	(e) *Detailed information has been given. Because client shows understanding, there is no need to repeat information.*
	4. Voice steady, not shaky.	4. Outcome met. Speaks in steady voice.		
	5. Respiratory rate of 12–22 per min.	5. Outcome not met. Rate 26–36 per minute.	(f) As client can tolerate, encourage her to express and expand on her concerns about her child and her work. Explore alternatives as needed.	(f) Awareness of source of anxiety enables client to gain control over it.
	6. Freely expresses concerns about work and parenting—places them in perspective in view of her illness.	6. Outcome partially met. Discussed only briefly on 3–11 shift. Not done on 11–7 shift because of client's need to rest. (Evaluated 4/17/01 JW).	(g) ~~Note whether husband returns as scheduled. If he does not, institute care plan for actual Altered Family Processes.~~ (4/17/01 Mr. Sanchez returned. JW).	(g) Husband's continued absence would constitute defining characteristic for this nursing diagnosis. It is important that this assessment be made right away so child care can be arranged if needed.

ETHICAL CONSIDERATIONS

Some say that because nursing affects people when they are most vulnerable, everything a nurse does has a moral aspect. Following this line of reasoning, the act of creating patient care plans has a moral dimension.

Conventional ethical principles are those that are widely held, expressed in practice, and enforced by sanctions. Among the basic conventional principles held by nurses are the following:

1. Nurses have an obligation to be competent in their work.
2. The good of the patient should be the nurse's primary concern.

A nurse who is careless and uncaring violates both principles. Other nurses on the unit may sanction her by avoiding her or perhaps even by reporting her behavior to a supervisor. These ethical principles suggest that nurses have a moral duty to promote client healing. A good nursing care plan aids healing by assuring that the client's needs are communicated and met. When all caregivers understand her needs and preferences, the client is reassured and less anxious and can conserve energy needed for healing.

Although not a conventional principle of nursing, the moral principle of **justice** (in the sense of fairness) is also supported by good planning. In this era of cost-containment and limited healthcare resources, it is important not to misuse human and material resources. A written care plan makes efficient use of the nurse's time, assuring that efforts will not be duplicated or time wasted in ineffective interventions. As previously mentioned, critical pathways have been shown to conserve resources by decreasing the length of hospital stays. However, nurses must always be careful not to overlook individual needs in their zeal to keep patients "on the pathway."

SUMMARY

A comprehensive care plan

- is a written guide for goal-oriented nursing action.
- provides the written framework necessary for individualized care and third-party reimbursement.
- includes a client profile, instructions for meeting basic needs, aspects of the medical plan to be implemented by the nurse, and a nursing diagnosis care plan for the client's nursing diagnoses and collaborative problems.
- may combine both standardized and individualized approaches.
- supports conventional ethical principles of nursing and the moral principle of justice.
- is replaced by a critical pathway for frequently occurring conditions in some institutions.

Nursing Process Practice

1. On the following form, construct a care plan (for one problem only) by placing the defining characteristics, nursing diagnosis, predicted outcomes, and nursing orders in the correct columns. Choose from the following scrambled list of items:

Verbally denies he is ill.

Patient will adhere to activity limitations.

Observed out of bed in spite of medical order for bed rest.

Encourage to express feelings and concerns about being hospitalized.

Give positive reinforcement for compliance (eg, staying in bed, taking meds).

Refused to take his 3 PM medication.

Patient will acknowledge consequences of not complying with treatment regimen.

Patient will agree to follow plans for care (eg, medications, bed rest).

Noncompliance (medical treatment plan) r/t denial of illness.

Develop a written contract with patient regarding bed rest and meds.

Evaluate patient's support system and need for emotional support from staff.

Defining Characteristics	Nursing Diagnosis	Predicted Outcomes	Nursing Orders

2. Use the "Guidelines for Writing Comprehensive Care Plans" in Box 10–2 on page 452 to evaluate the nursing care plan in Figure 10–13 on pp. 462–464. Use the following form. Comment on whether the care plan meets each of the guidelines (met/not met), or whether the guideline does not apply. If the guideline is not met, discuss or give an example to show how you arrived at that conclusion.

For Figure 10–13: Care Plan for Luisa Sanchez

Guideline 1:
Guideline 2:
Guideline 3:
Guideline 4:
Guideline 5:
Guideline 6:
Guideline 7:
Guideline 8:
Guideline 9:
Guideline 10:
Guideline 11:

3. Create a care plan for Mr. Cain, using the information in *(a)* through *(f)* and the instructions that follow *(f)*.

    a. Use the Patient Kardex (Figure 10–14 on page 471) for the patient profile, basic care needs, and collaborative aspects of care.

    b. Use the blank Nursing Care Plan (Figure 10–15 on page 472) for your patient's complete problem list.

    c. You have the following information from the patient's database.

Name: Harvey Cain	Age: 83	Birth date: 1/25/18
Marital Status: Married		
Home Phone: 555-1098	Religion: Catholic:	Wife's Name: Mildred Cain
	Father Wise, 555-0097	Vital Signs: Temp. 100°F
Allergies: codeine; states	No special rites.	BP 100/60, Pulse 90,
no food allergies		Resp. 20

Mr. Cain is a thin, older adult male being admitted to Room 426 for an intestinal obstruction and dehydration. He has not had a bowel movement for 5 days. His abdomen is distended and painful; bowel sounds are absent. He has been vomiting large amounts of green fluid. His skin turgor is poor; his sacrum and heels are reddened, but the skin is intact. His tongue and mouth are dry, and he complains he is a little bit thirsty. He says, "I really feel awful. Am I going to die?" He appears too weak to manage his own hygiene needs. He is oriented to place and person and able to follow second-level commands, but is drowsy and lethargic.

---

    d. The physician, Elton Hobbs, MD, has left the following orders:

IV D$_5$ lactated Ringer's, 125 mL/hr	Lab: CBC, electrolytes, SMA12
NPO	x-ray: Flat plate of abdomen, barium enema
Nasoenteric tube to continuous suction	Call Dr. Martin Botha for consult
Foley catheter to dependent drainage	Save any stools
Hourly urine measurements	Bedrest
Upper GI	

    e. Your nursing unit has the following resources available:

Standards of Care:	*Standardized Care Plans*:
Anorectal Abscess	Altered Oral Mucous Membrane
Appendicitis	Bowel Incontinence
Cholecystitis	Impaired Verbal Communication
Intestinal obstruction	Pain
Peritonitis	

Protocols for Care of Patients having:
- Barium enema
- Cholecystography
- Fiberoptic colonoscopy
- Liver biopsy
- Paracentesis

Policies and Procedures:
- Intravenous therapy
- Nasoenteric intubation and suction

f. Mr. Cain's complete problem list has already been developed for you:

Potential Complications of Bowel Obstruction:
- Dehydration
- Electrolyte imbalance
- Hypovolemic shock
- Necrosis → Infection

Risk for Altered Tissue Integrity (Pressure Ulcer) r/t decreased mobility, poor nutritional status, and poor skin turgor 2° dehydration

Abdominal Pain r/t abdominal distention

Altered Oral Mucous Membrane r/t fluid loss from vomiting 2° intestinal obstruction

Possible Fear of Dying r/t unknown outcome of illness and lack of information

Possible Fear or Anxiety r/t hospital environment, diagnostic tests, equipment & procedures

Potential Complications of IV Therapy: Phlebitis, Infiltration

Potential Complications of Nasoenteric Intubation: Ulceration→Hemorrhage

Potential Complications of Upper GI Endoscopy: Perforation, Aspiration

Potential Complications of Barium Enema

INSTRUCTIONS FOR PREPARING THE NURSING CARE PLAN

(Refer to "Comprehensive Care Plans" on pp. 434–439, and Step 5 of the Care Planning Guide on page 450.)

1. Put the client profile information on the Kardex (Figure 10–14).

2. Put the instructions for meeting basic needs (hygiene, etc.) on the Kardex.

3. Incorporate the medical orders on the Kardex.

4. On the blank form (Figure 10–15), write the problems in the appropriate columns. Write them in order of priority, the most urgent one first, or assign priority numbers, with 1 being the most urgent.

5. Indicate where the nursing interventions for each problem are to be found (review Table 10–1 on page 457 to see how this is done). Some of the problems would require the nurse to write the goals and nursing interventions. You do not need to do this; just write "Nurse will develop plan" beside those problems.

SHAWNEE MISSION MEDICAL CENTER

Date ord.	Radiology	Date Sch	DONE	Date ord.	Laboratory	Date Sch	DONE	Date ord.	Special Procedures	Date Sch	DONE
									Daily Tests		
		Ancillary Consults									
									Daily Weight		

Diet:

Food Allergies:

Hold:

Feeding/Fluids				**Activities**
☐ Self				☐ Bedrest
☐ Assist				☐ BRP
☐ Feeder				☐ Dangle
☐ Force				☐ Chair
☐ Restrict				☐ Commode
	meal	Ext	IV	☐ Up ad Lib
7-3				☐ Turn
3-11				☐ Ambulate
11-7				

☐ I&O
☐ IV
☐ Other_____

Transportation

per _____

Safety Measures

☐ Siderails
☐ Restraints
☐ Other_____

Hygiene
☐ Bedbath
☐ Assist
☐ Self Bath
☐ Shower
☐ Tub
☐ Vanity
☐ Oral Care

Bowel/Bladder
☐ Foley   IN _____
             OUT _____
☐ Cath care Bid
☐ Incontinent
☐ Colostomy
☐ Ileostomy
☐ Urostomy

Communication

Cardio-Pulmonary

Physical Therapy	Date	**Treatments**

Drug Allergies: _____

Isolation: In   Out

Emergency Instructions:

Relatives:

Phone:

Clergy:

Religion:

Religious Rites:

Code Blue

Diagnosis:

Surgery & Dates:

Consults & Dates

Room	Name		Adm Date	Age	Physician

Figure 10–14

Patient Kardex. *Source:* Courtesy of St. Luke's-Shawnee Mission Health System, Shawnee Mission, KS.

Problem List For Harvey Cain

Date and Initials	Nursing Diagnoses/Problems	Source for Goals and Nursing Orders

Figure 10–15
Nursing Care Plan (Problem List) Form

Critical Thinking Practice: Similarities and Differences

You note significant similarities and differences when you classify things (eg, grouping assessment data), when you make clincial judgments, and for other kinds of reasoning (eg, see Critical Thinking Practice in Chapter 5, "Comparing and Contrasting Ideals and Actual Practice"). The purpose of comparison is to make intelligent choices and decisions. Not all factors are equally important to our decisions. For example, if you had only $15 to spend on shoes, price would certainly be more important than style—and perhaps even more important than comfort. Critical thinkers know that things that are superficially alike may be different in significant ways.

You should avoid making **incomplete comparisons**—that is focusing on too few points. If you bought shoes based solely on the difference in price, they might be too uncomfortable to wear, and you would have wasted your money. A **selective comparison** occurs when you take a biased view: focusing only on the factors favoring one side and ignoring the factors favoring another. For example, suppose you are looking for a house and you want to live near your family. You might focus on the good points of the houses near your family and perhaps fail to notice that those houses are more expensive or need more repairs than houses you saw in other neighborhoods.

Learning the Skill

An **analogy** is a special kind of comparison that looks for ways in which things from *different categories* are similar to each other. For example, time and money are from completely different categories, but there is an expression that "Time is money." One way that time and money are similar is that everyone has only a limited amount of each.

1. List other ways in which time and money are similar.

Analogies assume that because the things are similar in some ways, they must be similar in other ways as well. For example, data from animal research are used to make decisions about drugs intended for human use.

2. How are animals and humans similar?

3. What assumptions must the researchers make about the similarities between animals and humans when recommending animal-tested drugs for human use?

Applying the Skill

A. Mari Winfrey, age 30, and Jin Li, age 85, each had a right mastectomy for breast cancer on the same day. Their nurse is planning care for both women, using a critical pathway for mastectomy patients. In addition to the usual complications of surgery (eg, pain, bleeding, and infection), the pathway addresses the nursing diagnoses of Altered Mobility and Risk for Ineffective Individual Coping.

1. What similarities do these two patients have?

2. What differences do they have?

3. What else does the nurse need to know about these women in order to know whether the critical pathway will effectively address the needs of both?

B. Two patients have a nursing diagnosis of Risk for Ineffective Management of Therapeutic Regimen related to Knowledge Deficit. Debby Minks is a 14-year-old girl who has recently been diagnosed with type 1 diabetes mellitus. She lives with her parents. Gloria Williams is an 82-year-old woman who has chronic congestive heart failure, being treated by medication and diet. She lives alone. The nurse has printed out a standardized care plan for Knowledge Deficit and wonders if she can use it to plan teaching for both patients.

1. List all the ways in which these patients are similar.

2. Do these similarities mean that the standardized plan will work for both?

3. In # 1, underline the similarities that are significant to Knowledge Deficit.

4. In what ways are these two patients different?

5. Why are these differences important when planning interventions for Knowledge Deficit?

APPENDIX A

American Nurses Association Code for Nurses

1. The nurse provides services with respect for human dignity and the uniqueness of the client, unrestricted by considerations of social or economic status, personal attributes, or the nature of health problems.
2. The nurse safeguards the client's rights to privacy by judiciously protecting information of a confidential nature.
3. The nurse acts to safeguard the client and the public when health care and safety are affected by the incompetent, unethical, or illegal practice of any person.
4. The nurse assumes responsibility and accountability for individual nursing judgments and actions.
5. The nurse maintains competence in nursing.
6. The nurse exercises informed judgment and uses individual competence and qualifications as criteria in seeking consultation, accepting responsibilities, and delegating nursing activities to others.
7. The nurse participates in activities that contribute to the ongoing development of the profession's body of knowledge.
8. The nurse participates in the profession's efforts to implement and improve standards of nursing.
9. The nurse participates in the profession's efforts to establish and maintain conditions of employment conducive to high-quality nursing care.
10. The nurse participates in the profession's effort to protect the public from misinformation and misrepresentation and to maintain the integrity of nursing.
11. The nurse collaborates with members of the health professions and other citizens in promoting community and national efforts to meet the health needs of the public.

Reprinted with permission from *Code for Nurses with Interpretive Statements*, © 1985. American Nurses Publishing, American Nurses Foundation/American Nurses Association, Washington, DC.

APPENDIX B

Portion of Nursing Data Base Based on Gordon's Functional Health Patterns

Patient Admission Assessment

Name: _____ Age: _____

Prefer to be called: _____ Date: _____

Next of Kin: _____ Relationship: _____ Phone: _____

Other contact person: _____ Phone: _____

Primary Language, if other than English: _____ Person completing form: _____

Why are you being admitted to the hospital? _____

List any previous hospitalizations and/or surgeries: _____

Do you have any of these health problems (please check)

___Alzheimers	___Dizziness	___Hepatitis	___Asthma	___Chest Pain
___Epilepsy	___High Blood Pressure	___Hiatal Hernia	___Cough	___Heart Flutter
___Seizures	___Diabetes	___Arthritis	___Mucous Production	___Congestive Heart Failure
___Numbness	___Thyroid	___Back Injury	___Shortness of Breath on Activity	___Heart Pounding
___Tingling	___Swelling		___Difficulty Breathing	___Pacemaker
			___Emphysema	___No Problems

If yes, please explain: _____

Are there any other medical problems of which we should be aware? _____

Do you have any eyesight and/or hearing difficulties? Yes ☐ No ☐

If yes, indicate use of: glasses contacts hearing aid other: _____

Do you wear dentures? Yes ☐ No ☐ If yes, what kind? Upper Lower Partial Full

Are you on a special diet? Yes ☐ No ☐ If yes, what kind: _____

ALLERGIES

Do you have any allergies to: Food: _____ Type of Reaction: _____

Medications: _____ Type of Reaction: _____

Anesthesia: _____ Type of Reaction: _____

Other (wool, tape, pollens): _____ Type of Reaction: _____

It is important that we are aware of the use of any of the following substances in order to keep you comfortable and to avoid interaction with other medication/anesthetic that might be prescribed. Do you use any of the following? (Please circle)

Alcohol	Tobacco	Amphetamines (uppers)	Barbiturates (downers)	Tranquilizers
Marijuana	Heroin	Cocaine	Caffeine (tea, coffee, pop)	Other: _____

Are you currently taking _any_ medications? Yes ☐ No ☐ Did you bring them with you? Yes ☐ No ☐

Are you taking your medications as ordered by your physician? Yes ☐ No ☐

Please list below, any medications you are taking (including prescription and over the counter medications)

MEDICATIONS

MEDICATION	DOSE	HOW OFTEN	REASON	PRESCRIBING PHYSICIAN

Form No. 102A (Revised 9/89)   PATIENT ADMISSION ASSESSMENT

476

APPENDIX B, CONTINUED

**PATIENT ADMISSION
ASSESSMENT
continued—Page 2**

NUTRITION/ METABOLIC

Any recent weight loss or gain?: Yes ☐ No ☐   If yes, how much:_____ ☐ Gain   ☐ Loss
Do you have?: (Please circle)   Nausea/Vomiting   Stomach Pains   Poor Appetite
                                Difficulty Chewing or Swallowing   Heartburn   No Problems
Comments:_____

ELIMINATION

Last bowel movement: _____
What is your usual bowel pattern?   Daily   Twice a day   Every other day   Other:_____
Do you have?   Constipation   Diarrhea   Hemorrhoids   Other: _____
Indicate any laxatives/enemas or "home remedies" that you use:_____
Have you been experiencing any urinary problems?:   Burning   Frequency   Urgency
     Bed Wetting   Bloody Urine   Problems holding urine   Difficulty starting to urinate   Last void: _____
     No Problems   Other:_____
How often do you urinate?:_____   Describe color: _____
Comments:_____

SEXUAL/ REPRODUCTIVE

FEMALE: Have you been through menopause?: Yes ☐ No ☐   Please explain your normal menstrual pattern:_____
Any recent problems or changes in your menstrual pattern?:   Yes ☐ No ☐   If yes, please explain:_____

Date of last normal period:_____   Could you be pregnant?: Yes ☐   No ☐
Do you take birth control pills?: Yes ☐ No ☐   Do you perform a monthly breast exam?: Yes ☐   No ☐
MALE: Have you experienced any?: (Please circle) Prostate problems   Sores on your penis   Testicular problems   Bleeding   Discharge
Do you perform a monthly testicular exam?:   Yes ☐   No ☐   No problems

SLEEP

How long do you sleep?:_____p.m. to_____a.m.   Is it adequate?: Yes ☐ No ☐   Do you nap? Yes ☐   No ☐
Do you have difficulty sleeping?:   Yes ☐ No ☐   If yes, what do you do to help yourself fall asleep?:_____

COGNITIVE/ PERCEPT

Do you have a history of chronic pain?:   Yes ☐ No ☐   If yes, please explain:_____

What do you do to relieve pain?:_____
How do you learn best?: (Please circle)   Reading   Listening   Demonstration

SELF. PERCEPT

How are you feeling about being hospitalized?:   Frightened   Calm   Angry   Worried   Relieved   Sad   Hopeful
Other:_____

ROLE/ RELATIONSHIP

Marital status: (Please circle)   Single   Married   Separated   Divorced   Widowed
Do you have children?:   Yes ☐   No ☐   List ages:_____
Are you presently employed?:   Yes ☐   No ☐   Occupation:_____
Are you presently in school?:   Yes ☐   No ☐   Will illness interfere?   Yes ☐ No ☐
Upon discharge, if needed, will you be able to afford: Medicine Yes ☐ No ☐   Supplies Yes ☐ No ☐   Medical Care Yes ☐ No ☐

COPING/ STRESS

Are you experiencing any stressful situations other than your illness/hospitalization?:   Yes ☐   No ☐
If yes, please describe:_____
How do you usually cope with tension or stress?:_____

VALUE/ BELIEF

Will illness/hospitalization interfere with any of the following?: (Please circle)
          Spiritual or Religious Practice   Family Traditions   Cultural Beliefs or Practice   Will not interfere
If yes, please explain:_____
Would you like your Clergy or Hospital Chaplain to be contacted?:   Yes ☐   No ☐
If yes, state name and number:_____

APPENDIX C

Multidisciplinary (Collaborative) Problems Associated with Diseases and Other Physiological Disorders

(*Source*: Wilkinson (1999), *Nursing Diagnosis and Interventions Pocket Guide*, 7th ed, Upper Saddle River, NJ: Prentice Hall Health)

*PC = Potential Complications

■ CANCER

*PC of Cancer:
Anemia
Bowel obstruction
Cachexia
Clotting disorders
Electrolyte imbalance
Fractures, pathological
Hemorrhage
Obstructive uropathy
Metastasis to vital organs (eg, brain, lungs)
Pericardial effusions, tamponade
Sepsis—septic shock
Spinal cord compression
Superior vena cava syndrome
Tissue anoxia→ necrosis

PC of Antineoplastic Medications:
Specify for each drug (eg, anemia, bone marrow depression, cardiac toxicity, CNS toxicity, congestive heart failure, electrolyte imbalance, enteritis, leukopenia, necrosis at IV site, pneumonitis, renal failure, thrombocytopenia)

PC of Narcotic Medications:
Depressed respirations, consciousness, and blood pressure; cardiovascular collapse, biliary spasm

PC of Radiation Therapy:
Increased intracranial pressure, myelosuppression, inflammation, fluid/electrolyte imbalances

* Also see specific disorders, such as Gastrointestinal Function Disorders, for effects of cancer on those patterns

■ CARDIAC FUNCTION DISORDERS

PC of Angina/Coronary Artery Disease:
Myocardial infarction

PC of Congestive Heart Failure:
Ascites
Cardiac decompensation, severe
Cardiogenic shock
Deep vein thrombosis
Gastrointestinal congestion→malabsorption
Hepatic failure
Pulmonary edema, acute
Renal failure

PC of Digitalis Administration:
Toxicity

PC of Dysrhythmias:

Decreased cardiac output→Decreased my-
   ocardial perfusion→Heart failure
Severe atrioventricular conduction blocks
Thromboemboli formation→Stroke
Ventricular fibrillation

PC of Myocardial Infarction:

Cardiogenic shock
Dysrhythmia
Infarct extension or expansion
Myocardial rupture
Pulmonary edema
Pulmonary embolism
Pericarditis
Thromboembolism
Ventricular aneurysm

PC of Pericarditis/Endocarditis:

Cardiac tamponade
Congestive heart failure
Emboli (pulmonary, cerebral, renal, spleen,
   heart)
Valvular stenosis

**PC of Reheumatic Fever/Rheumatic
Heart Disease:**

Congestive heart failure
Decreased ventricular function
Endocarditis
Pericardial effusion
Valvular changes

■ ENDOCRINE FUNCTION DISORDERS

PC of Adrenal Gland Disorders:

PC of Addison's Disease:
Addisonian crisis (shock, coma)
Diabetes mellitus
Thyroid disease

PC of Cushing's Disease:

Congestive heart failure
Hyperglycemia
Hypertension
Pancreatic tumors
Potassium and sodium imbalance
Psychosis

PC of Diabetes Mellitus:

Coma
Coronary artery disease
Hypoglycemia
Infections
Ketoacidosis
Nephropathy
Peripheral vascular disease
Retinopathy

PC of Parathyroid Gland Disorders:

PC of Hyperparathyroidism:
Hypercalcemia→Cardiac arrhythmias
Hypertension
Metaboic acidosis
Pathologic fractures
Peptic ulcers
Psychosis
Renal calculi, renal failure

PC of Hypoparathyroidism:
Hypocalcemia→Cardiac arrhythmias
Convulsions
Malabsorption
Psychosis
Tetany

PC of Pituitary Gland Disorders:

PC of Anterior Pituitary Disorders:
Acromegaly
Congestive heart failure
Seizures

PC of Posterior Pituitary Disorders:
Loss of consciousness
Hypernatremia
Seizures

PC of Thyroid Gland Disorders:

PC of Hyperthyroidism:
Exophthalmos
Heart disease
Negative nitrogen balance
Thyroid crisis

PC of Hypothyroidism:
Adrenal insufficiency
Cardiovascular disorders
Myxedema coma
Psychosis

■ GASTROINTESTINAL (GI) FUNCTION DISORDERS

PC of Esophageal Disorders:

PC of Esophageal Diverticula:
Obstruction
Pulmonary aspiration of regurgitated food

PC of Esophageal Surgery:
Reflux esophagitis
Stricture formation

PC of Hiatal Hernia:
Incarceration
Necrosis→Hemorrhage

PC of Gallbladder, Liver, and Pancreatic Disorders:

PC of Cirrhosis:
Ascites
Anemia
Diabetes
Disseminated intravascular coagulation (DIC)

Esophageal varices
GI bleeding/hemorrhage
Hepatic encephalopathy
Hyperbilirubinemia
Hypokalemia
Splenomegaly
Peritonitis
Renal failure

PC of Cholelithiasis and Cholecystitis:
Fistula
Gallbladder perforation
Intestinal ileus/obstruction
Obstruction of common bile duct→liver
  damage
Pancreatitis
Peritonitis

PC of Hepatic Abscess:
Fluid/electrolyte imbalance
Hyperbilirubinemia

PC of metronidazole or iodoquinol administration:
Bone marrow suppression

PC of Hepatitis:
Cirrhosis
Hepatic encephalopathy
Hepatic necrosis

PC of Pancreatitis:
Ascites
Cardiac failure
Coma
Delirium tremens
Diabetes mellitus
Hemorrhage
Hypovolemic shock
Hypocalcemia
Hyper/hypoglycemia
Pancreatic abscess
Pancreatic pseudocyst

Pleural effusion/respiratory failure
Psychosis
Renal failure
Tetany

PC of GI Infections:

PC of Appendicitis:
Abscess
Gangrenous appendicitis
Perforated appendix
Peritonitis
Pylephlebitis

PC of Bacterial or Viral Infections (eg, Food Poisoning):
Bowel perforation
Dehydration
Hemolytic uremic syndrome
Hypokalemia
Hypovolemic shock
Metabolic acidosis
Metabolic alkalosis
Peritonitis
Respiratory muscle paralysis
Thrombotic thrombocytopenic purpura

PC of Helminthic Infections:
Anemia
Bowel, biliary, or pancreatic duct obstruction
Migration to liver or lungs

PC of Peritonitis:
Hypovolemic shock
Septicemia
Septic shock

PC of GI Inflammatory Diseases (eg, diverticulitis, gastritis, peptic ulcer, ulcerative colitis):
Abscess
Anal fissure
Anemia
Colorectal carcinoma
Fistula

Fluid/electrolyte imbalances
GI bleeding/hemorrhage
Intestinal obstruction
Intestinal perforation
Peritonitis
Pyloric obstruction
Toxic megacolon

PC of Gastrectomy, Pyloroplasty:
Dumping syndrome

PC of Structural and Obstructive GI Disorders:

PC of Hemorrhoids and Anorectal Lesions:
Anemia
Infection
Thrombosed hemorrhoid
Sepsis

PC of Hernias:
Bowel infarction
Bowel perforation
Hernia incarceration and strangulation
Peritonitis

PC of Intestinal Obstruction:
Bowel wall necrosis
Gangrene
Fluid and electrolyte imbalance
Hypovolemic or septic shock
Intestinal perforation
Peritonitis

PC of Malabsorption Syndromes:
Anemia
Bleeding
Delayed maturity
Lack of growth
Muscle wasting
Rickets (and other nutrient deficiencies)
Tetany

■ HEMATOLOGIC DISORDERS

PC of Aplastic Anemia:
Congestive heart failure
Hemorrhage
Infections

PC of Coagulation Disorders:
Hemorrhage (Specific effects are determined by site of bleeding, eg, increased intracranial pressure in the brain, adult respiratory distress syndrome in the cardiovascular system.)
Joint deformity/disability

PC of Leukemias:
Anemia
Bleeding difficulties/internal hemorrhage
Bone infarctions
Coma
Hepatomegaly
Infections
Renal failure
Seizures
Splenomegaly
Tachycardia

PC of Nutritional Anemias:
Impaired neurologic functioning (eg, problems with proprioception)
Impaired cardiac functioning

PC of Iron Therapy:
Hypersensitivity
Toxicity (cardiovascular collapse, liver necrosis, metabolic acidosis)

PC of Cyanocobalamin Therapy:
Hypersensitivity
Hypokalemia
Peripheral vascular thrombosis
Pulmonary edema

PC of Polycythemia:
Bone marrow fibrosis
Gastrointestinal bleeding and ulcers
Splenomegaly
Thrombosis (various organs)

PC of Sickle Cell Anemia:
Multisystem organ failure (eg, congestive heart failure, hyperuricemia, hepatomegaly, hepatic abscesses/fibrosis, hyperbilirubinemia, gallstones, bone marrow aplasia, osteomyelitis aseptic bone necrosis, skin ulcers, vitreous hemorrhage, retinal detachment)
Sickle cell crisis

PC of Sickle Cell Crisis:
Aplastic crisis
Cerebrovascular accident
Hemosiderosis (from repeated transfusions)
Infections (eg, pneumonia)
Seizures
Splenic sequestration→circulatory collapse

■ IMMUNE FUNCTION DISORDERS

PC of Altered Immune Function:
Allergic reactions→Anaphylaxis
Autoimmune disorders (eg, systemic lupus erythematosus)
Delayed wound healing
Infections (eg, nosocomial, opportunistic)
Spesis→septicemia
Tissue inflammation, acute/chronic (eg, granulomas)
Transplant/graft rejection

PC of Autoimmune Deficiency Syndrome (AIDS):
HIV wasting syndrome
Malignancies: Cervical cancer, Kaposi's sarcoma, lymphomas
Neurologic: Dementia complex, meningitis
Opportunistic infections (eg, candida, cytomegalovirus, herpes, *Mycobacterium*

avium, Pneumocystis carinii pneumonia, toxoplasmosis, tuberculosis)

■ IMMOBILIZED PATIENT

PC of Immobility:
Contractures
Decreased cardiac output
Decubitus ulcers
Embolus
Hypostatic pneumonia
Joint ankylosis
Orthostatic hypotension
Osteoporosis
Renal calculi
Thrombophlebitis

■ MUSCULOSKELETAL DISORDERS AND TRAUMA

PC of Amputation:
Contracture
Delayed healing
Edema of the stump
Infection

PC of Fractures:
Compartment syndrome
Deep vein thrombosis
Delayed union
Fat embolism
Infection
Necrosis
Reflex sympathetic dystrophy
Shock

PC of Gout:
Nephropathy
Uric acid stones→renal failure

PC of Osteoarthritis:
Contractures
Herniated disk

PC of Osteomyelitis:
Cutaneous sinus tract formation
Necrosis
Soft tissue abscesses

PC of Osteoporosis, Osteomalacia:
Fractures
Neuropathies
Posttraumatic arthritis

PC of Paget's Disease:
Bone tumors
Cardiovascular complications (eg, arteriosclerosis, hypertension, CHF)
Degenerative osteoarthritis
Dementia
Fractures
Renal calculi

PC of Rheumatoid Arthritis:
Anemia
Bony and/or fibrous ankylosis
Carpal tunnel syndrome
Contractures
Episcleritis or scleritis of the eye
Felty's syndrome
Muscle atrophy
Neuropathy
Pericarditis
Pleural disease
Vasculitis

PC of Corticosteroid Intraarticular Injections:
Intraarticular infection
Joint degeneration

PC of Corticosteroid Systemic Administration:
Atherosclerosis
Cataract formation
Congestive heart failure
Cushing's syndrome

Delayed wound healing
Depressed immune response
Edema
Growth retardation (children)
Hyperglycemia
Hypertension
Hypokalemia
Muscle wasting
Osteoporosis
Peptic ulcers
Psychotic reactions
Renal failure
Thrombophlebitis

PC of Nonsteroidal Anti-inflammatory Medications:
Gastric ulcers/bleeding, nephropathy

■ NEUROLOGIC DISORDERS

PC of Organic Brain Diseases (eg, Alzheimer):
Aspiration pneumonia
Dehydration
Delusions
Depression
Falls
Malnutrition
Paranoid reactions
Pneumonia

PC of Brain Injury and Intracranial Hemorrhage:
Brain ischemia
Herniation
Increased intracranial pressure

PC of Brain Tumor:
Hyperthermia
Increased intracranial pressure
Paralysis
Sensorimotor changes

PC of Cerebrovascular Accident (CVA):
(NOTE: The manifestations and complications of a CVA vary according to the area of the brain affected. Also, it is difficult to determine which effects are manifestations/symptoms and which are actually complications. Furthermore, many of the complications of CVA are due to the resulting immobility rather than to the pathophysiology of the CVA itself. Refer to "Immobilized Patient.")

Behavioral changes
Brain stem failure
Cardiac dysrhythmias
Coma
Elimination disorders
Increased intracranial pressure
Language disorders
Motor deficits
Respiratory infection
Seizures
Sensory-perceptual deficits

PC of Increased Intracranial Pressure (eg, Cerebral Edema, Hydrocephalus):
CNS ischemic response (increased mean arterial pressure, increased pulse pressure, and bradycardia)
Coma
Failure of autoregulation of cerebral blood flow
Hyperthermia resulting from impaired hypothalamic function
Motor impairment (decorticate or decerebrate posturing)

PC of Intracranial Aneurysm:
Hydrocephalus
Hypothalamic dysfunction
Rebleeding
Seizures
Vasospasm

PC of Meningitis and Encephalitis:
Arthritis
Brain infarction
Coma
Cranial nerve damage
Hydrocephalus
Increased intracranial pressure
Seizures

PC of Multiple Sclerosis:
Pneumonia
Dementia
Sudden progression of neurological symptoms: convulsions, coma
Urinary tract infection

PC of Myasthenia Gravis:
Aspiration
Cholinergic crisis
Dehydration
Myasthenic crisis
Pneumonia

PC of Parkinson's Disease:
Depression and social isolation
Falls
Infections related to immobility (eg, pneumonia)
Malnutrition related to dysphagia and immobility
Oculogyric crisis
Paranoia and hallucinations
Pressure ulcers

PC of Seizure Disorder:
Accidental trauma (eg, burns, falls)
Aspiration
Head injury
Status epilepticus→Acidosis, hyperthermia, hypoglycemia, hypoxia

PC of Spinal Cord Injury:
Autonomic dysreflexia
Cardiac dysrhythmias

Complications due to Immobility (See "Immobilized Patient.")
Hypercalcemia
Necrosis of spinal cord tissue
Paralytic ileus
Respiratory infection secondary to decreased cough reflex
Spinal shock

◼ PERIPHERAL VASCULAR AND LYMPHATIC DISORDERS

PC of Aneurysms:

PC of Aortic Aneurysm:
Dissection
Hemiplegia and lower extremity paralysis (with dissection)
Rupture→hypovolemic shock

PC of Femoral and Popliteal Aneurysms:
Embolism
Gangrene
Rupture
Thrombosis

PC of Hypertension:
Aortic dissection
Cerebrovascular accident
Congestive heart failure
Hypertensive crisis
Malignant hypertension
Myocardial ischemia
Papilledema
Renal insufficiency
Retinal damage

PC of Lymphedema:
Cellulitis
Lymphangitis

PC of Peripheral Arterial Disease:
Arterial thrombosis
Cellulitis

Cerebrovascular accident
Hypertension
Ischemic ulcers
Tissue necrosis→gangrene

PC of Thrombophlebitis:
Chronic leg edema
Pulmonary embolism
Stasis ulcers

PC of Varicose Veins:
Cellulitis
Hemorrhage
Vascular rupture
Venous stasis ulcers

■ RESPIRATORY FUNCTION DISORDERS

PC of Asthma:
Atelectasis
Cor pulmonale
Dehydration
Pneumothorax
Respiratory infection
Status asthmaticus

PC corticosteroid therapy:
Hypertension, hypokalemia, hypoglycemia,
    immunosuppression, osteoporosis, ulcers

PC of methylxanthine therapy:
Toxicity (seizures, circulatory failure, respira-
    tory arrest)

PC of Chronic Obstructive Pulmonary Disease (COPD):
Hypoxemia
Respiratory acidosis
Respiratory failure
Respiratory infection
Right-sided heart failure
Spontaneous pneumothorax

PC of Pneumonia:
Bacteremia→Endocarditis, meningitis, peri-
    tonitis
Lung abscess and empyema
Lung tissue necrosis
Pleuritis

PC of Pulmonary Edema:
Cerebral hypoxia
Multi-system organ failure
Right-sided heart failure

PC of Pulmonary Embolism:
Pulmonary infarction with necrosis
Right ventricular heart failure
Sudden death

PC of Tuberculosis:
Bacteremia—extrapulmonary tuberculosis
    (eg, genitourinary tuberculosis, meningitis,
    peritonitis, pericarditis)
Bronchopleural fistula
Empyema

PC of medications for tuberculosis:
Hepatotoxicity, hypersensitivity, nephrotoxic-
    ity, peripheral neuropathy (isoniazid), optic
    neuritis (ethambutol)

■ SEXUALY TRANSMITTED DISEASES

PC of Chlamydial Infections:
Females: Abortion, infertility, pelvic abscesses,
    pelvic inflammatory disease, postpartum en-
    dometritis, spontaneous abortion, stillbirth
Males: Epididymitis, prostatitis, urethritis
Neonates: Ophthalmia neonatorum, pneumo-
    nia

PC of Genital Herpes:
All: Herpes keratitis
Females: Cervical cancer

Males: Ascending myelitis, lymphatic suppuration, meningitis, neuralgia, urethral strictures

Neonates: Potentially fatal infections; infections of eyes, skin, mucous membranes, and central nervous system

PC of Genital Warts:
All: urinary obstruction and bleeding

Females: Increased risk of cancer of the cervix, vagina, vulva, and anus; obstruction of the birth canal during labor; transmission to neonate

Neonates: Respiratory papillomatosis

PC of Gonorrhea:
All: Secondary infection of lesions, fistulas, chronic ulcers, sterility

Females: Abdominal adhesions, ectopic pregnancy, pelvic inflammatory disease

Males: Epididymitis, nephritis, prostatitis, urethritis

Neonates: Ophthalmia neonatorum

PC of Syphilis:
Blindness, paralysis, heart failure, liver failure, mental illness

■ SHOCK

PC of Shock:
Cerebral hypoxia→coma
Multiple organ system failure
Paralytic ileus
Pulmonary emboli
Renal failure

■ SKIN INTEGRITY DISORDERS

PC of Burns:
Airway obstruction (inhalation injury)
Curling's ulcer
Hypothermia
Hypovolemic shock

Hypervolemia
Infection secondary to suppression of immune system
Negative nitrogen balance
Paralytic ileus
Renal failure
Sepsis
Stress ulcers

PC of Skin Lesions/Dermatitis/Acne:
Cyst formation
Malignancy
Infection

PC of Herpes Zoster:
Dissemination→visceral lesions
Encephalitis
Loss of vision

PC of Pressure Ulcer:
Necrotic damage to muscle, bone, tendons, joint capsule
Infection
Sepsis

■ URINARY ELIMINATION DISORDERS

PC of Cystitis:
Bladder ulceration
Bladder wall necrosis
Renal infection

PC of Polycystic Kidney Disease:
Renal calculi
Urinary tract infection
Renal failure

PC of Pyelonephritis:
Bacteremia
Chronic pyelonephritis
Renal insufficiency
Renal failure

PC of Renal Failure, Acute:
Electrolyte imbalance
Fluid overload
Metabolic acidosis
Pericarditis
Platelet dysfunction
Secondary infections

PC of Renal Failure, Chronic:
Anemia
Cardiac tamponade, pericarditis
Congestive heart failure
Fluid and electrolyte imbalance
Gastrointestinal bleeding

Hyperparathyroidism
Infections
Medication toxicity
Metabolic acidosis
Pleural effusion
Pulmonary edema
Uremia

PC of Urolithiasis:
Hydronephrosis
Hydroureter
Infection
Pyelonephritis
Renal insufficiency

APPENDIX D

Multidisciplinary (Collaborative) Problems Associated with Surgical Treatments

(*Source*: Wilkinson (1999), *Nursing Diagnosis and Interventions Pocket Guide*, 7th ed, Upper Saddle River, NJ: Prentice Hall Health)

Type of Surgery	Potential Complications (Multidisciplinary Problems)
Potential Complications of:	
General Surgery (Complications that can occur regardless of type of surgery)	Atelectasis Bronchospasm or laryngospasm on extubation (with general anesthesia) Electrolyte imbalance Excessive bleeding→shock Fluid imbalance Headache from leakage of cerebrospinal fluid (with regional anesthesia) Hypotension (with regional anesthesia) Ileus Infection Stasis pneumonia Urinary retention→bladder distention Venous thrombosis→pulmonary embolism Wound dehiscence→evisceration
Instructions: Choose complications from "General Surgery" above; then choose those that apply to patient's particular type of surgery, following. The following are *in addition to* the complications for "General Surgery."	
Abdominal surgery	Dehiscence Fistula formation Paralytic ileus Peritonitis Renal failure Surgical trauma (eg, to ureter, bladder, or rectum)
Breast surgery	Cellulitis Hematoma Lymphedema Seroma

Type of Surgery	Potential Complications (Multidisciplinary Problems)

Chest surgery:
  Coronary artery
  bypass graft
	Cardiovascular insufficiency
	Renal insufficiency
	Respiratory insufficiency

Chest surgery:	Adult respiratory distress syndrome
Thoracotomy	Bronchopleural fistula Cardiac dysrhythmias Empyema of the chest cavity Hemothorax Infection at chest tube sites Mediastinal shift Myocardial infarction Pneumothorax Pulmonary edema Subcutaneous emphysema
Craniotomy	Cardiac dysrhythmias Cerebral/cerebellar dysfunction Cerebrospinal fluid leaks Cranial nerve impairment Gastrointestinal bleeding Hematomas Hydrocephalus Hygromas Hyperthermia/hypothermia Hypoxemia Increased intracranial pressure Meningitis/encephalitis Residual neurological defects Seizures
Eye Surgery	Endophthalmus Hyphema Increased intraocular pressure Lens implant dislocation Macular edema Retinal detachment Secondary glaucoma
Musculoskeletal Surgeries	Bone necrosis Fat embolus Flexion contractures Hematoma Joint dislocation/displacement of prosthesis Nerve damage Sepsis Synovial herniation
Neck Surgeries	Airway obstruction Aspiration Cerebral infarction

Type of Surgery	Potential Complications (Multidisciplinary Problems)
Neck Surgeries (continued)	Cranial nerve damage Fistula formation (eg, between hypopharynx and skin) Flap rejection (in radical neck dissection) Hypertension/hypotension Hypoparathyroidism (in thyroidectomy/parathyroidectomy) Local nerve damage (eg, laryngeal nerve) Respiratory distress Tetany (in thyroidectomy) Thyroid storm Tracheal stenosis Vocal cord paralysis
Rectal Surgery	Fistula formation Stricture formation
Skin Grafts	Edema Flap necrosis Graft rejection Hematoma
Spinal Surgery	Displacement of bone graft (in laminectomy/spinal fusion) Bladder or bowel dysfunction Cerebrospinal fistula Hematoma Nerve root injury Paralytic ileus Sensorineural impairments Spinal cord edema or injury
Urologic Surgery	Bladder neck constriction Bladder perforation (intraoperative) Epididymitis Paralytic ileus Retrograde ejaculation (in prostate resection/prostatectomy) Stomal necrosis, stenosis, obstruction (in urostomy/nephrostomy) Urethral stricture Urinary tract infection
Vascular Surgery: Aortic Aneurysm Resection	Congestive heart failure Myocardial infarction Renal failure Rupture of the suture line→hemorrhage Spinal cord ischemia
Vascular Surgery: Other	Cardiac dysrhythmia Compartmental syndrome Failure of anastomosis Lymphocele Occlusion of graft

ANSWER KEY for "Nursing Process Practice"

Chapter 1

1. *Caring for.* Stories will vary. Should include a nurse "doing" for a patient; for example, giving a bath, giving a medication, performing an assessment, etc. *Caring about.* Should include something about a nurse demonstrating feelings (eg, empathy, concern) for a patient. For example, a nurse stayed late to make telephone calls to a sitter for a patient who was worried about her children.

2. The appropriate phenomena of concern for the nurse are that the patient:
   a. smokes two packs of cigarettes a day
   b. coughs a lot
   c. becomes short of breath when climbing stairs
   d. is afraid that he has cancer (fear).

3. 1—c   4—d, c   7—e
   2—a   5—e   8—f
   3—d   6—e   9—b
                        10—b

4. a. Interpersonal skills
   b. Psychomotor skills
   c. Cognitive skills
   d. Creativity and curiosity
   e. Interpersonal skills

Chapter 2

1. Humility is **b**, because Patrick knew the limits of his knowledge. He took a psychology course, looked up a new medication, and reviewed the inflammatory process. The nurse in "a" did attend an inservice, where she could have acquired new knowledge. However, the situation says it was a "required" inservice, so you cannot be sure she knew the limits of her knowledge. Perhaps she thought she already knew all she needed to about the IV pump, and merely attended the meeting because it was required.

2. Independence is **d**, because Samantha thought for herself. She didn't just "follow the rules" about needle size, but adapted the procedure to the patient's needs. She didn't blindly follow visiting hours procedures, but adapted the rules to fit her patient's needs. She performed an independent nursing action for the patient with a low blood glucose level before calling the physician.

3. These actions represent clinical judgments:
   a. "*. . . helped resuscitate him and put him on a ventilator.*" This is the only action in this situation that probably was a result of the nurse's thinking. She could have been performing the neurological checks because they were a part of a standardized care plan. The medications were medical orders.
   b. No clinical judgments in this situation because no patient is involved.
   c. "*. . . turns his immobile patient at least every 2 hours.*" Based on his knowledge, Roberto made the judgment that the patient was at risk for pressure sores, and then made a judgment about what to do to prevent them. The situation presents this as though it represents Roberto's thinking.
   d. "*. . . chose to use a smaller-than-usual needle . . .*" "*. . . decided to let a patient's family stay past visiting hours . . .*" and "*. . . decided to give him some juice . . .*" The words *chose* and *decided* imply that these are all decisions resulting from Samantha's thinking about patient data and nursing actions.

4. *Nursing is an applied discipline*—**C.** The nurse applied principles of nursing to the care of a particular patient. *D* may match too. The nurse probably applied principles in making the decision about the needle size, although the case doesn't say so. She may have based her decisions on what the other nurses had been doing, on habit, on some rules she was aware of, or on her emotions. This case doesn't demonstrate application of principles as clearly as does case *C*. In *A*, the nurse is active, but the case doesn't mention application of principles. In *B*, the nurse is acquiring knowledge, but not applying it.

   Nursing draws on knowledge from other subjects and fields—**B.** The nurse is acquiring knowledge from the fields of psychology, pharmacology, and physiology. In *A*, it appears the nurse will need knowledge from other subjects, but the case doesn't point out which fields, nor that such knowledge is actually being used by the nurse. *C* would be correct if the knowledge clearly came from a field other than nursing (such as physics). This case clearly demonstrates the application of principles, but it isn't clear that the principles are from a field other than nursing. In *D*, the nurse may have used knowledge from other fields to make the decisions, but the case doesn't say so. She could just as easily have based her decisions on what the other nurses had been doing, on habit, on some rules she was aware of, on her emotions, etc.

Nurses deal with change in stressful environments— **A** is the best example of change and stress: the client stopped breathing, the nurse had three IVs to keep track of, she had to interrupt her care to go to a meeting, the schedule for neurological checks was changed, and the patient's medication was changed. All of these changes are stressful, as would be the workload of 15-minute neurological checks and three IVs. *B* does not necessarily indicate change or stress. This nurse may not find all that reading stressful—perhaps it is even relaxing. *C* indicates neither change nor stress. Perhaps this is the only patient the nurse has to care for, and he finds it relaxing to deal with immobile patients. *D* demonstrates that the nurse made several decisions, probably based on some principles. You might interpret these as stressful, but the situation doesn't make that clear. Nothing is said about change in this example.

Nurses make frequent, varied, and important decisions in their work—**D** demonstrates a series of decisions the nurse made. *C* represents only one decision made by the nurse, not "frequent or varied" decisions. In *A*, it isn't clear that it was *the nurse's* decision to resuscitate the patient, although it is possible that it was. Still, there is only one patient-care decision in *A*. In *B* the nurse made no decisions "in his work"; that is, no patient-care decisions. It is, however, implied that he decided to improve his knowledge base.

5. *Nurse C* demonstrated critical thinking.
6. *Nurse A* did not have an attitude of inquiry. She blindly accepted the night nurse's advice for therapy (authority) without any evidence that Mr. Stewart was really hypoglycemic. The night nurse's description of Mr. Stewart could indicate almost anything— not necessarily diabetes. *Nurse A* may also have failed to reflect, jumping to the conclusion that Mr. Stewart was hypoglycemic.

Nurse B made the same thinking errors as *Nurse A*—even more so, because she had no plans of her own to assess Mr. Stewart (as far as we can tell from the case). She did not look up diabetes in a text in order to make her own judgments about Mr. Stewart's symptoms. She appears to have no confidence in her ability to make judgments.

Nurse D did not reflect before giving the orange juice. She passively and unquestioningly accepted the night nurse's advice to give orange juice without any evidence that it was needed. She certainly jumped to the conclusion that Mr. Stewart had a hypoglycemic reaction when she initiated a care plan without first assessing the patient.

7. The following are some answers you may have given. There may be others, depending on your reasoning.
   a. *Creative thinking.* Because the thinking resulted in a new approach.
   b. *Rational, reasonable thinking.* Although the nurse may have reflected, the situation doesn't indicate it. Getting an aide to help probably doesn't indicate a new approach.
   c. *Conceptualization.* The nurse realized that the cues (tense facial expression, trembling hands) represented her concept of anxiety. You might also have chosen *rational/reasonable thinking* for this situation.
   d. *Reflective thinking.* The nurse took time to ponder Ms. Ginsburg's situation. She drew on her own past experience. She did not, however, consider a broad array of possibilities in deciding what action to take.

8. a. **(E)**   c. **(S)**
   b. **(E)**   d. **(P)**

   Actually, (a) and (b) might also demonstrate practice wisdom *(P)*. In the absence of ethical knowledge, the nurse in (a) might have said what she did because her nursing instructor told her this was the proper behavior, or because agency policies specify that patient data are confidential. The nurse in (b) might have heard another nurse say that families should not look at the charts; if her action is based on this, it is practice wisdom. If it is based upon her understanding of the principles of autonomy and confidentiality, then it is ethical knowledge.

CHAPTER 3

1. These meet the standard and should be checked: *a, d, f*. They demonstrate that data collection is "systematic, accessible, communicated, and in a retrievable form" and do not violate any of the other criteria. In *b*, data collection is not "continuous." In *c*, data collection is not "systematic." In *e*, data collection did not involve the patient or family, as there are no subjective data.
2. a. C   c. I   e. C   g. I   i. C
   b. C   d. I   f. C   h. C   j. I

3.

Subjective Data	Objective Data	Primary Source	Secondary Source
f, j, n, r	a, b, c, d, e, g, h, i, k, l, m, o, p, q	c, e, f, i, j, k, l, m, n, o, q, r	a, b, d, g, h, p

4. Either way is correct. If you chose to read the chart first, your reasons should include the following:
   a. It would give me at least some information about her so I would feel more comfortable.
   b. It might help me think of some initial questions to ask.
   c. It would prevent me from repeating examinations or questions that had already been covered.
   d. It would assure that I review the chart early in the data collection process. I might forget to do it later.

If you chose not to read the chart first, your reasons should be as follow:
   a. I prefer not to have any preconceived ideas or biases about her when I interview her. This will help me be more objective.
   b. I might not have time to read the chart and still be sure of getting the interview and examination finished in time for surgery. I will do those first to be sure I finish on time.

5. a. The nurse who recorded the B/P on the chart used examination *(E)*. The nurse reading the chart really used none of these. You might say she used observation, because she used her sense of sight to read the numbers on the chart—but that is a stretch!
   b. I
   c. O
   d. O
   e. E
   f. O
   g. I
   h. E
   i. I
   j. *E* (Auscultation does use the sense of hearing, but it is a special examination skill that requires the use of a stethoscope to aid that sense.)
   k. *I* (In a sense, the nurse obtained the data by interview (I) from the anesthetist; the anesthetist used the sense of touch, or observation (O).)

6. a. C
   b. O
   c. C
   d. O
   e. O
   f. C
   g. O
   h. C
   i. O
   j. O

7. Some examples of questions the nurse might ask follow:
   a. *Closed questions*: "Is it sharp or dull?" "Is it continuous or does it come and go?" "How long have you had it?" "Do you take any medication for it?"
   b. *Open-ended questions.* "Tell me more about it." "Would you describe it for me?" "Tell me how it began." "What do you do to relieve it?" "What makes it worse?"

8. a. To prepare for the interview you should do the following:
   (1) Form your goals for the interview.
   (2) Decide on a time to do it. You will need 15 to 20 minutes when you do not have treatments and other tasks to do for other patients. You will need to be sure she isn't scheduled to leave the unit for tests or treatments, that it isn't too close to mealtime, and so on.
   (3) Ask her family to leave for awhile.
   (4) Ask her if she needs anything for pain, and allow enough time for the medication to work if you give it.
   (5) Be sure she has water; ask if she needs to go to the bathroom.
   (6) Assess her emotional status/anxiety level. Deal with that as needed before beginning.
   (7) Turn down TV; turn off phone.
   (8) Pull the curtain around the bed; shut the door.
   (NOTE: You should not have listed "review her chart," because the scenario says this has already been done.)
   b. To elicit from Ms. Contini *her* understanding of "Reason for Hospitalization," you might say, "Tell me why you are here," or "Why did you come to the hospital?" Because the chart tells you she is here for knee surgery, it is more open and honest to say something like, "I see you're having knee surgery. I'd like to hear how you made that decision."
   c. In a comprehensive assessment you should ask the questions about sexual functioning. You cannot assume she is celibate or uninterested in sex because she is too old, single, or in too much pain. In fact, if the patient does have a sexual partner, one of the nurse's roles is to help the patient adapt to diseases/disabilities in order to preserve sexual functioning. This might be important to this patient if her arthritis pain is interfering with her sexual functioning.

9. You should validate the following data:
   (1) Because subjective and objective data do not match: *a, b, f*
   (2) The subjective information is not the same at both times: *d*
   (3) You will repeat the earlier questions to be sure the client was giving reliable data. If he answers the same way both times and he seems lucid, it is probably valid: *e*
   (4) There may be factors that interfere with the accuracy of the data: *g.* The client may be saying this because he is looking for an excuse to not

obtain treatment for his addiction. Or perhaps he is just not well informed of the resources in his community.

The data in item *c* do *not* need to be validated. You would expect some staining of the fingers and teeth from a heavy smoker.

10. a. *Neither.* This action contributes to the patient's autonomy. Both veracity and confidentiality can affect the patient's autonomy, but neither of those is involved in this situation.
    b. *Veracity*
    c. *Veracity*
    d. *Confidentiality*
    e. Both *veracity* and *confidentiality.* Confidentiality, because the nurse does not intend to keep the information confidential; veracity, because she is being honest with the client about what she intends to do with the information.

11. (Note that your text does not say specifically what you should do in this event.) If you expect the nurse to return very soon, you might give her the information. However, it is usually best for the nurse who makes the assessment to record it, because there is less chance for misinterpretation and error. Also, as a rule, you should record data in the client's record as soon as possible after you obtain it.

12. Health perception/Health management: none

    Nutrition/Metabolism: *h, j, l*

    Elimination: *g, l, n*

    Energy Maintenance: *a, b, c, d, e, f, g, i, k, o, p, q*

    Cognition/Perception: *f, j, r*

    Self-Perception/Self-Concept: none

    Role Relationships: *b (possibly)*

    Sexuality/Reproduction: none

    Coping/Stress tolerance: *b, f*

    Values/Beliefs: none

    Safety/Protection: *h, m, s*

    Comfort: *j, n, r*

13. A. Both assess some things about family functioning and structure (eg, coping, family roles, communication). Both assess physical health and activities of daily living.
    B. Family assessment is only one part of the home health assessment (Box 3–6) and it is done in less detail than in Box 3–7. The home health care assessment looks at the physical assessment of an individual; Box 3–7 looks at the health status of all family members. The family assessment assesses the overall health of the family, whereas the home health assessment assesses the family only as it relates to the functioning and support of the individual patient.

CHAPTER 4

1. The patient problems are *c, e, h,* and *i.*
   a. Appendicitis is a response occurring at the organ (appendix) level. Cell and organ responses, however, are usually medical diagnoses. Appendicitis is a stressor that causes problem responses at the whole person level (eg, pain).
   b. Catheter obstruction is a nursing problem. It could be the etiology for a problem of urinary retention or infection.
   d. Asthma is a medical diagnosis (see *a*).
   f. Bowel resection is a treatment. It may be the source of several patient problems.
   g. NPO is a medical order. It can cause thirst, dry mouth, and other human responses.
   j. Skin care is stated as a need. The problem might be risk for impaired skin integrity.
   k. Low white blood cell count is a laboratory test value and a cellular- or system-level response (see *a*). It may be the symptom of a problem.
   l. Lack of cooperation is a problem for the nurse, not necessarily for the patient.
   m. Constant need for attention is a problem for the nurse, not necessarily for the patient. The problem is whatever is causing the symptom (the need for constant attention).

2. You might discuss with her how nursing diagnosis can: (a) help to individualize patient care, (b) actually make care planning easier, (c) improve her care by providing a focus for planning goals and interventions, (d) help define her job to patients and other healthcare professionals, (e) help in staffing, budgeting, and work load, (f) improve communication among nurses, (g) increase nursing autonomy and accountability, and (h) help her prepare for computerizing patient records.

3. Stressors: blood clot in right thigh; intravenous catheter; heparin drip (although this is a therapy for the blood clot, it is also a stressor in other ways because of its possible side effects); complete bedrest (if you are not aware of the physiological and psychological effects of immobility, ask your instructor to recommend some references, or look in a fundamentals of nursing text).
   Responses: thigh swollen and warm, also slightly red; she rang for a nurse several times; asking to have her leg checked; requesting pain medication; observed reading her Bible. . . ; her clotting time returned to normal.

4.

Response	Level	Dimension
Thigh swollen	Organic	Physical
Thigh warm	Organic	Physical
Thigh red	Organic	Physical
Rang for nurse several times	Whole person	Interpersonal; probably caused by a psychological response (eg, anxiety, fear)
Requesting pain medication	Whole person	Interpersonal
Observed reading Bible	Whole person	Spiritual
Clotting time returned to normal	Systemic	Physical

5.

For a client with a medical diagnosis of:	Problem	r/t Etiology
Fractured femur	a. Acute Pain	r/t edema and tissue trauma
	b. Risk for Impaired Skin Integrity: pressure sores or excoriation	r/t pressure from cast, immobility
Pneumonia	a. Ineffective Breathing Patterns	r/t obstructed airways and decreased chest excursion
	b. Activity Intolerance	r/t decreased oxygenation 2° ineffective breathing patterns

6.

a. C	d. C	g. C	j. N
b. N	e. N	h. N	k. N
c. C	f. C	i. C	l. C

7.

a. A (Actual Pain)

b. Pot (Risk for injury: falls)

c. Pot

d. Pot

e. Pot

f. A

g. Pos

h. Pot

i. A

j. Pos

k. A (She has symptoms of pain)

l. Pot (Her medical diagnosis and the signs of inflammation lead you to think she will develop pain, if it is not already present. You might choose *possible*, but she really has no symptoms of pain at this time.)

m. Pos (Limping is a sign of pain, but not enough for positive diagnosis, as it could be caused by weakness or joint stiffness.)

8. The nursing diagnoses are *b, c, d,* and *e.*

a. This is a collaborative problem; the nurse cannot independently treat or prevent either arrhythmia or myocardial infarction.

In the nursing diagnoses, the parts you should have circled follow:

b. Low Self-Esteem and Perceived Sexual Inadequacy

c. Skin Breakdown

d. Perineal Rash and Excoriation; and perhaps Urinary Incontinence. The cause of the incontinence determines whether the nurse can intervene independently.

e. Confusion and Disorientation

9.

Cluster 1	***Health-Perception/***
B/P 190/100 mm Hg	***Health-Management***
Hasn't been taking B/P pills	
because "don't make me feel	
any better."	
Forgets to take B/P pills	
Cluster 2	***Nutrition/Metabolism***
50 lb. overweight	
Eats fast food; snacks a lot	
Sedentary job	
No physical exercise	
Eats out for fun	
Cluster 3	***Energy Maintenance***
B/P 190/100 mm Hg	
Hasn't been taking B/P pills	
regularly	
50 lb overweight	
Sedentary job	
No physical exercise	
Eats fast food; snacks a lot	

There are at least three themes running through these cues: her failure to take pills, her obesity, and her hypertension. Because hypertension is a medical problem, the best way to handle it would be to use it as one of the cues in the "pills" and "obesity" groups. Students often identify it as a problem, so it is included as a cue group (Cluster 3) here to show you how to deal with it if you have done that.

Step 1: Clustering cues. In Cluster 1, not taking the pills is related to the high blood pressure. In Cluster 2, the cues are related in that they all have something to do with eating, exercise, and weight. Cluster 3 is similar to Cluster 1, but includes all cues that may be related to blood pressure, not just the medication cues.

Step 2: Identify problem and etiology. To determine which pattern the problem represents, you must first decide which is the problem and which is the "cause." In Cluster 1, the problem is that she hasn't been taking the pills. This is because she lacks knowledge about whether they are helping her and because she forgets. A problem of "noncompliance" fits best in the Health-Perception/Health-Management category. You might have chosen "knowledge deficit" or "forgetting" as the problem; but remember that everyone lacks knowledge about some things, and everyone forgets sometimes. The nurse needs to be concerned about those facts only if they are causing a problem for the patient in some way.

In Cluster 2, the best explanation is that she is overweight because she consumes too many calories and burns too few with exercise. "Overweight" is identified as a separate problem. Because it is only a *part* of the etiology of Cluster 3, it may not receive the attention it needs; therefore, a separate problem is listed for it. "Overweight" fits in the Nutrition/Metabolism category.

In Cluster 3 the best explanation is that she is hypertensive—a physiological problem. The exact etiology of essential hypertension is unknown, but obesity, improper diet, lack of exercise, and failure to take her pills are all contributing factors. The problem is a medical one (hypertension) that fits into the Energy Maintenance category; thus, you would not include this on a care plan. For nurses, hypertension is merely a cue to other nursing diagnoses (such as the problems identified in Clusters 1 and 2, both of which contribute to her hypertension).

10. *Cluster 1.* Using your own terms you might have written something like "Failure to take blood pressure medications r/t lack of knowledge about benefits of medication and forgetting." Using NANDA labels you would write, "Noncompliance (blood-pressure meds) r/t knowledge deficit (therapeutic effects) and forgetfulness."

Cluster 2. In your own words you might write, "Obesity r/t improper eating habits and lack of exercise." Using NANDA labels: "Altered Nutrition: More than Body Requirements r/t improper eating habits and lack of exercise."

Cluster 3. A medical diagnosis: hypertension. You do not need to write a statement for this cluster.

11. a. (3). The nurse may be generalizing from past experience, if she has previously cared for elderly people. Stereotypes may also be based on very limited experience with members of a group; so if the nurse's experience with the elderly is limited, this might represent stereotyping.

b. (2)

c. (4) and (5). It may also be premature data collection. Susan could have asked, "Why is that?" It is not stereotyping because stereotypes are based on *lack* of experience with a group.

d. (6). Actually, this case does not fully demonstrate that a diagnostic error was made. We are inferring that because the nurse was immobilized, she would miss important diagnoses.

12. a. Possible explanations:
The client has a pressure sore on his sacrum because the paralysis keeps him from moving about in bed and because his age causes his tissues to be fragile. Or, the client has broken skin on his sacrum because (1) he is elderly, (2) he is immobile secondary to being paralyzed on his left side. If you said, "Unable to move about in bed because of paralysis," this is an incomplete explanation because it does not explain the broken skin.

b. Possible explanations:
• Larry may become dehydrated because (1) he is losing fluids from diarrhea and vomiting and (2) he cannot take in fluids because of the vomiting.
• Possible fluid volume deficit because of excess fluid loss and inadequate fluid intake.
• Insufficient fluids in body because of diarrhea and vomiting.

You might have said: "losing fluids because of vomiting and diarrhea," but that is an incomplete explanation because it addresses only fluid loss and does not consider insufficient fluid intake nor the possible results (fluid deficit).

CHAPTER 5

1. a. Label   c. Label   e. Related factors
   b. Risk   d. Qualifying
      factors   term

2. a. 2   c. 4   e. 5
   b. 1   d. 3

3. The correctly written diagnoses are *a, d, e, g, h.*
   b—Both parts of the statement mean the same thing.
   c—Elevated temperatrue is a symptom, not a combination of cues.
   f—Problem needs more specific descriptor; the nurse cannot alter the problem or the etiology.
   i—Problem needs more specific descriptor; etiology is legally questionable.
   j—Crying is a symptom, not a problem.

4. Risk factors: possibility of going blind, post-operative NPO. Related factors: progessive loss of vision, effects of surgery, recent loss of job.
5. a. Nonadherance to medication regimen r/t lack of understanding of effects of the medication and forgetting to take it. (This is not a NANDA label.)
   b. Impaired skin integrity: pressure sore on coccyx r/t inability to move about in bed (or r/t immobility)
   c. Altered Nutrition: More Than Body Requirements r/t irregular schedule, emotional eating pattern, and insufficient exercise
   or
   Altered Nutrition: More Than Body Requirements r/t excess calorie intake and inadequate exercise
   d. Potential Complication of Hysterectomy: Hemorrhage
   e. Risk for Infection Transmission r/t communicable nature of the disease
   or
   Possible Self-Esteem Disturbance r/t social implications of the disease
   or
   Risk for Altered Sexuality Patterns r/t pain, infectious nature of the disease, and implications for relationships
6. Altered Nutrition: More Than Body Requirements
   Diarrhea   Constipation
   Risk for Infection   Altered Protection
   Risk for Aspiration   Activity Intolerance
   Social Isolation
7. *a, c, d, e*
8. *Examples:*
   a—Activity Intolerance (**Level II**)
   c—Sensory-Perceptual Alteration (**Visual**)
   d—**Moderate** Chronic **Back** Pain
   e—Impaired Physical Mobility (**Inability to sit up**)
9. a. Bowel incontinence
   b. Diarrhea
   c. Fatigue
   d. Risk for aspiration
   e. Ineffective airway clearance
10. 1. *a*   2. *c*   3. *d*
    4. *b*   5. *e*   6. *f*
11. a. Ineffective Denial
    b. Dressing/Grooming Self-Care Deficit +2
    c. Unilateral Neglect
    d. Stress Incontinence
    e. Urge Incontinence
    f. Altered Tissue Perfusion (Peripheral)
    g. Risk for Fluid Volume Deficit
    h. Parental Role Conflict
    i. Decisional Conflict (whether to have abortion)
    j. Activity Intolerance

12. Long-term stress, Loss of belief in God, Prolonged activity restriction creating isoation.
13. a. Ms. Petrie   b. Jill   c. Mr. A
14. a. Perceived Constipation r/t impaired thought processes A.M.B. overuse of laxatives and suppositories, and expectation of a daily bowel movement
    b. Constipation r/t unknown etiology
    c. Constipation r/t inadequate fluid and fiber intake and inadequate physical activity 2° weakness from chronic lung disease
    d. Ineffective Individual Coping r/t complex etiology A.M.B. verbalizing inability to cope and observed inability to problem solve
    e. Potential Complication of IV Therapy: phlebitis, infiltration, infection
    f. Possible Risk for Violence to Self, possibly r/t toxic reaction to medication
    g. Health-Seeking Behaviors (Exercise)
15. a. Low   e. High   i. Low
    b. Low   f. Medium
    c. High   g. Medium
    d. Medium   h. Low
16. a. 4   c. 1   e. 1   g. 1   i. 2
    b. 5   d. 3   f. 3   h. 3

CHAPTER 6

1. The observable goals are: *b, c, d, g, h, i, j, n*
2. Some suggested responses are provided. You may have thought of others that are slightly different. However, they should be similar.
   b. Absence of redness or swelling at site. Skin intact. Wound edges intact if healing by primary intention. Granulation tissue present if healing by secondary and tertiary intention.
   c. Temperature at least 98.0°F. Skin warm, dry, and pink. No shivering.
   d. Able to dress self. Able to dress self without assistance.
   e. Mucous membranes pink, moist, without lesions (intact). No bleeding.
3. Examples of expected outcomes using the opposite responses in exercise.

Subject	Action Verb	Special Conditions	Performance Criteria
a. (client)	will have	(none)	regular, soft, formed BM.
b. Skin	will be	(none)	without redness or swelling at site.
Skin	will be	(none)	intact.
Wound edges	will be,	if healing by primary intention,	intact.

Granulation	will be,	if healing by secondary and tertiary intention,	present.
c. Temperature	will be	(none)	at least 98.0° F.
Skin	will be	(none)	warm, dry, and pink.
(Client)	will not	(none)	shiver.
d. (Client)	will dress	(unassisted)	self.
e. Mucous membranes	will be	(none)	pink, moist, without lesions or bleeding.

4. *Back Pain r/t incision of recent spinal fusion and muscle stiffness from decreased mobility.*

Good outcomes are individualized to fit the patient. For instance, you would not say "VS within normal limits," but would list the patient's usual pulse, B/P, etc. Some ideas for outcome criteria follow:

a. Experiences adequate pain relief, as evidenced by
  (1) States pain is less than 3 on a 1–10 scale, within 20 minutes after IM analgesic
  (2) Will have no need for analgesics by postoperative day 5
  (3) After medication, will have no facial grimace or muscle tension; VS within normal limits for client (you should state actual numbers)
b. Relief of muscle stiffness, as evidenced by
  (1) Verbalizes he feels relaxed after being turned and repositioned

5. Possible outcomes:
- Pain Level acceptable, as indicated by: slight reported pain, no oral expressions of pain, or restlessness, or
- Pain Level—indicators:
  Reported pain = 4
  Oral expressions of pain = 5
  Restlessness = 5

6. Maintains skin integrity as evidenced by (a) no redness over bony prominences, (b) skin intact, (c) good skin turgor.

7. The correctly written goals are *b, c, f, i, m, n,* and *o.* Errors are as follows:

Predicted Outcome	Errors (Guideline Violated)
a. Ct will develop adequate leg strength by 9/1	*Develop* and *adequate* are not observable; should think but not write *client.*
b. . . . VS-WNL, Hct and Hbg WNL	"Within normal limits (WNL)" is not specific; but we do not know who the patient is, so we cannot individualize norms—thus, *b* is acceptable in this instance.
d. Will feel better by morning	*Feel better* is not specific, observable, or measurable.
e. Improved appetite	No verb; no special conditions or performance criteria; not observable/measurable.
g. On a 30-bed unit with only 2 wheelchairs . . .	Not realistic.
h. Client will discuss expectations . . .	Should not write *client.* Too long and complex. Derived from more than one nursing diagnosis (one relates to expectations of hospitalization, one to diet).
j. Injects self w/insulin	No performance criteria (eg, using sterile technique).
k. Will state adequate pain relief . . . and will take . . .	Derived from more than one nursing diagnosis (pain and fluids)
l. IV will remain patent . . .	A nursing goal, not a statement of desired client response.

8 and 9. In order of priority: *b, *d, a, c.

* You must address Chronic Pain and Noncompliance today.
  Rationale:
  Diagnosis *b* must have first priority because the chronic pain must be under control in order to accomplish interventions for *d,* teaching about NPO. Pain interferes with learning, Also, Pain is an immediate physical need (Maslow's hierarchy).
  Diagnosis *d* would be second. You would not want to teach about NPO after you had given pre-operative medications, which depress the central nervous system and hinder learning.
  Diagnosis *a* would probably come before *c* because (1) it may be more amenable to short-term intervention, and (2) poor self-esteem might make the pattern of "emotional" eating worse. Teaching could be done for *d* while the client is in the hospital, but the problem does not seem to be caused by lack of knowledge; so about all the nurse could do for this problem is make referrals.

10. Underline: Risk for Situational Low Self-Esteem, Chronic Pain, Altered Nutrition: More than Body Requirements for calories, and Risk for Noncompliance with NPO order.

11. Examples of goals for the two top-priority diagnoses follow. You may think of others.

Nursing Diagnosis	Goals/Desired Outcomes
Chronic Pain r/t inflammation of knee 2° rheumatoid arthritis	Will be able to carry out ADLs before surgery. States that pain is within acceptable limits before surgery at all times
Risk for Noncompliance with NPO Order r/t lack of understanding of its importance for anesthesia	Will remain NPO After teaching, will relate side effects of anesthesia to need for NPO

12. (1) Signs and symptoms:

Inflammation: Localized diffuse redness of skin around insertion site; tender to touch; skin warm at area of redness. Possibly pus at insertion site.

Phlebitis: Hardness along vein, usually above insertion site; redness of vein and surrounding vein; warmth and tenderness at insertion site and along vein.

Infiltration: Swelling at site; painful to touch or to infusion of fluids; absence of blood return when bag lowered or tubing aspirated; skin around site hard, cold, pale; fluid not running well.

(2) Predicted outcomes for each complication:

Sign/Symptom	Goals/Outcomes
Inflammation	• No redness, warmth, or pus at insertion site • States not tender • Temp. <100°F
Phlebitis	• No hardness, redness or warmth along or around vein and site • States not tender • Pulse and temp. WNL for patient
Infiltration	• Skin not cool, pale, hard, or swollen at insertion site • States not tender to touch • No complaint of pain on infusion of fluid or meds • Infusing at prescribed rate

CHAPTER 7

1. A. (1) Turn q2h around the clock. This intervention compensates for the patient's lack of mobility.

B. (1) Keep sheets taut and wrinkle-free; check bed at each turning for foreign objects; (2) Assess skin over bony prominences with each turning; (3) Encourage balanced diet, with protein and vitamin C; (4) Don't use soap to bathe; use lotion & light massage after bath. These interventions do nothing to change the etiology, but they address the problem either by assessing for signs and symptoms or by measures to preserve skin integrity, regardless of etiology.

2. A. *Observation orders*: (1) Inspect site 24h for signs of inflammation, phlebitis, or infiltration; (2) Check site for tenderness; (3) Check IV rate hourly.

B. *Prevention orders for inflammation*: (1) Wash hands before IV care; (2) Do not leave IV bag hanging for >8 hrs; (3) Change dressing & tubing q24h, on 3 to 11 shift; use aseptic technique per agency procedure; (4) Do not disconnect tubing to change gown, etc.

Prevention orders for phlebitis: (1) Check site for tenderness; (2) pulse and temp q8h; retake in 1 hr if elevated;

(You may have written orders such as, "If symptoms noted, DC IV and notify physician" or "If symptoms occur, remove IV, restart at new site, and notify physician." These are not, strictly speaking, preventive, as they would be done only after symptoms occur.)

C. *Patient teaching orders*: (1) Teach pt. to avoid touching site; (2) Teach pt. to call for help if any discomfort, if container nearly empty, or if flow changes.

3. Intervention #1. Most likely: *b* and *e*. Both mention exercise, and *b* specifically mentions strength. NIC label *d* does involve exercise, but is specifically directed to joint mobility, not increasing strength. The other interventions seem unrelated to exercise and strength, although they may help with Activity Intolerance in other ways.

Intervention #2. Although *f* might be useful, item *g* refers *specifically* to weight management. Nutrition Management probably includes nutrition for other purposes, such as preventing vitamin deficiency.

You would, of course, need to look up NIC label definitions and activities in the NIC book to know for certain what the labels mean and which to use.

4. The nursing orders are: *c, d, e, h,* and *i*.

5. a. *P* c. *A* e. *A* g. *C*
   b. *C* d. *C* f. *P* h. *P*

6. Independent: *a, b, e, f, g, h, i, j, k, l, m*
   Dependent: *c, d*
   Observation: *h, i; f* might be considered an observation order, since it states specifically *how* the assessment is to be made.
   Treatment: *a, b, e, g,* and *m* could be either treatment or prevention, depending on the problem status (*m* is most likely health promotion). *c* and *d* are treatment only.

Prevention: *a, b, e, g,* and *m* could be either prevention or treatment, depending on problem status. Orders *j, k,* and *l* are prevention only. Order *f* is preventive in the sense that it would prevent injury to rectal mucosa.

Health
Promotion: Order *b* might be considered health promotion, if Ms. Adkin's grief work is progressing normally and she has no problem in that area. It would more likely be used to treat the etiology of a problem. Order *m* is really the only nursing order that is clearly for health promotion.

Physical Care: *c, d, f, g, h, i, j,* possibly *e*

Teaching: *a, k, m*

Counseling: *b.* Possibly *l* if persuasion or help with decision making is needed.

Referral: *l*

Environment
Management: *e, g, j*

7. a. ok
   b. #1–Unclear, imprecise. #3–Incomplete. #4–Not specific. Might read, "Encourage fluids, 100 mL/hr while awake." If the patient has a fluid preference, you would specify that as well.
   c. #3–Incomplete. Needs specific times, ie, "Monitor serum potassium levels *daily* and report levels < 3.5."
   d. #2–Not concise. "Change dressing daily. Refer to unit procedures."
   e. ok
   f. #1–Unclear. #3–Incomplete. #4–Not specific. Example: "Encourage patient to *walk to the end of the hall 3 ×/day (can walk independently).*"

8. Correct: *a, c, e. b* is redundant and unnecessary because the patient is already on bed rest. *d, f,* and *g* all say "instruct," which is inappropriate at this time because of the patient's mental status. If that improves, they might be appropriate.

CHAPTER 8

1. Because they are within the scope of practice for both nurses and UAPs, you could delegate the enema and the pHisohex shower. You could have the UAP remind the patient that she is NPO and remove any water from the room; however, Ms. Atwell's compliance is ultimately the nurse's responsibility.

2. The enema is the most obvious threat to privacy and dignity. Her privacy should also be respected during the shower. She may also be embarrassed that she has difficulty walking. She may be uncomfortable talking about the hysterectomy because it involves reproductive matters. She will have her hip exposed for the pre-operative injection.

3. a. Possibilities: Refer Ms. A. to a home health agency; arrange for outpatient physical therapy.
   b. One possibility: Talk with Ms. A. about alternative ways to manage household chores, such as sitting down to iron or not ironing at all.

4. She should tell her that the shower is meant to assure general cleanliness, and to have Ms. A. use soap and rinse well. Soap and water will mechanically remove some microorganisms that could contribute to infection. Germicidal substances will be used in the operating room to destroy microorganisms in the area of the incision. If the nurse does not know the rationale, she should look it up before explaining.

5. First assess whether she still needs a sleeping pill. If she is asleep, do not wake her to give it. If she does need it, tell her what it is and what it is expected to do for her. Explain how she can make it more effective (eg, by turning off the lights and staying in bed).

6. Therapeutic communication examples: (a) Talk to her to help her identify and relieve anxiety. She says she is not anxious about surgery, but she might have other anxieties (eg, loss of childbearing function, how she will manage at home). (b) Communication could help you identify whether she is grieving over loss of childbearing ability. (c) Assess her understanding of the importance of NPO. (d) Doing preoperative teaching.

7. a. *Determine that the action is appropriate.* The turning was postponed because one need takes priority over another, not because the action would be less successful if performed at this time. You might also have chosen *provide for privacy and comfort*—Ms. Bates might not like to have her visitor see her in pain.
   b. *Be sure you know the rationale for the action. Question any actions you do not understand. Improve your knowledge base.*
   c. *Provide for privacy and comfort. Perform interventions according to professional standards.* The ANA Code of Ethics requires that you maintain client dignity.
   d. *Perform interventions according to professional standards of care . . .* Most agencies have a policy requiring insulin dose to be checked by two professional nurses. The nurse in this case does not lack knowledge of the action; she is simply guarding against error.
   e. *Perform interventions according to professional standards* (which include safety).
   f. *Determine that the action is still needed and appro-*

priate. The medication may not be needed if the patient's blood pressure is now lower than normal.

8. a. 8/6/01, 8:00 PM
   D—Says his head hurts and light makes his eyes hurt. Eyes shut tightly.—L. Nye, RN
   A—Cool cloth placed on head; door closed. Tylenol #3, tabs I, given p.o. at 6 PM (see medication record). Plan: Disturb as little as possible, keep room dark, notify Dr. King if headache unrelieved after second dose of Tylenol #3.—L. Nye. RN
   R—At 7 PM stated "My head still hurts."—L. Nye, RN

   b. 8/6/01, 6:00 PM
   D—Says his head hurts and light makes his eyes hurt. Eyes shut tightly.—
   A—Cool cloth placed on head; door closed. Tylenol #3, tabs I, given p.o. (see medication record).—L. Nye, RN
   8/6/01, 7:00 PM
   R—States head still hurts.————
   A—Plan: Disturb as little as possible, keep room dark, notify Dr. King if headache unrelieved after second dose of Tylenol #3.—L. Nye, RN
   (Did you remember to date, time, and sign your entry, and to draw lines through blank spaces?)

9. 12/9/02, 9:00 AM
   Problem: Risk for Noncompliance with Pre- and Post-operative Instructions r/t lack of knowledge.
   S—States she understands preoperative teaching, including need for NPO.————
   O—All preoperative teaching done (see unit policies and procedures). Explained NPO, including rationale.—
   A—No knowledge deficit regarding pre-op procedures.—
   P—Remind pt. periodically not to drink anything. Place NPO sign in room. Remind any visitors that the pt. cannot eat or drink.—L. Nye, RN
   (Did you remember to date, time, and sign your entry?)

10. A. You *could* delegate everything except the medication and the skin assessment, depending on the situation. If the assistant is "medication certified," you might even delegate administration of the p.o. stool softener.
    B. You might say, "Please give Mrs. A. a complete bed bath today. Be gentle with her skin; rinse and dry her well, because she may be developing a bedsore. Let me know in report if her sacral area is still red, or if the skin is breaking down—or if you see any other red spots. You can probably turn her yourself, but let me know if you need someone to hold her so you can give good back and perineal care."
    C. You could most easily assess her skin while giving the bath—and you might choose not to delegate this task, because you *must* make a skin assessment anyway. You might perform the assessment when you turn and reposition Mrs. A., but you would have to adjust her clothing to expose the skin over bony prominences.
    D. Possible plans for evaluating delegated activities:
       —*vital signs*: See that they are recorded every 4 hours; retake 1 set of VS yourself and compare with the assistant's results.
       —*bed bath/linen change*: Inspect the linen; ask the patient, "Did Sue change your sheets and give you a bath?" Examine the patient: Is she clean between her toes? Are her eyes free of matter? Are there any odors (eg, mouth, perineum)?
       —*turn/reposition*: Check throughout the day to see if Mrs. A. is in different positions and positioned/supported correctly.
       —*feeding Mrs. A.*: Check flowsheet; ask assistant how much/what Mrs. A. ate; look at Mrs. A.'s tray after lunch; ask Mrs. A. what she ate.
    E. You would *not* delegate the feeding. For a new diagnosis caused by Impaired Swallowing, you would need to feed Mrs. A. yourself in order to assess her ability to swallow and to be sure she does not aspirate. An RN should be there during the feeding to intervene in case Mrs. A. does aspirate.
    F. If you must delegate this task, you would (1) find out what experience the assistant has had feeding patients, (2) explain the risk for aspiration, including the signs, and tell the assistant what to do if it occurs, (3) tell the assistant how to position the patient and how to decrease the risk of aspiration while feeding, and if at all possible, (4) demonstrate how to feed her. If you cannot demonstrate the techniques, try to find another RN or an experienced aide to do so. Check on the progress of the feeding, if possible; or ask someone else to do so.

CHAPTER 9

1. The specific, measurable or observable criteria are *b*, *c*, and *d*.
   a. "Safe" is not observable. "Side rails up" would demonstrate safety.
   e. "Adequate number" is not measurable. "Three w/c on each unit" would demonstrate "adequate."

f. "Systematic" is not measurable. "A complete abdominal assessment is recorded in the chart once per shift" is measurable.

2. 1. *b* and *c*
   2. *a* (The data would come from the manual in structure evaluation. In process evaluation, one might note whether a nurse is following some procedures, but the data would come from observing the nurse's activities.)
   3. *c* (possibly *b*—client might report whether nurse has done required teaching, etc.)
   4. *c*
   5. *b*
   6. *a*
   7. *b*
   8. *a*

3. 1. c   5. a
   2. b   6. a (possibly b)
   3. a   7. a
   4. c

4. a. Possible outcome criteria: (1) Oral mucosa pink, moist, intact; (2) States no oral pain; (3) No inflammation or ulcerations in oral cavity; (4) Able to swallow without difficulty when no longer NPO.
   b. Examples of methods for obtaining data for the criteria:
   Examine the patient's oral cavity. Ask the client if his mouth is sore. Observe the patient swallowing or ask him if he is having difficulty. (If you were performing a retrospective audit, you would look for this evidence in the chart—probably in the progress notes.)

5. Hint: Look up the defining characteristics for Anxiety in a nursing diagnosis handbook—or in a mental health nursing text.
   a. The following are examples. You may have thought of other cues. Verbal cues that would indicate achievement of the objective might be: "I'm confident everything will go all right. I certainly don't have any experience with this kind of thing, but I know you will tell me what I need to know. I feel pretty relaxed."
   b. Nonverbal cues that would indicate achievement of the goal: Client shows no facial tension; hands folded loosely in lap; sitting quietly; no fidgeting.
   c. Verbal cues that would indicate the objective has not been achieved: "I'd really rather not talk about it now." "I'm still pretty scared."
   d. Nonverbal cues that would indicate the objective has not been achieved: Moving restlessly in bed; perspiring heavily; not making eye contact; voice is shaky and tremulous; tearful; pale; facial muscles tense; wringing hands; elevated pulse.

6. *Risk for Anxiety.* Goal met. Ct. verbalizes understanding of procedure and effects of surgery; exhibits no physical signs of anxiety. (Could also quote progress notes verbatim as evidence of goal achievement.)
   Risk for Grief. Goal partially met. Expressed feelings of relief at no longer having menses, but avoided discussion of inability to bear children. Will need to follow up after surgery.
   Risk for Noncompliance with NPO. Goal partially met. Client verbalized reasons for NPO and verbalized intent to comply with restriction; however, she did drink some water at 1130, stating "I forgot."

7. *Risk for Anxiety.* The problem has been resolved. Discontinue this entire section of the plan: nursing diagnosis, goals, and nursing orders.
   Risk for Grief. This is still a potential problem. Keep the nursing diagnosis and goal.
   Risk for Noncompliance. Because the goals are only partially met, you should keep the diagnosis. You should mark off the first goal, because the ct. has already done this.

8. *b.* Even though the client does not actually have Impaired Skin Integrity, risk factors are still present because of the client's immobility. If the nursing interventions are discontinued, the client will probably develop Impaired Skin Integrity.

CHAPTER 10

1. Column 1, Defining Characteristics:
   Verbally denies he is ill.
   Observed out of bed in spite of medical order for bedrest.
   Refused to take his 3 PM meds.
   Column 2, Nursing Diagnosis:
   Noncompliance (Medical Treatment Plan) r/t denial of illness
   Column 3, Predicted Outcomes:
   Pt. will adhere to activity limitations.
   Pt. will acknowledge consequences of not complying with treatment regimen.
   Pt. will agree to follow plans for care (eg, meds, bedrest).
   Column 4, Nursing Orders:
   Encourage to express feelings and concerns about being hospitalized.
   Give positive reinforcement for compliance (eg, staying in bed, taking meds).
   Develop a written contract with pt. regarding bedrest and meds.
   Evaluate pt.'s support system and need for emotional support from staff.

2. *Box 10–2 and Figure 10–13, Care Plan for Luisa Sanchez.*

Guideline 1: Does not apply. This care plan is for nursing diagnoses only and is not intended to address the client's medical plan of care nor her routine basic needs. It does, however, include some client-profile information (name, admitting date, and diagnosis) and some medical orders.

Guideline 2: Not met. Problems are dated but not signed.

Guideline 3: Met. The problems are numbered in order of priority.

Guideline 4: Probably met. The plan does not indicate that the nursing orders are listed in order of priority, but they appear to be.

Guideline 5: Met, for the most part. Plan occasionally fails to abbreviate.

Guideline 6: Met. Written legibly, typed (not in ink).

Guideline 7: Met. Refers to other sources for detailed treatments (eg, IV therapy).

Guideline 8: Partially met. Considers physiological and psychological (self-esteem) needs. Does not address spiritual needs. However, Ms. Sanchez's database does not indicate that she has any special needs in these areas.

Guideline 9: The problem list is individualized. There are not enough data about Ms. Sanchez to adequately individualize her nursing orders. For instance, we do not know what kinds of fluids and high-fiber foods she likes.

Guideline 10: Some collaborative aspects are included (eg, IV therapy, heparin administration). Laboratory tests, x-ray, etc. would probably be in another section.

Guideline 11: This plan does not show any discharge planning. However, it may be included in the Unit Standards of Care for Pneumonia.

3. The care plan for Harvey Cain appears in the figures below and on the following page.

Problem List For Harvey Cain

Date and Initials	Nursing Diagnoses/Problems	Source for Goals and Nursing Orders
1-1-01 JW	Potential complications of bowel obstruction	Refer to Standards of Care for Intestinal Obstruction.
1-1-01 JW	Risk for Altered Tissue Integrity (Pressure Ulcer) r/t decreased mobility, poor nutrition …	Nurse will develop goals and nursing orders.
1-1-01 JW	Abdominal Pain r/t abdominal distention	Refer to standardized care plan for Pain.
1-1-01 JW	Altered Oral Mucous Membranes r/t fluid loss from vomiting 2° intestinal obstruction	Refer to standardized care plan for Altered Oral Mucous Membrane.
1-1-01 JW	Possible Fear or Anxiety r/t hospital environment, diagnostic tests, equipment, and procedures	Nurse will develop goals and nursing orders.
1-1-01 JW	Possible Fear of Dying r/t unknown outcome of illness and lack of information	Nurse will develop goals and nursing orders.
1-1-01 JW	Potential Complications of Upper GI endoscopy Perforations …	Nurse will develop goals and nursing orders.
1-1-01 JW	Potential Complications of IV Therapy …	See "Policies and Procedures for IV Therapy."
1-1-01 JW	Potential Complications of Nasoenteric Intubation: Ulceration → Hemorrhage	See "Policies and Procedures for Nasoenteric Intubation and Suction."
1-1-01 JW	Potential Complications of Barium Enema	See "Protocol for Barium Enema."

SHAWNEE MISSION MEDICAL CENTER

Date ord.	Radiology	Date Sch	D O N E	Date ord.	Laboratory	Date Sch	D O N E	Date ord.	Special Procedures	Date Sch	D O N E
1-1	Upper GI	1/1		1-1	CBC, Lytes	1-1	✓				
1-1	Flat plate abd.	1/1			SMA12						
									Daily Tests		
	Ancillary Consults										
									Daily Weight		

Diet: NPO

Food Allergies: none stated

Hold:

Feeding/Fluids NPO

- ☐ Self
- ☐ Assist
- ☐ Feeder
- ☐ Force
- ☐ Restrict

	meal	Ext	IV
7-3			
3-11			
11-7			

- ☒ I&O (hourly)
- ☒ IV D₅ LR 1250 c/hr
- ☐ Other_____

Safety Measures

- ☒ Siderails
- ☐ Restraints
- ☐ Other_____

Activities

- ☒ Bedrest
- ☐ BRP
- ☐ Dangle
- ☐ Chair
- ☐ Commode
- ☐ Up ad Lib
- ☒ Turn
- ☐ Ambulate

Transportation
per cart

Hygiene

- ☒ Bedbath
- ☐ Assist
- ☐ Self Bath
- ☐ Shower
- ☐ Tub
- ☐ Vanity
- ☐ Oral Care

Bowel/Bladder

- ☒ Foley   IN 1-1   OUT
- ☒ Cath care Bid
- ☐ Incontinent
- ☐ Colostomy
- ☐ Ileostomy
- ☐ Urostomy

Communication

1-1 Save any stools

Physical Therapy	Date	Treatments
	1/1	Nasoenteric tube to Gomco
Cardio-Pulmonary		

Drug Allergies: Codeine.

Isolation: In   Out

Emergency Instructions:
Relatives: Mildred Cain (wife)
Phone: 631-1098

Clergy: Fr. Wise 842-0097
Religion: Catholic

Surgery & Dates:

Religious Rites: No Special   Code Blue

Diagnosis: Intestinal Obstruction; Dehydration

Consults & Dates
Martin Botha, M.D.

Room	Name	Adm Date	Age	Physician
426	Cain, Harvey	1-1-01	78	ELTON HOBBS, M.D.

Kardex for Harvey Cain. Courtesy of Shawnee Mission Medical Center, Merriam, KS

Answer Key for "Critical Thinking Practice" Exercises

There is usually no single, correct answer for these exercises because the intent is to have you practice *thinking*, not recall facts. The nature of a critical thinking problem is that it has more than one solution, and that there may not be a "best" solution. You should compare your answers with your classmates—both your solutions and the thinking you used. Discussing your thinking processes is one way to help improve your thinking. Also, it is important for you to begin collaborating with your peers. During your nursing career, the thinking of other nurses will be an important resource to you, just as your thinking can be for them.

Chapter 1

1. The qualities to be ranked are: Cognitive/intellectual skills (including decision making and critical thinking), creativity and curiosity, interpersonal relationships (including verbal and nonverbal communication), cultural competence, psychomotor skills, and technological skills.
2–4. No correct answers. Will vary with individuals.
5. Plan should include experiences needed, a plan for practicing/rehearsing the qualities, and a time frame.

Chapter 2

Reminder: Discuss answers with peers or instructors. Answers may vary. Also, you will learn as much from the discussion as you do from the exercises.

A. **Using Language Precisely**
   1. Examples of answers you might use to clarify.
      (b) *tolerated fluids well because*: she drank 50 mL of fluids every hour with no nausea or vomiting.
      (c) *ambulated with no difficulty because*: he walked to the end of the hall by himself with no shortness of breath; he rated his pain as 3 on a scale of 1–20 when turning in bed; he ambulated to the bathroom with nurse's help, with no change in vital signs.
   2. You should have underlined: elderly, patient, moderate amount of distress, and heroic measures or treatment.
   3. One possible answer: 80-year-old man admitted to Room 212 in moderate respiratory distress. States, "I can't seem to get enough air." He is pale, but not cyanotic. States that if he becomes terminally ill, he does not wish any heroic measures or treatments. States that he will accept IVs and antibiotics, but does not want cardiopulmonary resuscitation and does not want to be put on a ventilator under any circumstances.

B. **Jargon, Clichés, and Euphemisms:** You should have underlined and identified the following. You could rewrite the sentences in many ways; a few examples are given.
   1. E—kind of stocky (eg, change to "50 lbs overweight")
   2. E—passed away (eg, change to "died")
   3. No jargon, euphemism, or cliché in this statement.
   4. E—full-figured (eg, change to, "Can you find me a gown that will cover my hips?")
   5. J—tubes (eg, change to "myringotomy tubes, to allow his ears to drain." This one is difficult because just labeling the tubes more specifically doesn't remove the jargon; you need to add an explanation.)
   6. E—check your tummy (eg, "check your uterus," "feel your abdomen")
      E—have your blessed event (eg, "have your baby," "deliver your baby")
   7. E—little girls' room (eg, "restroom, bathroom")
   8. C—it's always darkest just before dawn (eg, "what can I do to help you?" or "recovery from this surgery is usually slow, but results are almost always good" or "it usually takes 6 to 8 weeks of physical theapy before you see any results, but they *will* come.")
   9. J—get you ambulating (eg, "help you walk a bit")
   10. J—I & O ("intake and output," "fluids taken and urine passed"); voided ("urinated"), residual (urine left in your bladder); cath ("catheterization," "putting the tube in your bladder")

11. C—Healthcare is a right. (You might say, "I believe that all people have an equal right to healthcare." That makes it your own opinion instead of a cliché. You might, then, be asked to justify your opinion.)

12. J—"stick, gas, and lytes." You might say, "Lab will be here soon to draw blood to check your oxygen and electrolytes."

13. J—vital signs ("blood pressure, temperature, and pulse"); ECG ("test for your heart," "electrocardiogram"; what you say depends on the patient's level of understanding).

Chapter 3

Reminder: Discuss answers with peers or instructors. Answers may vary. Also, you will learn as much from the discussion as you do from the exercises.

Part I (Facts and Interpretations)

A. Fact. You could verify it in a textbook.

B. Interpretation. The term "professional" means different things to different people. It cannot be observed.

C. Fact

D. Fact. The patient's subjective feeling can be confirmed by asking the patient.

E. Fact

F. Interpretation

G. Interpretation

H. Interpretation—unless you ask Ms. Benitez and confirm that it is a fact.

I. Fact

J. Judgment. States "a *good* idea"—a value statement. Without "are a good idea," the statement might be a fact; you could see if there is any research to support it. Or it might just be something that sounds like a fact but is untrue, if the research does not support it.

K. Fact. Look up in a textbook or research articles.

L. Belief or opinion. A conclusion that is drawn from observations and stated as though it were a fact. It is inaccurate because babies whose parents change them often also get diaper rash.

M. Fact. Look at the ANA Standards.

N. Judgment. "Good" is the conclusion; based on the values (criteria) of "systematic, timely, and retrievable."

O. Fact. The nurse's statement is a fact; you could check with Mrs. Brady to see if she did say that.

P. Personal preference.

Q. Belief/opinion.

R. Probably a judgment, based on the nurse's idea of what a "good" Christian is. Could be an inference, too, based on the nurse's observations of the patient's religious behaviors.

S. Fact. The Bible does say that, or you could check to see if it does.

T. Belief/opinion. There is no way to check the accuracy of the statement.

Part II (Inferences). Learning the Skill

1. A cloud has come over the sun. There is an eclipse. A spaceship is hovering over your house.

2. Yes; it might be raining. Rain comes from clouds, so the first inference in #1 was probably correct.

3. I infer it is raining. However, someone might be on the roof with a garden hose, so I can't be sure unless I go outside and look.

Part II (Inferences). Applying the Skill

1. Circle *c* and *d*. For *c* you might ask what Mr. Jiminez said. For *d* you might ask the nurse what the incision looked like.

2. a–Fact   c–Fact   e–Fact
   b–Inference   d–Inference

3. Underline the following:
   Had . . . surgery, returned to her room at 4:00 PM, drowsy, responding to her name, Foley catheter in place, draining clear pale yellow urine, IV patent, 1,000 mL of D_5LR running at 75 mL/hr, B/P 124/75–130/82, pulse 72–86, resp 12–20, sat on side of bed for 15 min, moved slowly, complained of incisional pain, rated 10, administered own morphine by PCA, rated pain "about 5" lying still, abd. dressing dry and intact, had sips of carbonated drink, complained of nausea.

4. The cues were:
   a. Ms. G. had had surgery; nurse observed drowsiness.
   b. Catheter was draining clear pale yellow urine; skin turgor was good; vital signs given were in normal range.
   c. IV patent, running at 75 mL/hr; skin turgor good; vital signs given were in normal range; dressing dry; no vomiting.
   d. Patient complained of pain, rated 10 before and 5 after morphine; moved slowly
   e. Patient rated pain 10 before and 5 after morphine
   f. Mrs. G. had had surgery, had sips of carbonated drink, complained of nausea

5. a. Nurse assumed the drowsiness was from anesthetic. But perhaps Ms. G. had spinal anesthesia, which would not cause drowsiness. Perhaps it was the pain medication, maybe she was just sleepy, or maybe there was a neurological problem.

e. Ms. G's pain was improved after the morphine; however, it was a 5 only when lying still. In order to conclude "effective," the nurse might want her to rate pain while moving.

f. The nausea is a fact. The inference is about what caused the nausea. Without knowing the kind of anesthesia, the nurse cannot conclude that is the cause. Both morphine and pain can also cause nausea.

6. a. *Cues*: Do not circle anything. All statements were or could be verified. Underline "bowel sounds absent," "drank 100 mL of fluid," "immediately vomited," and "complained of nausea." *Explanation*: Underline "nausea and vomiting." Underline "decreased gastrointestinal activity." Circle "caused by decreased GI activity secondary to general anesthetic."

b. *Cues*: Circle none. All statements are facts, so you could underline everything. *Explanation*: Circle "anxious" and "due to being in a strange environment."

c. *Cues*: You might have circled "poor" skin turgor. Underline "just been admitted," "palms cool and damp," and "speaking rapidly." *Explanation*: Circle "fluid volume deficit" and "caused by being unable to drink and by diarrhea and vomiting." Underline "unable to drink" and "diarrhea and vomiting."

7. The inferences are:
a. *Patient's N&V were caused by decreased GI activity secondary to anesthetic.* Adequate. Absent bowel sounds do indicate that there is decreased GI activity. Patient did have general anesthetic, so it is appropriate to infer that as a cause of N&V; however, you cannot directly observe it as the cause. Remember, inferences can't be "proven" in the same way as facts.

b. *Patient is anxious* is an inference. That the anxiety is *due to being in a strange environment* is a second inference. The first inference has adequate evidence. For the second inference, you need to know if the hospital *is* strange to him; and need to ask him if that is the source of his anxiety. If the patient states that he is anxious due to being in a strange environment, then that changes your inference to a fact.

c. *Fluid volume deficit* is first inference. *Caused by being unable to drink and by diarrhea and vomiting* is second inference. Both have adequate evidence. The patient has observable signs of fluid volume deficit. You cannot observe that those factors (eg, unable to drink) *caused* the fluid volume deficit; however, the literature associates them closely, so that too is a valid inference.

Chapter 4

Reminder: Discuss answers with peers or instructors. Answers may vary. You should learn as much from the discussion as you do from the exercises.

Analysis

1. Did you underline the same key words as your peers? If not, what was your reasoning?
2. Did you define any of the words differently than others? Did your discussion cause you to change your mind about your definitions?
3–6. One assumption the author would have had to make in order to make that statement is that nurses and other healthcare professionals "speak the same language." That is, that a statement of, for example, Ineffective Airway Clearance, written by one nurse, will be understood in the same way by other nurses—and other professionals. That assumes that diagnostic statements are clear, accurate, and unambiguous.
7. One question you should have asked is: Is it *possible* to keep one's values from influencing decisions and judgments?

Synthesis

A. You could diagnose a problem of Risk for Pain in Lower Legs. After working through questions A1–6, you should synthesize the explanation that because Mr. Dupree has a constant state of reduced blood flow to his legs, he will probably experience pain whenever his legs experience an increased need for oxygen (combining the idea of "oxygen availability" and "oxygen need").

B. The etiology (risk factor) for Risk for Pain in Lower Legs for Mr. Dupree is "exercise." You do not have enough information to know how much or what kind of exercise it would take to produce pain, nor how severe the pain would be. But you can reasonably conclude that exercise puts him at risk for pain.

Chapter 5

Reminder: Discuss answers with peers or instructors. Answers may vary. You should learn as much from the discussion as you do from the exercises.

I. Clarifying
   A1. Responses will vary.
   A2. Responses will vary.
   A3. Beliefs are personal and will vary.
   A4. For example, he may believe the clinic visits are a waste of time, especially if he has to miss work

to go there. Answers will vary widely because you were asked to speculate; there is no way to really know his perspective.

B1. You might need to clarify "impaired coordination" and "watched closely," for example.

B2. Responses will vary. You would need to ask the reporting nurse a few questions.

B3. Responses will vary.

B4. Ms. Harris might believe that the nurses will not take care of her, for example. Or she might believe that people should be independent and take care of themselves. This is speculation only, as is B5, the beliefs of the reporting nurse.

II. Comparing and Contrasting

A1–3. These are all completely individual, and will vary.

B1. You should list the formats shown in the margin boxes in Chapter 5.

B2. You should list qualities such as: stated clearly, concise, acurate and valid, etc., taken from items 1–12 on pages 219 through 222.

B3. Answers will vary.

B4. Answers will vary.

Chapter 6

Only a few suggestions are provided. Discuss in class or with your peers.

A1. These will vary in different communities.

A2. A possible grouping (grapefruit, tennis ball, marble) (envelope, $1 bill, sheet of construction paper) (grass, snow)

A3. Other possible grouping characteristics: shape, natural vs. man-made

A4. The items in A2 are grouped on the basis of shape: round versus rectangular; grass and snow fit in the "other" category.

A5. Discuss with peers.

B1. Discuss with peers. Discuss *why* items were grouped as they were when your groupings are not the same.

B2. Discuss with peers. You may find this exercise difficult because some of the models are not explained in great detail in Chapter 3.

Chapter 7

Only a few suggestions are provided. Discuss in class or with your peers.

Learning the Skill. The definition of Fear includes "apprehension and fright." You might have written a rule such as, "If the patient reports only vague uneasiness

rather than outright fright, diagnose Anxiety." Continue in the same manner for #2 and #3. For #4, one clue is that his diagnosis of pneumonia is relevant. This is because it is a known specific threat to him.

Applying the Skill. (1) Probably the 2 most obvious complications are infiltration and inflammation (or phlebitis). You should be able to find symptoms in your textbooks. (2) Look up Impaired Tissue Integrity and Risk for Impaired Tissue Integrity in your *Nursing Diagnosis Guide*. (3) You should *not* have included nutrition, level of consciousness, or mobility assessments. They are relevant because they can contribute to Impaired Skin Integrity.

Chapter 8

Only a few suggestions are provided. Discuss in class or with your peers.

I.A. There is no "exactly right" spot to mark on the lines.

1. You would evaluate the credibilty of both the nurse and Ms. Alexander. The two sources do conflict. Unless you have reason to do otherwise, you usually assume another nurse is believable. On the other hand, all things being equal, the patient is the best source of information about her own pain. You need to know if the nurse has been reliable in the past (you could base this on your own experience, or ask other team members). You also need to know specifically what Ms. Alexander's pain symptoms are (you could ask the nurse, look in the chart, or observe/ask Ms. A). Based just on the information given, you should mark both people somewhere in the middle of the credibility line.

2. Sister confirms what Mrs. Domingo said. Apparently she observed directly that Mrs. D. did not needlepoint. Her purpose is probably to obtain pain relief for Mrs. D. Sister has no reason to lie, but could be over-interpreting because of anxiety/sympathy. Mark high on credibility line.

3. Mrs. Laurent is probably highly credible with regard to everything she said. However, it may *not* be the pain medications that are causing her dizziness and nausea. You need to know what kind of medication she is taking and the specifics of her "kidney disease" (both can be obtained from the chart). You can confirm her dizziness and nausea by observation; or another nurse may have charted that information.

4. The CNS is completely credible, if you assume she knows the patient and knows about kidney

diseases. If you wanted to be sure, you could look up the drug in a pharmacology book.

5. To mark this line, you should understand that the pharmaceutical company has a vested interest in convincing healthcare professionals to prescribe and use their new medication.

I.B. Possibilities: Do a literature search for other articles on exercise and beta-endorphins. Search the Internet. Contact the author(s) of the article. Contact authors of other articles on the topic.

II.A. (1) implication, (2) consequence, (3) consequence, (4) implication.

II.B. (1) Therapeutic effect might be pain relief. Undesirable effect might be liver damage or toxicity.

(2) Cold cloth and visualization might relieve headache, for example.

(3) Implies that you don't think the cold cloth and visualization would be adequate for relieving his pain—or that you think they would not be acceptable to Mr. X.

II.C. (1) Implies that you believe her symptoms include delusional thinking, even though the etiology of the diagnosis is not given. Implies that you believe the husband capable of understanding the teaching and dealing with Mrs. B's delusions.

(2) You need to find out if Mrs. B is, indeed, delusional; and what are Mr. B's capabilities.

(3) Ask, for example, "Has it worked in the past?" "What are its advantages/disadvantages?"

(4) Orienting. The fact that she is confused, alone, means she will need constant reorientation (refer to the NANDA definition of Chronic Confusion). You need to know more about Mrs. B's symptoms and the etiology of her confusion in order to judge the usefulness of the other two activities.

Chapter 9

The best learning occurs when you discuss your answers with colleagues.

Learning the Skill

1. All blood glucose entries are 80 mg/dL or lower. All readings are within normal limits—not dangerously low.
2. Yes.
3. Yes, *if* the data is accurate. There is *enough* data.
4. Two sources are involved: Ms. James, a frail, elderly woman who cannot see well; and the glucose meter, which she used to get her readings.

5. Because nothing in the case establishes the reliability of either, you should consider the possibilities for error.

6. Other explanations for *inaccurate readings* may include:
   (a) the monitor needs to be recalibrated
   (b) Ms. James' glasses were dirty, or for some other reason she couldn't see to read it correctly or to do the procedure correctly.
   (c) Ms. James' cognitive functioning might be impaired. She is drowsy and a little disoriented today, so perhaps she was even more so last week. A variety of factors could cause that: her blood glucose may have been high enough to impair her thinking; she may have had a mild stroke; she may have mild senile dementia, with intermittent cognitive difficulty; she may have a urinary tract infection, with confusion resulting from urosepsis.

7. Calibrate the machine. Check her preprandial (premeal) blood glucose levels yourself.

8. No. Although the data indicate goal achievement, and there are enough data, you cannot be certain enough of its accuracy.

9. You need to know whether the glucose monitor is working properly. You need to know how well Ms. James can see. You need more information about her mental status.

10. No. Your reading is clearly outside the goal range. You are sure it is accurate because you calibrated the machine and did the test properly.

11. No. Not necessarily. Something other than incorrect readings or a faulty machine may have caused Ms. James' blood glucose levels to be unusually low last week.

12. Ms. James may not have performed the procedure correctly, or she may have read the machine incorrectly (see #6c, preceding). Or her blood glucose may have been unusually low that week because she (a) didn't eat much or (b) gave herself too much insulin.

13. You can conclude that the goal was probably met, although some of the readings were lower than the goal range. You cannot be certain about goal achievement until you have more data.

14. Yes. That is still probably the "normal" range for her. Even if you find that she cannot perform the finger-stick test accurately, you still need this goal for regulating her glucose—regardless of who does the test. If her readings continue to be in the 60s, however, you may want to write a goal that focuses on the lower limit as well as the upper one (eg, ". . . will not be below 70 mg/dL").

15. (a) Yes. You will need to see her more often in the next few days to assure that her blood glucose levels don't become dangerously low, and to assess her ongoing mental status. Some of the necessary assessments will need to be made more than once to assure consistent performance.

(b) You will need to find out whether she can perform the fingerstick test and read the machine correctly. You will need to watch her administer her insulin a few times. You need to assess her mental status more fully. You need to observe and have her keep a record of what she is eating, and see whether she is having difficulty preparing food. You will need to observe her more than once because of possible changes in her mental status—she may perform well at some times and not at others.

Applying the Skill

1A. Probably, but not definitely. There are enough objective data, but what about the reliability of the subjective data? What factors might make it difficult to perceive pain in her legs, even if thrombophlebitis were present?

1B. Even if you charted "goal met," you should retain the problem on the care plan. This complication could still develop, and you must continue to assess for it and take preventive measures (eg, ambulation).

2A. No. Although the patient voided an adequate amount and her temperature is within normal limits, the nursing assistant didn't tell you whether the patient experienced burning on urination nor about the odor of the urine. Additionally, because the patient is drowsy and taking morphine, she may not experience burning if it is mild. It is probably too soon to know whether the patient is having urinary frequency, especially because she is receiving morphine and may not notice urethral and bladder sensations that would cause frequency.

2B. You should not conclude "goal met." Even if you did, you should retain the problem on the care plan (see 1B, preceding).

3A. First goal is met. You cannot conclude that the second goal has been met, even though the patient states she had a BM. There is evidence that she did *not* have a BM, and the patient's mental status (drowsy, disoriented) creates doubt about the accuracy of her statement. It is too soon to conclude second goal is "not met," because the target time is day 3 (today is day 2). Conclude "Too soon to evaluate." Chart what patient says and chart mental status and contrary evidence.

3B. Retain the problem. Only one of the two goals has been met, so you cannot discontinue it.

Chapter 10

Only a few suggestions are given. The best learning occurs when you discuss your answers with colleagues.

Learning the Skill

1. (a) Not everyone has an equal amount of both: some people live longer than others; some have more money than others. (In one sense, everyone does have the same amount of time—24 hours a day—but some people have more *free* time.)

(b) Both time and money are precious.

(c) Not having enough of either can create difficulty.

2. Animals and humans both have hearts that circulate blood through their body. Both are warm blooded. Both breathe oxygen. Many other physiological similarities.

3. Must assume that the drug would be absorbed and excreted in similar ways and would produce same pharmacological effects.

Applying the Skill

A1. Both are female; both had the same surgery, on the same side; both are in the hospital (we assume); they have the same nurse.

A2. There is an age difference, we know. There may be a cultural difference, based on the names, but there really aren't enough data to be sure about this.

A3. Need to know if they are right- or left-handed (especially relevant to the mobility problem). Need to know their feelings about the surgery; can't assume that because Ms. Winfrey is 30 years old, she will be more upset by loss of a breast. Need to know the mental status of both; can't assume that Ms. Li is cognitively impaired or disoriented just because she is 85 years old (although she is at higher risk of being disoriented by the anesthetic and narcotic analgesics).

B1. Both are women. Both have chronic diseases. Both have the same nurse. Both are being treated by medication and dietary alterations. Both have Knowledge Deficit.

B2. No.

B3. It is significant to their nursing diagnosis that they have Knowledge Deficit and need to learn about their medication and diet.

B4. Different ages. Different medical diagnoses; different medications; different diets. Debby has a new diagnosis (diabetes), whereas Gloria has probably had CHF for a long time.

B5. Without making too many assumptions, it is safe to assume that the approach to teaching would be different for a teenager than for an elderly woman, simply because of their developmental stages (eg, the need of teens to be like their peers). In addition, sight or hearing deficits may occur with aging. Because Debby's diagnosis is new, there will proba-

bly be a need to deal with the emotional problems (eg, shock, disbelief, anger). Emotional responses require energy and distract from concentration and learning. Gloria may have more difficulty changing her eating habits than Debby; lifelong dietary and activity habits are difficult to change. Also, Debby's parents will probably provide support for her, whereas Gloria lives alone.

Answer Key for "Case Studies: Applying Critical Thinking and Nursing Process"

Chapter 1

1. I—settled her comfortably in bed
   A—interviewed her
   A—obtained a temperature
   A—examined Ms. Boiko's chart
   I—administered oxygen
   A—performed the physical examination
   D—wrote a diagnosis
   Po—chose an outcome

   Pi—wrote nursing orders for skin care
   I—bathing Ms. Boiko
   E—observed that her coccygeal area was still red (this could also be *A*, for ongoing assessment)
   E—concluded the outcome had not been achieved
   E—changed the order on the care plan

2. Client data are as follows: Temp 101°F, pulse 120, resp. 32, B/P 100/68, reddened area over coccyx, unable to move about in bed, coccyx still red, a small area of skin was peeling off, there was some serous drainage. (Juan also obtained data that Ms. Boiko had been turned every 2 hours, except for 6 hours each night. These data are about care that was given to Ms. Boiko, but not data about her human responses.)

3. You should have circled the following as examples of reexamination of the nursing process phases (dynamic/cyclic):
   (1) . . . *concluded that the outcome had not been achieved.* This shows that Juan reexamined his original outcome.

   (2) *He was sure his data were adequate and that his nursing diagnosis was accurate.* This shows reexamination of the database *and* the original nursing diagnosis.
   (3) *The other staff members assured Juan that they had carried out the 2-hour turning schedule.* This shows that he checked to see if the nursing orders were properly implemented.
   (4) *He changed the order on the care plan.* This shows *revision* of the plan of care.

4. The nursing orders are:
   (1) to give skin care
   (2) a schedule for turning every 2 hrs except at night
   (3) frequent, continued observation
   (4) to turn every 2 hrs around the clock
   Because the case states that Juan was bathing Ms. Boiko, you may have assumed that he wrote a nursing order for that; however, the case study does not say so, and you must use only the information provided. Juan did perform some other nursing activities, such as settling the client in bed; however, we do not know that they were written as nursing orders. Don't confuse nursing interventions/actions (carried out) with nursing orders (written).

5. This is the most obvious example of overlapping phases: "Two days later, when bathing Ms. Boiko, Juan observed that her coccygeal area was still red, a small area of skin was peeling off, and there was

some serious drainage." In this example, Juan was implementing (bathing) at the same time he was assessing or evaluating (observing her coccygeal area).

You might also have chosen: "Juan Apodaca, RN, settled her comfortably in bed and briefly interviewed her about her symptoms." *Settled* is implementation, while *interviewed* is assessment. As written, it isn't certain that these occurred at the same time; however, if you think they did, then this is also a case of overlapping phases.

6. Juan demonstrated creativity by not continuing to use the turning schedule that was routinely used on his unit. He was not content to do what was usually done, but reasoned that in this case something more was needed (he also used his cognitive skills here).

7. You should have chosen *planned and outcome oriented*: The nurse based interventions on the patient's needs, not on unit routines. You should also have chosen *flexible*, because Juan did not adhere rigidly to his initial plan, but changed it as needed.

Chapter 2

1. Examples of factors that may affect Mrs. Lutz's *ability* to consent: She is probably taking pain medications; the nurse needs to know what they are and how Mrs. Lutz responds to them. Mrs. Lutz may be depressed because of her illness. Her thinking may be affected by her weakened, malnourished state. She may be thinking of refusing treatment because it will present a financial burden to her family.

2. The nurse should ask Mrs. Lutz to verbalize the purpose of the treatment, its risks, and its benefits; what she can expect to feel during the treatment; and the advantages and disadvantages of the alternative treatments that are available.

3. The nurse's approach was not appropriate. The nurse seems to be pressuring Mrs. Lutz into signing the form; she did not explain the risks of the procedure (she could have asked the physician if Mrs. Lutz had been informed about the risks); she did not explain what Mrs. Lutz would feel during the procedure, and she may even have been dishonest about that; she minimized the patient's fear by ignoring what she said.

4. Assessment

5. Item 1 asks the nurse to apply the standard of accuracy: Will the data obtained from Mrs. Lutz be correct and accurate? Item 2 asks for the standards of breadth (Does she have the *patient's* true point of view?); and accuracy (Is that true? How could we check it?).

Chapter 3

Only a few suggestions are given. The best learning comes from discussion of the case.

1. You may have listed: Is his disorientation continuous or just occasional? Is he just confused about where he is, or is his judgment poor about other things? Does he have a history of wandering about at night? What is his physical condition (eg, strength, balance, ability to walk)? What is the facility's policy regarding patient safety and restraints?

2. For a patient with a fractured hip, for example, you would need to know what pain medications he is taking (they may be causing the disorientation). You would do a focused pain assessment. You may not need as thorough a mental status assessment.

3. To do a mental status examination, you must use primary source, subjective data obtained by interviewing Mr. Brown. You will use observation and physical examination. You will use secondary sources, such as the chart and the person bringing him to the hospital.

4. Refer to Chapter 3, "Interviewing Elderly Patients," and "Cognitive Deficits."

5. For example, you used comparing and contrasting (data for senile dementia and fractured hip).

Chapter 4

Only a few suggestions are given. Discuss the case with your peers.

1. Examples of feelings are fear, anger, happiness.

2. You may have thought, "He's doing this to himself," or many other things.

3. A value that "people should want to get well" or that "nurses should help people to get well" would certainly affect the way you see this situation.

4. What you say is highly individual and depends on Items 1–3.

5. He might be feeling anger, embarrassment, guilt, or . . .

6. For example, many nurses may have already urged him to quit smoking; but maybe no one has ever focused on his feelings and how difficult it is to quit.

7. Noncompliance won't be a useful diagnosis unless you can find the reasons that the client continues to smoke. But the only etiology you can infer from these data is that he has an addiction to nicotine. You might speculate other reasons, such as "he doesn't care about his health," or "he is weak willed," but there are no data to suggest that.

8. There are no data to suggest that he smokes because of a lack of knowledge.

9. Based just on the data provided, you might consider Activity Intolerance r/t inadequate oxygenation. Or

perhaps Self-Care Deficit (Bathing/Hygiene, Feeding) r/t Activity Intolerance. Based on his outburst, you might consider a "possible" diagnosis of Ineffective Denial or Ineffective Individual Coping—but there are not enough data to confirm these as actual diagnoses.

Chapter 5

Only a few suggestions are given. Discuss the case with your peers.

1. Correct. The data do not explain why Mr. Gomez is in denial (if he actually is).
2. Incorrect. There are no data to suggest that Mr. Gomez lacks knowledge about anything—although, that could be the case. It would be correct to say *possibly* r/t lack of knowledge.
3. Incorrect. Failure to change lifestyle is a defining characteristic for that NANDA label, not a related factor. It is a symptom of the problem, not a cause.
4. Probably Ineffective Individual Management of Therapeutic Regimen. Mr. Gomez has the defining characteristics for Noncompliance; however, that NANDA definition requires "an *agreed-upon* . . . treatment plan." This situation does not say whether Mr. Gomez ever actually agreed to his prescribed treatment plan. This question is certainly open to discussion!
5. You may have written something like: Ineffective Individual Management of Therapeutic Regimen (diet, smoking, work pattern) possibly r/t denial of seriousness of illness A.M.B. working 60 hours/week, high-fat diet, smoking, exacerbation of physical symptoms, and statement ". . . working too hard . . . just need pills." Mr. Gomez's statement is the strongest cue that he is in denial, but by itself is not proof. His behaviors may be caused by something other than denial. The most important issue in this question is it is probably most useful to use denial in the etiology rather than as a problem.
6. This would depend on the framework you use. In a preservation of life framework, the collaborative problem would have highest priority.
7. Your perspective will affect your speculations about Mr. Gomez's priority. However, it appears, from the data, that he is probably most concerned about fatigue.
8. Answers are completely individual.

Chapter 6

Only a few suggestions are given. Remember that answers will vary based on knowledge, experience, and values. The most meaningful learning comes from discussing the case with others.

1. Items a–e should have helped you work through this question. If not, read more about diabetes and insulin. If you are still having trouble, see your instructor for help.
2. Poor peripheral circulation is one risk factor.
3. General goal would be that the foot would heal at an optimum rate; evidence of that would be approximation of edges and a clean, dry incision, for example.
4. To answer this question, ask: (a) Can the nurse provide most of the care to prevent delayed wound healing? (b) Are there factors that put this patient at higher risk for delayed wound healing than the "norm"? If so, you may want to write a nursing diagnosis. This is a difficult question, because "a" is probably No and "b" is Yes.
5. Example: Will state the signs and symptoms of infection.
6. Answers will vary, depending on your perspective. Is it possible to give culturally competent care to someone of a different race/culture/sex than the nurse? Are there situations in which someone of the same race/culture/sex might be more effective or increase the patient's comfort in some way?
7. Probably not. For example, his nutritional needs are different because of the surgery, and he is probably less able to shop and cook; his appetite may not be good because of the antibiotic side effects, or because of his probable decreased activity.
8. Examples: Will maintain present weight. Will state that he cooks and eats at least three meals per day.
9. To determine how his care needs can be managed at home and make those arrangements. Second to that, to assure that he knows the signs and symptoms of infection and antibiotic reactions.
10. Perhaps monitoring the diabetes to be sure it remains stable, because of the effect that can have on wound healing. Or perhaps to teach and give care to prevent infection of the wound. It depends on the framework you are using to prioritize. For example, the *most likely* problem is that he will fall; the *most serious* is either that his diabetes will not be controlled or his wound will become infected. Because the diabetes is controlled at present, the main focus should probably be wound care to prevent infection. However, none of these is an actual problem. If you identified an actual problem (such as inability to buy and prepare food), that might receive a higher priority.

Chapter 7

Note: Answers do not contain comprehensive information. Only a few suggestions are given.

1. Respiratory complications such as pneumonia and atelectasis.
2. Anesthesia, incisional pain, obesity, fatigue. Obese persons may have decreased alveolar expansion related to a sedentary lifestyle. She may be taking shallow breaths to decrease the pain—also because she is tired.
3. Has she recently received medication for pain? If so, is it adequately relieving her pain?
4. To prevent respiratory complications.
5. First, be sure pain relief is optimal. Then you may, for example, teach her to splint her incision with a pillow while doing the exercises, to minimize tension on the incision. Explain that consistent performance of the exercises will actually decrease her fatigue (by increasing the availability of oxygenated blood).
6. One action would be to demonstrate the exercises, then breathe along with her while she performs them. Verbal feedback (eg, "Well done") would support her efforts. Communicate the plan to other caregivers; check often to see if she is complying.
7. She will have no respiratory complications. Assess vital signs (especially temperature and respirations), lung sounds, skin color, etc.

Chapter 8

Note: Other answers may be possible. Only a few suggestions are given.

1. *Actual Diagnoses*: Functional Urinary Incontinence; Bathing/Hygiene Self-Care Deficit, Toileting S-CD, Dressing/Grooming S-CD (You could write Total Self-Care Deficit instead of these).
   Potential Diagnoses: Risk for Body Image and/or Self-Esteem Disturbance; Risk for Disuse Syndrome (a complication of immobility that includes Risk for Constipation, Altered Urinary Elimination, Disorientation, Body-Image Disturbance, and Powerlessness); Risk for Altered Thought Processes.
2. (a) No; not based on the information given. (b) He does have risk factors: decreased self-care abilities, incontinence, body changes, and inability to communicate all may be damaging to his self-esteem.
3. Add urinary incontinence as an etiology, because the dampness increases the risk for skin breakdown. There is also a possibility of inadequate nutrition related to his illness and his inability to feed himself. Inadequate nutrition is a risk factor for impaired skin integrity. It is important to add these etiological factors because they suggest nursing interventions.
4. Monitor for redness, breakdown, edema, excessive dryness or moistness, color and temperature, and hydration.

5. This is just the list of activities.
6. Refer to Box 2–9 on page 60.
7. (a) All activities are appropriate, except for "provide trapeze . . ." Mr. W. is probably not yet able to use the trapeze; this may be appropriate later. You might have drawn a line through "fecal" in the first activity because he has not been incontinent of stool. In the second activity, draw a line through "as appropriate." In the third activity, draw a line through "at least daily"—that is not often enough. In the last activity, draw a line through "as appropriate." (b) The last activity should specify the type of "specialty" bed/mattress (eg, foam, air, sheepskin).
8. Bleeding/hemorrhage
9. Use a soft bristle toothbrush. Use electric razor only. Bathe gently. Tell the nurse if you see any bleeding (eg, nose, mouth, or urine) or bruises.
10. Keep linens dry, taut, and wrinkle-free. Because he is immobile, wrinkled or damp linens will contribute to skin breakdown.
11. Example: Will be able to feed himself with his right hand within 3 weeks.
12. (a) Because of his Impaired Verbal Communciation, he cannot call for help. Also, he cannot tell the nurse of any subjective symptoms that are developing. (b) Place the call light/bell where he can reach it with his right hand. Ask "yes/no" questions about any symptoms of complications that you may be concerned about (eg, dizziness, disorientation).
13. Speech therapist, to practice speech-therapy activities and find alternative methods of communication. Nutritionist, to suggest high-protein menus to promote healthy skin, and high-fiber menus to prevent constipation; also, foods that he can feed himself. Physical therapist, for range-of-motion and muscle-strengthening exercises. Occupational therapist, for assistive devices for eating and other self-care; and for training in self-care.
14. One nursing order might be: Provide passive range-of-motion exercises for left arm and leg, and active range-of-motion exercises for right arm and leg every 4 hours while awake.

Chapter 9

1. Probably not. Ms. Jackson doesn't have the necessary defining characteristics to diagnose either Dysfunctional Grieving (duration too short) or Ineffective Individual Coping. She appears to be experiencing a normal grief process, for which there is no NANDA diagnosis. However, because her grief seems to be affecting her nutrition, the nurse should

find a way to include it in the description of her health status.

2. Do the defining characteristics fit Ms. Jackson? Is the etiology specific/descriptive enough to provide direction for the nursing interventions?

3. For example, you might add "as manifested by . . ." or add "secondary to grief over loss of husband."

4. Item #1 is vague and not observable. What *is* "optimal" daily caloric intake? For example, you might write, "Will decrease calorie intake by 500 calories/day." Need to add a fourth goal that would indicate resolution of the problem: that she will lose weight. State specifically how much weight and by when (eg, "Will lose 1 lb/week.")

5. c. Need to know how many calories it takes to produce a 1-lb weight loss; otherwise, you might set an impossible goal (eg, 10 lbs/week would mean she has to reduce her intake by 5,000 calories/day—probably more than her total intake has been). Principle *a* is the only one that does not apply. *b* explains the reason for dietary changes (to lose weight); *c* also explains relationship between calories and weight; *d* explains the concern for a "well-balanced" diet.

6. Refer her to support groups; for example, a grieving support group.

7. Outcome #1—This goal is impossible to evaluate because it is stated in broad, nonspecific terms. Her dietary log indicates she is eating well-balanced meals, but is that "optimal" intake? It is impossible to judge by her weight loss, because there was no goal to specify what that was to be. She lost less than 1 lb/week, however, so probably she is still consuming too many calories.

Outcome #2—Not met. She is only walking 20 minutes/day, not 30.

Outcome #3—Partially met. She realizes that she eats when she is bored and depressed; but there are probably other, more specific activities that are associated with her eating (eg, watching TV).

8. 2b—Because there is no evidence that this has ever been done.

3a—Because there is no evidence that this has been done, except for verbalizing that she eats when she is bored.

3b—Because there is no evidence that this has been done; it is important as motivation. The nurse should do all of these things at this clinic visit.

9. a. For example, when she watches TV, she might start doing something that requires her to use her hands: perhaps sewing, ironing, working on a photo album. "Stop watching TV" doesn't apply this principle; nor would "Stop snacking."

   b. She has not stopped smoking, but she has substituted better quality, healthier (and we assume lower-calorie) foods.

10. No suggestions. Answers will be unique to each person.

Index

Underscored terms indicate nursing diagnoses.